PEDIATRIC BEHAVIORAL NUTRITION FACTORS

Environment, Education, and Self-Regulation

PEDIATRIC BEHAVIORAL NUTRITION FACTORS

Environment, Education, and Self-Regulation

Edited by

Areej Hassan, MD, MPH

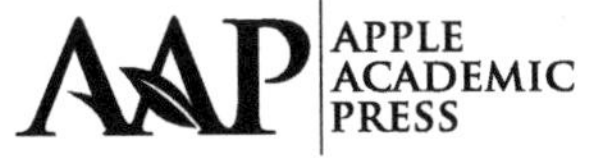

Apple Academic Press Inc.
3333 Mistwell Crescent
Oakville, ON L6L 0A2
Canada

Apple Academic Press Inc.
9 Spinnaker Way
Waretown, NJ 08758
USA

First issued in paperback 2021

Exclusive worldwide distribution by CRC Press, a member of Taylor & Francis Group

ISBN 13: 978-1-77-463686-2 (pbk)
ISBN 13: 978-1-77-188495-2 (hbk)

Library and Archives Canada Cataloguing in Publication

Pediatric behavioral nutrition factors : environment, education, and self-regulation / edited by Areej Hassan, MD, MPH.

Includes bibliographical references and index.
Issued in print and electronic formats.
ISBN 978-1-77188-495-2 (hardcover).--ISBN 978-1-315-36573-2 (PDF)

1. Children--Nutrition. 2. Diet therapy for children. 3. Nutrition--Social aspects. 4. Obesity in children--Social aspects. 5. Obesity in children--Prevention. I. Hassan, Areej, editor

RJ206.P43 2016 615.8'54083 C2016-907785-3 C2016-907786-1

Library of Congress Cataloging-in-Publication Data

Names: Hassan, Areej, editor.
Title: Pediatric behavioral nutrition factors : environment, education, and self-regulation / editor, Areej Hassan.
Description: Toronto ; New Jersey : Apple Academic Press, 2017. | Includes bibliographical references and index.
Identifiers: LCCN 2016054723 (print) | LCCN 2016055224 (ebook) | ISBN 9781771884952 (hardcover : alk. paper) | ISBN 9781771884969 (eBook) | ISBN 9781315365732 (ebook)
Subjects: | MESH: Child Nutritional Physiological Phenomena | Feeding Behavior | Sociological Factors
Classification: LCC RJ206 (print) | LCC RJ206 (ebook) | NLM WS 130 | DDC 362.19892--dc23
LC record available at https://lccn.loc.gov/2016054723

Apple Academic Press also publishes its books in a variety of electronic formats. Some content that appears in print may not be available in electronic format. For information about Apple Academic Press products, visit our website at **www.appleacademicpress.com** and the CRC Press website at **www.crcpress.com**

About the Editor

Areej Hassan, MD, MPH

Areej Hassan, MD, MPH, is an attending in the Division of Adolescent/ Young Adult Medicine at Boston Children's Hospital and Assistant Professor of Pediatrics at Harvard Medical School. She completed her residency training in Pediatrics at Brown University before her fellowship at BCH. In addition to primary care, Dr.Hassan focuses her clinical interests on reproductive endocrinology and global health. She also maintains an active role in medical education and has particular interest in building and developing innovative teaching tools through open educational resources. She currently teaches, consults, and is involved in pediatric and adolescent curricula development at multiple sites abroad in Central America and Southeast Asia.

Contents

List of Contributors

Jean Adams
Centre for Diet & Activity Research, MRC Epidemiology Unit, University of Cambridge, School of Clinical Medicine; Institute of Health & Society, Newcastle University

Ashley J. Adamson
Institute of Health & Society, Newcastle University; Human Nutrition Research Centre, Newcastle University

Wilke J. C. van Ansem
IVO Addiction Research Institute; Erasmus Medical Centre

Olga H. van der Baan-Slootweg
Merem Treatment Centers

Rachel Bachner-Melman
Psychiatry, Hadassah University Medical School, Jerusalem, Israel; Psychology, Hebrew University of Jerusalem, Israel

Ana Baylin
Department of Epidemiology, School of Public Health, University of Michigan

Ashley D. Beck
Washington State University

Maria del Mar Bibiloni
University of the Balearic Islands

Laura M. Bolten
Department of Health Sciences and the EMGO+ Institute for Health and Care Research, VU University Amsterdam

Kerri Boutelle
Department of Pediatrics, School of Medicine, University of California, San Diego; School of Medicine, Department of Psychiatry, University of California, San Diego

Tamara Brown
Wolfson Research Institute, Durham University, Queen's Campus, University Boulevard

Johannes Brug
Department of Epidemiology & Biostatistics and the EMGO+ Institute for Health and Care Research, VU University Medical Center

Nancy F. Butte
Baylor College of Medicine, USDA/ARS Children's Nutrition Research Center, Department of Pediatrics

Franco Cavallo
Department of Public Health and Pediatrics, University of Torino

Dawn Contreras
Department of Human Development and Family Studies, Michigan State University; Health and Nutrition Institute, Michigan State University

Karen W. Cullen
Professor of Pediatrics-Nutrition, Baylor College of Medicine

Paola Dalmasso
Department of Public Health and Pediatrics, University of Torino

Julianna Deardorff
Division of Community Health and Human Development, School of Public Health, University of California at Berkeley

Veronika Dolar
Department of Economics, Long Island University

Susan Dickstein
Department of Psychiatry and Human Behavior, Brown University Medical School

J. Andrea Jaramillo Duran
Children's Nutrition Research Center, Baylor College of Medicine

Elena Flores
Counseling Psychology Department, School of Education, University of San Francisco

Leslie A. Frankel
University of Houston

Mariano Vincenzo Giacchi
CREPS—Center of Research for Health Education and Promotion, Department Molecular and Developmental Medicine, University of Siena

Louis Goffe
Institute of Health & Society, Newcastle University; Human Nutrition Research Centre, Newcastle University

Moria Golan
Shahaf, Community Services for Eating Disorders, Department of Nutrition, Israel; Tel-Hai Academic College, Upper Galilee and the Hebrew University of Jerusalem, Israel

L. Suzanne Goodell
North Carolina State University

Louise C. Greenspan
Kaiser Permanente

Steven E. Gregorich
Department of Medicine, University of California at San Francisco

Cynthia L. de Groat
Department of Psychiatry, University of California at San Francisco

Jutka Halberstadt
Department of Health Sciences and the EMGO Institute for Health and Care Research, VU University Amsterdam

Holly E. Brophy Herb
Department of Human Development and Family Studies, Michigan State University

Mildred A. Horodynski
College of Nursing, Michigan State University

Sheryl O. Hughes
Children's Nutrition Research Center, Baylor College of Medicine

Kathy K. Isoldi
Department of Nutrition, Long Island University

Anita Jansen
Faculty of Psychology and Neuroscience, Department of Clinical Psychological Science, Maastricht University

Elissa Jelalian
Department of Psychiatry and Human Behavior, Brown University Medical School

Susan L. Johnson
University of Colorado Denver

Niko Kaciroti
Center for Human Growth and Development, University of Michigan

Pam J. Kaspers
Medical Library, VU University Amsterdam

Leonie F. M. Kohl
Department of Health Promotion, NUTRIM School for Nutrition and Translational Research in Metabolism, Maastricht University Medical Center+

Stef P. J. Kremers
Department of Health Promotion, NUTRIM School for Nutrition and Translational Research in Metabolism, Maastricht University Medical Center+

Willemieke Kroeze
Department of Health Sciences and the EMGO+ Institute for Health and Care Research, VU University Amsterdam

Amelia A. Lake
Wolfson Research Institute, Durham University, Queen's Campus, University Boulevard

Anna Lamberti
National Center for Epidemiology, Surveillance and Health Promotion, National Institute of Health

Giacomo Lazzeri
CREPS—Center of Research for Health Education and Promotion, Department Molecular and Developmental Medicine, University of Siena

Julie C. Lumeng
Center for Human Growth and Development, University of Michigan; Department of Pediatrics, University of Michigan

Sabine Makkes
Department of Health Sciences and the EMGO Institute for Health and Care Research, VU University Amsterdam

Suzanna M. Martinez
Department of Pediatrics, University of California at San Francisco

Dike van de Mheen
IVO Addiction Research Institute; Erasmus Medical Centre; Department of Health Education and Promotion, Maastricht University

Alison L. Miller
Center for Human Growth and Development, University of Michigan; School of Public Health, University of Michigan

Rana H. Mosli
Department of Nutritional Sciences, School of Public Health, University of Michigan; Clinical Nutrition Department, Faculty of Applied Medical Sciences, King Abdulaziz University

Paola Nardone
National Center for Epidemiology, Surveillance and Health Promotion, National Institute of Health

Chantal Nederkoorn
Faculty of Psychology and Neuroscience, Department of Clinical Psychological Science, Maastricht University

Andrea Pammolli
CREPS—Center of Research for Health Education and Promotion, Department Molecular and Developmental Medicine, University of Siena

Lauri A. Pasch
Department of Psychiatry, University of California at San Francisco

Karen E. Peterson
Center for Human Growth and Development, University of Michigan; School of Public Health, University of Michigan

Carlos Penilla
School of Public Health, University of California at Berkeley

Jordi Pich
University of the Balearic Islands

Veronica Piziak
Division of Endocrinology, Scott & White Healthcare, The Texas A&M Health Science Center College of Medicine

Antoni Pons
University of the Balearic Islands

Thomas G. Power
Washington State University

Kyung E. Rhee
Department of Pediatrics, School of Medicine, University of California, San Diego; Division of Academic General Pediatrics, Developmental Pediatrics, and Community Health, University of California, San Diego, School of Medicine

Betty del Rio-Rodriguez
Assistant Professor of Pediatrics, Baylor College of Medicine

Gerda Rodenburg
IVO Addiction Research Institute; Erasmus Medical Centre

Katherine Rosenblum
Center for Human Growth and Development, University of Michigan; Department of Psychiatry, University of Michigan

Carola T. M. Schrijvers
IVO Addiction Research Institute; Erasmus Medical Centre

Jacob C. Seidell
Department of Health Sciences and the EMGO Institute for Health and Care Research, VU University Amsterdam

Ronald Seifer
Department of Psychiatry and Human Behavior, Brown University Medical School

Ester F. C. Sleddens
Department of Health Promotion, NUTRIM School for Nutrition and Translational Research in Metabolism, Maastricht University Medical Center+

Angela Spinelli
National Center for Epidemiology, Surveillance and Health Promotion, National Institute of Health

Julie Staples-Watson
Center for Human Growth and Development, University of Michigan

Carolyn Summerbell
Wolfson Research Institute, Durham University, Queen's Campus, University Boulevard

Jeanne M. Tschann
Department of Psychiatry, University of California at San Francisco

Josep A. Tur
University of the Balearic Islands

Elizabeth Velema
Department of Health Sciences and the EMGO+ Institute for Health and Care Research, VU University Amsterdam

Emely de Vet
Department of Health Sciences and the EMGO Institute for Health and Care Research, VU University Amsterdam

Martin White
Centre for Diet & Activity Research, MRC Epidemiology Unit, University of Cambridge, School of Clinical Medicine; Institute of Health & Society, Newcastle University

Kimberly Williams
University of Colorado Denver

Rena Wing
Department of Psychiatry and Human Behavior, Brown University Medical School

Wendy Wrieden
Institute of Health & Society, Newcastle University; Human Nutrition Research Centre, Newcastle University

Acknowledgments and How to Cite

The editor and publisher thank each of the authors who contributed to this book. Many of the chapters in this book were previously published elsewhere. To cite the work contained in this book and to view the individual permissions, please refer to the citation at the beginning of each chapter. The editor carefully selected each chapter individually to provide a nuanced look at how environment, education, and self-regulation impact pediatric nutrition.

Introduction

We still don't know all the various factors that intertwine with and influence nutrition. Often, we assume that poor nutrition is a socioeconomic issue, but the articles in this compendium make clear that this simplistic assumption is not accurate. This is a massive, multifaceted topic. The articles included here were chosen to present as accurate a total image as possible, based on recent research. The final chapters offer innovative interventions that should become the foundation for ongoing investigation.

—Areej Hassan, MD

The literature on determinants of dietary behavior among youth is extensive and unwieldy. The authors of chapter 1 conducted an umbrella review or review-of-reviews to present a comprehensive overview of the current knowledge. Therefore, the authors included systematic reviews identified in four databases (i.e. PubMed, PsycINFO, The Cochrane Library and Web of Science) that summarized determinants of observable child and adolescent dietary behaviors. Data extraction included a judgment of the importance of determinants, strength of evidence and evaluation of the methodological quality of the eligible reviews. In total, 17 reviews were considered eligible. Whereas social-cognitive determinants were addressed most intensively towards the end of the 20th century, environmental determinants (particularly social and physical environmental) have been studied most extensively during the past decade, thereby representing a paradigm shift. With regard to environmental determinants, mixed findings were reported. Sedentary behavior and intention were found to be significant determinants of a wide range of dietary behaviors in most reviews with limited suggestive evidence due to the cross-sectional study designs. Other potential determinants such as automaticity, self-regulation and subjective norm have been studied in relatively few studies, but results are promising. The multitude of studies conducted on potential determinants of dietary behaviors found significant associations between some variables and behaviors. However, because of concern of weak research designs in the studies included, the evidence for true determinants is suggestive at best.

The USDA summer food service program (SFSP) provides free lunches during the summer. Chapter 2 examined the foods selected and consumed by participating children. Three hundred and two children were observed in 14 schools during a 4-week period in June, 2011; 50% were male; 75% were in elementary school. Dietary intake was observed and recorded; selected and consumed foods were entered into nutrient analysis software to obtain selected and consumed nutrients. Meals offered to students met the National School Lunch Program (NSLP) meal patterns. However, students selected meals that were low in Vitamin C, and did not include the two servings of fruit and/or vegetable allowed in the meal pattern. Elementary students consumed a mean of 63% of energy selected and 0.57 serving of fruit+ vegetables (0.29 cup); intermediate students consumed 73% of energy selected and mean a 0.39 serving of fruit+ vegetables (0.20 cup). Food waste was high (>30%) for fruit, vegetables and s. The SFSP as offered to children met the USDA lunch standards but interventions are needed to improve student food selection and consumption.

Parental feeding practices are thought to influence children's weight status, through children's eating behavior and nutritional intake. However, because most studies have been cross-sectional, the direction of influence is unclear. Moreover, although obesity rates are high among Latino children, few studies of parental feeding practices have focused on this population. The 2-year longitudinal study in chapter 3 examined mutual influences over time between parental feeding practices and children's weight status, in Mexican American families with children 18 years old at baseline. Mothers (n = 322) and fathers (n = 182) reported on their feeding practices at baseline, 1-year follow-up, and 2-year follow-up. Weight status, defined by waist-height ratio (WHtR) and body mass index (BMI), was ascertained at all assessments. Cross-lagged panel models were used to examine the mutual influences of parental feeding practices and child weight status over time, controlling for covariates. Both mothers' and fathers' restriction of food predicted higher subsequent child weight status at Year 1, and for fathers this effect was also found at Year 2. Mothers' and fathers' pressure to eat predicted lower weight status among boys, but not girls, at Year 1. Child weight status also predicted some parental feeding practices: boys' heavier weight predicted mothers' less pressure to eat at Year 1, less use of food to control behavior at Year 2, and greater restriction at Year 2; and girls' heavier weight at Year 1 predicted fathers' less pressure to eat and less positive involvement in child eating at Year 2. Chapter 3 provides longitudinal evidence that some parental feeding practices influence Mexican American children's weight status, and that children's weight status also influences some parental feeding practices.

Feeding practices of both mothers and fathers were related to children's weight status, underscoring the importance of including fathers in research on parental feeding practices and child obesity.

There is growing interest in the relationship between general parenting and childhood obesity. However, assessing general parenting via surveys can be difficult due to issues with self-report and differences in the underlying constructs being measured. As a result, different aspects of parenting have been associated with obesity risk. The authors of chapter 4 developed a more objective tool to assess general parenting by using observational methods during a mealtime interaction. The General Parenting Observational Scale (GPOS) was based on prior work of Baumrind, Maccoby and Martin, Barber, and Slater and Power. Ten dimensions of parenting were included; 4 were classified in the emotional dimension of parenting (*warmth and affection, support and sensitivity, negative affect, detachment*), and 6 were classified in the behavioral dimension of parenting (*firm discipline and structure, demands for maturity, psychological control, physical control, permissiveness, neglect*). Overweight children age 8–12 years old and their parent (n = 44 dyads) entering a weight control program were videotaped eating a family meal. Parents were coded for their general parenting behaviors. The Mealtime Family Interaction Coding System (MICS) and several self-report measures of general parenting were also used to assess the parent-child interaction. Spearman's correlations were used to assess correlation between measures. The emotional dimensions of warmth/affection and support/sensitivity, and the behavioral dimension of firm discipline/structure were robustly captured during the family meals. Warmth/affection and support/sensitivity were significantly correlated with affect management, interpersonal involvement, and communication from the MICS. Firm discipline/structure was inversely correlated with affect management, behavior control, and task accomplishment. Parents who were older, with higher educational status, and lower BMIs were more likely to display warmth/affection and support/sensitivity. Several general parenting dimensions from the GPOS were highly correlated with similar family functioning constructs from the MICS. This new observational tool appears to be a valid means of assessing general parenting behaviors during mealtimes and adds to our ability to measure parent-level factors affecting child weight-related outcomes. Future evaluation of this tool in a broader range of the population and other family settings should be conducted.

Being a last-born child and having a sister have been associated with higher body mass index (BMI). Encouragement to eat that overrides children's self-regulation has been reported to increase the risk of obesogenic eating behaviors.

The study in chapter 5 sought to test the hypothesis that encouragement to eat during mealtime from older siblings and sisters mediates associations of being last-born or having a sister with higher BMI. Children aged 4–8 years ($n = 75$) were videotaped while eating a routine evening meal at home with one sibling present. Encouragement to eat (defined as direct prompts to eat or general positive statements about food) delivered to the index child (IC) from the sibling was coded from the videotape. Path analysis was used to examine associations between IC's birth order, sibling's sex, encouragement counts, and IC's measured BMI z-score (BMIz). Being the younger sibling in the sibling dyad was associated with the IC receiving more encouragements to eat from the sibling (β: 0.93, 95% confidence interval (CI): 0.59, 1.26, $p < 0.0001$). The IC having a sister compared with a brother was not associated with the IC receiving more encouragements to eat from the sibling (β: 0.18, 95% CI: −0.09, 0.47, $p = 0.20$). The IC receiving more encouragements to eat from the sibling was associated with lower IC BMIz (β: −0.06, 95% CI: −0.12, 0.00, $p = 0.05$). Children were more likely to receive encouragements to eat from older siblings than younger siblings. Being the recipient of encouragements to eat from a sibling was associated with lower, not higher, child BMIz, which may reflect sibling modeling of maternal behavior. Future longitudinal studies are needed to examine whether encouragements to eat from siblings lead to increase in BMI over time. Encouragements from siblings may be a novel intervention target for obesity prevention.

Food prepared out-of-home tends to be less healthful than food prepared at home, with a positive association between frequency of consumption and both fat intake and body fatness. There is little current data on who eats out-of-home food. The authors of chapter 6 explored frequency and socio-demographic correlates of eating meals out and take-away meals at home, using data from a large, UK, population representative study. Data were from waves 1–4 of the UK National Diet and Nutrition Survey (2008–12). Socio-demographic variables of interest were gender, age group, and socio-economic position. Self-reported frequency of consuming meals out and take-away meals at home was categorised as: less than once per week and once per week or more. Analyses were performed separately for adults (aged 18 years or older) and children. Data from 2001 adults and 1963 children were included. More than one quarter (27.1%) of adults and one fifth (19.0%) of children ate meals out once per week or more. One fifth of adults (21.1%) and children (21.0%) ate take-away meals at home once per week or more. There were no gender differences in consumption of meals out, but more boys than girls ate take-away meals at home at least weekly.

The proportion of participants eating both meals out and take-away meals at home at least weekly peaked in young adults aged 19–29 years. Adults living in more affluent households were more likely to eat meals out at least once per week, but children living in less affluent households were more likely to eat take-away meals at home at least once per week. There was no relationship between socio-economic position and consumption of take-away meals at home in adults. One-fifth to one-quarter of individuals eat meals prepared out-of-home weekly. Interventions seeking to improve dietary intake by reducing consumption of out-of-home food may be more effective if tailored to and targeted at adults aged less than 30 years. It may also be important to develop interventions to help children and adolescents avoid becoming frequent consumers of out-of-home food.

Despite a growing consensus on the feeding practices associated with healthy eating patterns, few observational studies of maternal feeding practices with young children have been conducted, especially in low-income populations. The aim of the study in chapter 7 was to provide such data on a low income sample to determine the degree to which observed maternal feeding practices compare with current recommendations. Eighty low-income mothers and their preschool children were videotaped at dinner in their homes. Mothers were chosen from a larger study to create a 2 X 2 X 2 design: maternal ethnicity (African American vs. Latina) by child gender by child weight status (healthy weight vs. overweight/obese). Observers coded videotapes for a range of maternal feeding strategies and other behaviors. Many mothers spent considerable time encouraging eating—often in spite of the child's insistence that he or she was finished. Mothers talked little about food characteristics, rarely referred to feelings of hunger and fullness, and made more attempts to enforce table manners than to teach eating skills. Latina mothers showed higher levels of teaching eating skills and encouraging their children to eat; African American mothers showed higher levels of enforcing table manners and getting children to clear their plates. Mothers of boys used more unelaborated commands and less questions/suggestions than mothers of girls. Finally, compared to mothers of overweight/obese children, mothers of healthy weight children showed higher levels of encouraging eating and lower levels of discouraging eating. Most of the mothers in this study did not engage in feeding practices that are consistent with current recommendations. They did this, despite the fact that they knew they were being observed. These results should be used to inform future research about the motivations behind mothers' feeding practices and the development of interventions by helping identify areas in greatest need of change.

The international increase in overweight and obesity among children and adolescents over the past three decades confirms that childhood obesity is a global 'epidemic'. The World Health Organization considers childhood obesity to be a major public health concern. Childhood obesity is associated with cardiovascular, endocrine, musculoskeletal and gastrointestinal complications, and may have psycho-social consequences. The aim of chapter 8 is to examine overweight (including obesity) prevalence and its association with geographic area of residence, parental education and daily breakfast consumption in Italian students aged 11–15 yrs. A nationally representative sample of 11–15 year old students from 20 Italian Regions (Italian Health Behaviour in School-aged Children 2010-HBSC) was randomly selected (2,504 schools and 77,113 students). Self-reported anonymous questionnaires, prepared by the international HBSC network, were used to collect the data. BMI was calculated using self-reported weight and height and the International Obesity Task Force cut-offs. Multiple logistic regressions were performed to assess the relationship between the risk of overweight and parental education, area of residence and breakfast consumption in each age group and gender. Boys were more likely to be overweight or obese than girls (28.1% vs. 18.9% at 11 yrs-old, 24.8% vs. 16.5% at 13 yrs and 25.4 vs. 11.8% at 15 yrs). The prevalence of overweight and obesity was lower among the older girls. Overweight and obesity rates increased from the North of Italy to the South in both boys and girls and in all age groups. Boys 11-15 yrs living in southern Italy had an OR=2.05 (1.77-2.38) and girls 2.04 (95% CI 1.70-2.44) for overweight (including obesity) compared with those living in the North. Parent's low educational level and no daily breakfast consumption were also associated with overweight including obesity ($p<0.05$). The prevalence of obesity and overweight in Italian school-children 11-15 yrs old are high, in particular in the South and in boys. These findings suggest appropriate interventions are needed, at the community as well as the individual level, in particular in the southern regions. However, more research is warranted on intermediary factors to determine which interventions are likely to be most effective.

The aims of chapter 9 are 1) to investigate the association between maternal educational level and healthy eating behaviour of 11-year-old children (fruit, vegetables and breakfast consumption), and 2) to examine whether factors in the home food environment (parental intake of fruit, vegetables and breakfast; rules about fruit and vegetables and home availability of fruit and vegetables) mediate these associations. Data were obtained from the Dutch INPACT study. In total, 1318 parent-child dyads were included in this study. Multilevel regression models were used to investigate whether factors of the home food environment mediated the association between maternal educational level and children's healthy eating behaviour. Children of mothers with a high educational level consumed more pieces of fruit per day (B = 0.13, 95% CI: 0.04-0.22), more grams of vegetables per day (B = 23.81, 95% CI = 14.93-32.69) and were more likely to have breakfast on a daily basis (OR = 2.97, 95% CI: 1.38-6.39) than children of mothers with a low educational level. Home availability, food consumption rules and parental consumption mediated the association between maternal education level and children's fruit and vegetable consumption. Parental breakfast consumption mediated the association between maternal education level and children's breakfast consumption. Factors in the home food environment play an important role in the explanation of socio-economic disparities in children's healthy eating behaviour and may be promising targets for interventions.

The prevalence of early childhood obesity has increased dramatically particularly among the Mexican American population. Obesity leads to earlier onset of related diseases such as type 2 diabetes. The Head Start population of Texas is largely Mexican American. Dietary intake in this population demonstrated a diet very low in fiber, high in salt, and containing excessive calories with a low intake of fruit and vegetables. The study in chapter 10 was performed in a Texas Head Start population to evaluate a bilingual pictorial nutrition education game. Acceptance of the bilingual concept and the game had been previously studied in a Head Start population in five Texas counties. The effectiveness in producing a change in eating habits was studied as a pilot project 413 children and their parents at the Bastrop County Head Start. Parents were asked to supply data about at home food frequency at the beginning and the end of the school year and the results compared. The parents were given a demonstration of the educational objectives and the students played the game throughout the year. By the end of the school year there was a statistically significant increase in the vegetables offered to this population both during the week at home ($p = 0.009$) and on the weekends ($p = 0.02$).

The objective in the study in chapter 11 was to reduce intake of sugar-sweetened beverages (SSBs) in youths as a means to reduce obesity risk. To that end, youths 5–14 years old attending a summer program were given a two-hour workshop addressing the sugar content in SSBs, the health risks from drinking SSBs, and hands-on preparation as well as tastings of low-sugar beverage alternatives. Data on usual intake of SSBs was obtained at baseline, and pre- and postprogram surveys were conducted to gauge change in knowledge and/or attitudes regarding SSBs. There were 128 participants (63% male) in the program.

SSBs were commonly consumed with over 80% reporting regular consumption (mean daily intake 17.9 ounces). Significant increase in knowledge regarding the sugar content of commonly consumed SSBs was achieved; however change in attitudes was not significant. The large majority of youths reported enjoying the workshop and intention to reduce intake of SSBs following program participation. SSBs are commonly consumed by youths. Knowledge regarding the sugar content of SSBs is easier to impart to youths than influencing attitudes held about these beverages. The authors of chapter 11 conclude that long-term interventions that reach out to parents and address the widespread availability of SSBs are needed to influence resistant attitudes and beverage choosing behaviors in youths.

Failure in self-regulation has been proposed as a moderator in the development of overweight and obesity, primarily through its effects on deregulated eating behavior. As a result, it might cause regulatory problems in the energy balance, as well as rapid weight gain from early childhood through adolescence. Self-control is the exertion of control over the self by the self. Self-control occurs when a person (or other organism) attempts to change the way he or she would otherwise think, feel, or behave. Thus, self-control may be view as part of self-regulation. Parents and health care providers face the challenge of helping children practice regulation and develop coping skills alongside the ability to take care of their own well-being. Chapter 12 attempts to bridge the gap between self-control theories and interventions for the management of childhood obesity. The dietary restriction approach will be compared with the trust paradigm, which emphasizes children's internal hunger, satiety cues and a division of responsibilities between parents and children.

Adolescents' self-control weight behaviors were assessed (N = 1961; 12–17 years old; 2007–2008) in the Balearic Islands, Spain. The study in chapter 13 analyzed the relationships between body weight status, body image, and self-weight concern, and actual attempts to lose weight by restrained eating and/or increased exercising. In terms of regulatory focus theory (RFT), the authors considered that efforts to lose or to maintain weight (successful or failed) would be motivated either by a "promotion focus" (to show an attractive body), or a "prevention focus" (to avoid social rejection of fatness), or both. Results showed that 41% of overweight boys and 25% of obese boys stated that they had never made any attempt to lose weight, and 13 and 4% in females. Around half of overweight boys and around a quarter of obese boys stated that they were "Not at all" concerned about weight gain, and girls' percentages decreased to 13 and 11%, respectively. By contrast, 57% of normal weight girls monitored their weight and stated that they had tried to become slim at least once. Weight self-regulation in females attempted to combine diet and exercise, while boys relied almost exclusively on exercise. Apparent lack of consciousness of body weight status among overweight boys, and more important, subsequent absence of behaviors to reduce their weight clearly challenges efforts to prevent obesity. The authors argue that several causes may be involved in this outcome, including unconscious, emotional (self-defense), and cognitive (dissonance) mechanisms driven by perceived social stigmatization of obesity. The active participation of social values of male and female body image (strong vs. pretty), and the existence of social habituation to overweight are suggested. A better knowledge of psychosocial mechanisms underlying adolescent weight self-control may improve obesity epidemics.

Adequate treatment of severe childhood obesity is important given its serious social, psychological and physical consequences. Self-regulation may be a crucial determinant of treatment success. Yet, little is known about the role that self-regulation and other psychosocial factors play in the long-term outcome of obesity treatment in severely obese children and adolescents. In chapter 14, the authors describe the design of a study that aims to determine whether the ability to self-regulate predicts long-term weight loss in severely obese children and adolescents. An additional objective is to identify other psychosocial factors that may modify this relation. The study in chapter 14 is designed as a prospective observational study of 120 severely obese children and adolescents (8–19 years) and their parents/caregivers undergoing an intensive combined lifestyle intervention during one year. The intervention uses behavior change techniques to improve the general ability to self-regulate. Measurements will be taken at three points in time: at baseline (start of treatment), at the end of treatment (1 year after baseline) and at follow-up (2 years after baseline). The primary outcome measurement is the gender and age-specific change in SDS-BMI. The children's general self-regulation abilities are evaluated by two behavioral computer tasks assessing two distinct aspects of self-regulation that are particularly relevant to controlling food intake: inhibitory control (Stop Signal Task) and sensitivity to reward (Balloon Analogue Risk Task). In addition to the computer tasks, a self-report measure of eating-specific self-regulation ability is used. Psychosocial factors related to competence, motivation, relatedness and outcome expectations are examined as moderating factors using several questionnaires for the patients and their parents/caregivers. At the conclusion of the study, the authors hope to provide knowledge about the relation between self-regulation and long-term weight loss after intensive lifestyle interventions over a two-year period in severely obese children and adolescents, a growing but often overlooked patient group. The authors aim to investigate to what extent (changes in) the general ability to self-regulate predicts weight loss and weight loss maintenance. The results may contribute to the development of more successful interventions.

Nearly one in five 4-year-old children in the United States are obese, with low-income children almost twice as likely to be obese as their middle/upper-income peers. Few obesity prevention programs for low-income preschoolers and their parents have been rigorously tested, and effects are modest. The authors in chapter 15 are testing a novel obesity prevention program for low-income preschoolers built on the premise that children who are better able to self-regulate in the face of psychosocial stressors may be less likely to eat impulsively in response to stress. Enhancing behavioral self-regulation skills in low-income children may be a unique and important intervention approach to prevent childhood obesity. The Growing Healthy study is a randomized controlled trial evaluating two obesity prevention interventions in 600 low-income preschoolers attending Head Start, a federally-funded preschool program for low-income children. Interventions are delivered by community-based, nutrition-education staff partnering with Head Start. The first intervention (n = 200), Preschool Obesity Prevention Series (POPS), addresses evidence-based obesity prevention behaviors for preschool-aged children and their parents. The second intervention (n = 200) comprises POPS in combination with the Incredible Years Series (IYS), an evidence-based approach to improving self-regulation among preschool-aged children. The comparison condition (n = 200) is Usual Head Start Exposure. The authors hypothesize that POPS will yield positive effects compared to Usual Head Start, and that the combined intervention (POPS + IYS) addressing behaviors well-known to be associated with obesity risk, as well as self-regulatory capacity, will be most effective in preventing excessive increases in child adiposity indices (body mass index, skinfold thickness). The authors will evaluate additional child outcomes using parent and teacher reports and direct assessments of food-related self-regulation. They will also gather process data on intervention implementation, including fidelity, attendance, engagement, and satisfaction. The Growing Healthy study may shed light on associations between self-regulation skills and obesity risk in low-income preschoolers. If the project is effective in preventing obesity, results can also provide critical insights into how best to deliver obesity prevention programming to parents and children in a community-based setting like Head Start in order to promote better health among at-risk children.

PART I
Pediatric Dietary Behaviors

CHAPTER 1

Determinants of Dietary Behavior Among Youth: An Umbrella Review

Ester F. C. Sleddens, Willemieke Kroeze, Leonie F. M. Kohl, Laura M. Bolten, Elizabeth Velema, Pam J. Kaspers, Johannes Brug, and Stef P. J. Kremers

1.1 BACKGROUND

Dietary behaviors have been found to track from childhood into adulthood [1]. Unhealthy food habits in childhood, therefore, can have a tremendous health impact later in life. Given the high prevalence of nutrition-related disease and mortality in Western countries [2], it is necessary to develop effective behavioral interventions to improve diet quality. But which factors determine a person's dietary behavior? Interventions to improve health-related behaviors should be tailored to the most important and changeable determinants of these behaviors, preferably applying behavior change theories [3]. To facilitate improvement of relevant, effective programs and policies promoting healthy eating targeting dietary behavior it is important to identify the various factors that may influence children's and adolescents' food consumption.

Socio-cognitive models of (health) behavior and behavior change, such as the Theory of Planned Behavior [4], Social-Cognitive Theory [5], and the Health Belief Model [6] have been applied frequently in development of nutrition education interventions. In very general terms -and not paying attention to the richness of and also differences between these models—these theories regard nutrition behavior to be determined by beliefs and conscious decisions, rational considerations of pros and cons of the behavior, perceived social influences, and assessment of personal efficacy and control. In additional fields of research, the physiological and affective influences on dietary behaviors have been studied, providing evidence for such basic factors as hunger and satiety, sensory perceptions, and perceived palatability of foods [7] as important drivers of food choice and dietary behaviors. And somewhat more recently, the so-called food environment that defines the availability and accessibility (i.e. physical environment), affordability (i.e. economic environment), social appropriateness or support (social-cultural environment), as well as rules, regulations and policies (i.e. political environment) regarding food choice and dietary behaviors has been studied in relation to food intake and dietary behaviors, as informed by (social) ecological behavior models [8-12]. Kremers and colleagues [13] proposed to integrate these insights in their Environmental Research framework for weight Gain prevention (EnRG; Figure 1). EnRG is a dual-process model and regards dietary behavior and physical (in) activity to be the result of direct 'automatic' responses to environmental cues (e.g. meal patterns and routines) as well as of more rational decision making based on cognitions such as intentions and beliefs. Furthermore, EnRG includes mediating pathways between environment and cognitions as well as potential moderators of the impact of these determinants such as habit strength and self-regulation skills.

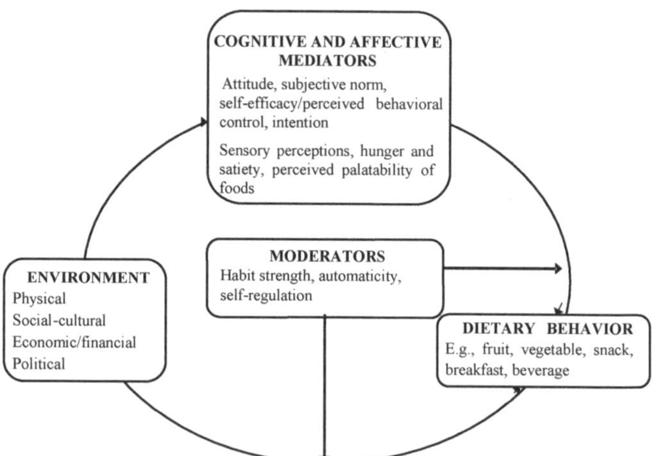

FIGURE 1.1 Environmental research framework for weight gain prevention (EnRG), adapted from Kremers et al. [13].

The purpose of this study was to get a comprehensive and systematic overview of the scientific literature on correlates (referred to as potential determinants) and determinants of dietary behavior among children and adolescent (referred to as youth) to facilitate the improvement of effective healthy eating promoting interventions and identify gaps for future research initiatives. Because the scientific literature on this topic is unwieldy and has been documented in a number of systematic reviews in recent years, we aimed to conduct a review-of-reviews to provide a more comprehensive overview. We were interested in the association of all determinants that are potentially modifiable (social-cognitive, environmental, sensory and automatic processes) with observable dietary behavior (actual consumption behaviors like fruit consumption, beverage intake, snacking) among youth. By conducting a review-of-reviews, the so-called umbrella review, we aimed to (a) explore which determinant-behavior relationships have been studied so far, and (b) assess the importance and strength of evidence of potential determinants. The EnRG framework served to categorize the findings. Parallel to this umbrella review, a separate review-of-reviews of studies among adults was conducted by the same team with the same methodology [14]. Some parts of these two reviews -especially the description of the methodology—are therefore very similar.

1.2 METHODS

1.2.1 Search Strategy and Eligibility Criteria

To identify all relevant systematic reviews, we conducted systematic searches in the bibliographic databases PubMed, PsycINFO (via CSA Illumina), The Cochrane Library (via Wiley) and Web of Science for articles published between January 1, 1990 and May 1, 2014. The search terms included controlled terms, e.g. MeSH in PubMed, Thesaurus in PsycINFO, as well as free text terms (only in The Cochrane Library). Search terms expressing 'food and dietary behavior' were used in combination with search terms comprising 'determinants', 'study design: (systematic) review', 'study population: humans' and 'time span (January 1, 1990 to May 1, 2014)'. The PubMed search strategy can be found in Table 1. The search strategies used in the other databases were based on the PubMed strategy.

Studies were included if they met the following criteria: (i) systematic reviews on observable food and dietary behavior (i.e. consumption behaviors like fruit intake and snacking consumption, not purchasing behavior); (ii) studies describing potential behavioral determinants; (iii) study design: (systematic) review; (iv) study population: humans and (v) time span: January 1, 1990 to May 1, 2014. We excluded: (i) studies that were not written in English; (ii) studies in which dietary behavior was not an outcome of the study; (iii); studies about dietary behaviors in disease management and treatment; (iv) studies that focused on specific population groups (e.g. chronically ill, pregnant women, cancer survivors); (v) studies not published as peer reviewed systematic reviews in scientific journals, e.g. theses, dissertations, book chapters, non-peer reviewed papers, conference proceedings, reviews of case studies and qualitative studies, design and position papers, umbrella reviews; (vi) reviews of studies on not directly observable dietary behavior (e.g. nutrient or energy intake, appetite); (vii) reviews of studies on non-modifiable determinants (e.g. physiological, neurological or genetic factors); (viii) reviews of studies on the effect of interventions (but reviews of experimental manipulation of single determinants were included); (ix) reviews not conducted systematically (search strategy including keywords and databases used not identified, and/or with too little information of the included studies presented). The current umbrella review focuses on youth (<18 years). A second umbrella review using the same methodology about determinants of dietary behavior in adults is published elsewhere [14].

TABLE 1.1 Search strategy in PubMed: January 1st, 1990 to May 1st, 2014 (bottom-up): N = 13,156

Set	Search terms
#6	#1 AND #2 AND #3 AND #4 NOT #5
#5	("addresses" [Publication Type] OR "biography" [Publication Type] OR "case reports" [Publication Type] OR "comment" [Publication Type] OR "directory" [Publication Type] OR "editorial" [Publication Type] OR "festschrift" [Publication Type] OR "interview" [Publication Type] OR "lectures" [Publication Type] OR "legal cases" [Publication Type] OR "legislation" [Publication Type] OR "letter" [Publication Type] OR "news" [Publication Type] OR "newspaper article" [Publication Type] OR "patient education handout" [Publication Type] OR "popular works" [Publication Type] OR "congresses" [Publication Type] OR "consensus development conference" [Publication Type] OR "consensus development conference, nih" [Publication Type] OR "practice guideline" [Publication Type])
#4	"review" [tiab]
#3	"humans" [Mesh]

TABLE 1.1 *(Continued)*

Set	Search terms
#2	("food and beverages" [Mesh] OR "food" [tiab] OR "beverage" [tiab] OR "beverages" [tiab] OR "diet" [Mesh] OR "diet" [tiab] OR "eating" [Mesh] OR "eating" [tiab] OR "feeding behavior" [Mesh] OR "feeding behavior" [tiab] OR "feeding behaviour" [tiab] OR "drink" [tiab] OR "sodium chloride, dietary" [Mesh] OR "dietary sodium chloride" [tiab] OR "carbohydrates" [Mesh:noexp] OR "food habit" [tiab] OR "food habits" [tiab] OR "meal" [tiab] OR "meals" [tiab] OR "meal pattern" [tiab]) NOT "dietary supplements" [Mesh]) NOT "food additives" [Mesh]) NOT "micronutrients" [Mesh]) NOT "cannibalism" [Mesh]) NOT "carnivory" [Mesh]) NOT "herbivory" [Mesh]) NOT "bottle feeding" [Mesh]) NOT "breast feeding" [Mesh]) NOT "mastication" [Mesh])
#1	("association" [Mesh] OR "association" [tiab] OR "associations" [tiab] OR "determinant" [tiab] OR "determinants" [tiab] OR "correlation" [tiab] OR "correlations" [tiab] OR "correlated" [tiab] OR "correlates" [tiab] OR "relation" [tiab] OR "relations" [tiab] OR "relationship" [tiab] OR "relationships" [tiab] OR "relate" [tiab] OR "related" [tiab] OR "relates" [tiab] OR "factor" [tiab] OR "factors" [tiab] OR "predict" [tiab] OR "predicted" [tiab] OR "prediction" [tiab] OR "predictive" [tiab] OR "predicts" [tiab] OR "predictor" [tiab] OR "associate" [tiab] OR "associates" [tiab] OR "associated" [tiab] OR "influence" [tiab] OR "influences" [tiab] OR "influencing" [tiab] OR "influenced" [tiab] OR "effect" [tiab] OR "effects" [tiab])

Note: Filters review; Publication data from 1990/01/01 to 2014/05/01; English.

1.2.2 Selection Process

Figure 2 summarizes the manuscript selection process. In total, 17714 citations were obtained using PubMed (n = 13156), PsycINFO (n = 961), The Cochrane Library (n = 920), and Web of Science (n = 2677). The subsequent screening of the citations was performed by multiple reviewers (all citations were screened by ES and WK; some were screened by LB, SK, and EV). All titles of the citations were independently screened for relevance by two reviewers (ES and WK). Any disagreement was resolved by including the citation into the abstract screening process. Subsequently, abstracts of the remaining 1031 citations were retrieved for further screening. Another 729 citations were removed, resulting in 292 articles for full-text assessment for eligibility. In case of doubt, potential inclusion was discussed with a third reviewer (SK). Studies that did not meet the inclusion criteria (n = 257) were removed. Figure 2 displays the reasons for exclusion. Additionally, duplicates (n = 10) were removed. Thereafter, the reference lists of all review papers selected for inclusion (n = 25) were scanned for further relevant references. This reference tracking technique resulted in one additional review article appropriate for inclusion. In total, 26 reviews were considered eligible. However, of these reviews, 9 were only focused on determinants of adult dietary behavior (references reported in the umbrella review about determinants of dietary behavior in adults of Sleddens et al. [14]). Five reviews assessed dietary behavior of both youth and adults [15-19]. Therefore, 17 reviews were considered eligible for our umbrella review on determinants of youth dietary behavior [15-31].

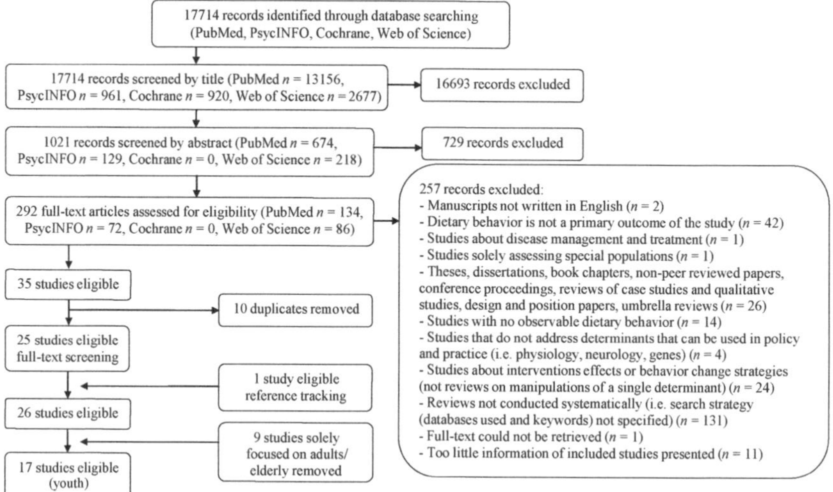

FIGURE 1.2 Flow diagram of literature search by database.

1.2.3 Data Extraction Including Rating of Methodological Quality

Four authors (ES, WK, LK, and LB) extracted data from the selected reviews. The extracted data included search range applied, total number of studies included in the reviews and number of studies included in the reviews that are eligible for the current umbrella review, total number of participants of included studies in the reviews and number of participants of the included studies that are eligible for the current umbrella review, and age and continent of included eligible studies. For a description of the results, correlate and outcome measures were extracted, as well as overall results of the reviews and overall limitations and recommendations of reviews. Additionally, the methodological quality of the reviews was evaluated using quality criteria adapted from De Vet, De Ridder, & De Wit [32] and based on the Quality Assessment Tool for Reviews [33]. In total, a review was scored on eight criteria (with a total quality scoring ranging from 0–8) (see Table 2); 0 when the criteria was not applicable for the included review; 1 when the criteria was applicable for the included review. Disagreement between the reviewers on individual items were identified and solved during a consensus meeting. The quality of the reviews could be labeled as weak (quality scores ranging from 0 to 3), moderate (quality scores ranging from 4 to 6) or strong (quality scores ranging from 7 to 8). Furthermore, we judged the importance of included determinants in the reviews and judged its strength of evidence. The importance of a determinant refers to the statistical significance of a potential determinant and/or effect size estimate in relation to a particular type of dietary behavior. It refers to the amount of reviews (or eligible studies within the reviews) that did or did not find statistically significant results. For a particular determinant to receive the highest ranking (highest level of importance), all eligible studies in each review should have found a significant relationship and/or reported a (non)-significant effect size larger than 0.30. The strength of evidence represents the consistency between study findings and designs of the studies. Longitudinal observational studies and -where relevant—experimental studies of sufficient size, duration and quality showing consistent effects were given prominence as the highest ranking study designs. For this judgment we applied two coding schemes, see Tables 3 and 4 respectively. The criteria for grading evidence were adapted from those of the World Cancer Research Fund [34]. The data extraction method is similar to the study of Sleddens et al. [14].

1.3 RESULTS

1.3.1 Description of Reviews

Quality assessment ratings are presented in Table 2. One review received a quality rating of 2 (weak). The other reviews were rated as moderate (n = 9) or strong (n = 7). In all reviews, the inclusion and exclusion criteria were clearly stated and the review did integrate findings beyond describing or listing findings of primary studies. Clearly defined search strategies were absent in more than half of the reviews (9 out of 17 reviews), as usually a flow chart of the data screening process was missing.

Table 5 provides an overview of the characteristics of the included reviews. In three reviews [22-24] all included studies were eligible for our current study.

TABLE 1.2 Quality assessment of reviews of determinants of dietary behavior among youth

Quality assessment criteria	Was there a clearly defined search strategy?[1]	Was the search strategy comprehensive?[2]	Are inclusion/exclusion criteria clearly stated?	Are the designs and number of included studies clearly stated?	Has the quality of primary studies been assessed?	Did the quality assessment include study design, study sample, outcome measures or follow-up (at least 2 of 4)	Does the review integrate findings beyond describing or listing findings of primary studies?	Has more than one author been involved in the data screening and/or abstraction process?	Sum quality score
Williams [31]	1	1	1	1	1	1	1	1	8
Gardner [17]*	1	1	1	1	1	1	1	0	7
Pearson & Biddle [19]*	0	1	1	1	1	1	1	0	6
Adriaanse [15]*	0	1	1	1	0	0	1	1	5
McClain [24]	0	1	1	1	1	1	1	1	7
Van der Horst [29]	0	1	1	1	0	0	1	1	5
Pearson [25]	1	1	1	1	0	0	1	0	5
De Craemer [21]	1	1	1	1	0	0	1	1	6
Pearson [26]	1	1	1	1	1	1	1	0	7
Verloigne [30]	1	1	1	1	1	1	1	0	7
Ford [22]	1	1	1	1	1	1	1	1	8
Caspi [16]*	0	0	1	0	0	0	1	0	2
Moore & Cunningham [18]*	1	1	1	1	0	0	1	1	6
Lawman & Wilson [23]	0	1	1	1	1	1	1	0	6
Sleddens [28]	0	1	1	1	0	0	1	1	5

TABLE 1.2 *(Continued)*

Quality assessment criteria	Was there a clearly defined search strategy?[1]	Was the search strategy comprehensive?[2]	Are inclusion/exclusion criteria clearly stated?	Are the designs and number of included studies clearly stated?	Has the quality of primary studies been assessed?	Did the quality assessment include study design, study sample, outcome measures or follow-up (at least 2 of 4)	Does the review integrate findings beyond describing or listing findings of primary studies?	Has more than one author been involved in the data screening and/or abstraction process?	Sum quality score
Berge [20]	0	0	1	1	1	1	1	0	5
Rasmussen [27]	0	1	1	1	1	1	1	1	7
	8/17	15/17	17/17	16/17	10/17	10/17	17/17	9/17	

Note: [1]A search is rated clearly defined if at least search words and a flow chart is presented; [2]A search is rated as comprehensive if at least two databases and the reference lists of examined papers were searched.

[*]Reviews also including adults; weak (score ranging from 0–3) n = 1 (5.88%), moderate (score ranging from 4–6) n = 9 (52.94%), strong (score ranging from 7–8) n = 7 (41.18%).

TABLE 1.3 Importance of a determinant

Five categories of importance are defined: ++ / + / 0 / - / —	
The categories are defined as follows:	
++	The variable has been found to be a statistically significant determinant in all identified reviews, without exception. This could mean that only one review has included a particular variable, and showed that this was a significant correlate and/or reported a (non)-significant effect size larger than 0.30, but it could also mean that a number of reviews were conducted that included this variable and all of them concluded that the variable was significantly related to the particular behavioral outcome.
+	The variable has been found to be a statistically significant determinant and/or reported a (non)-significant effect size larger than 0.30 in most reviews or studies within the review, with some exceptions. This implies that > 75% of the available reviews concluded the variable to be related, or the separate reviews report that 75% or more of the original studies concluded the factor to be related. This could therefore mean that only one review has included a particular variable, and showed that this was a significant correlate in > 75% of studies. But it could also mean that a number of reviews were executed towards this variable and most, but not all, concluded that the variable was significantly related to the particular behavioral outcome.
0	The variable has been found to be a determinant and/or reported a (non)-significant effect size larger than 0.30 in some reviews (25% to 75% of available reviews or of the studies reviewed in these reviews), but not in others. This could mean that only one review has included a particular variable, and showed 'mixed findings', but it could also mean that results are mixed across reviews.
-	The variable has been found not to be a determinant, with some exceptions. This implies that <25% of the available reviews or of the original studies in the included reviews concluded that the variable was related. This could thus mean that only one review has included a particular variable, and generally showed 'null findings', with some exceptions. But it could also mean that a number of reviews were executed towards this variable and most, but not all, concluded that the variable was not significantly related to the particular behavioral outcome.
—	The variable has been found not to be related to this particular outcome. The absence of a relation was identified in all identified reviews, without exception. This could mean that only one review has included a particular variable, and showed that this correlate was not related to the behavior in question, but it could also mean that a number of reviews were executed towards this variable and all of them concluded that the variable was unrelated to the particular behavioral outcome.

TABLE 1.4 Criteria for grading evidence, see World Cancer Research Fund [34] for the full list

Strength of evidence:	
Ideally the definition of the strength of evidence should be based on a relationship that has been established by multiple randomized controlled trials of manipulations of single isolated variables, but this type of evidence is often not available.	
The following criteria were used to describe the strength of evidence in this report. They are based on the criteria used by the World Cancer Research Fund (World Cancer Research Fund, 2007 [34]), but have been modified for the research question at hand. Four categories were defined: convincing/probable/limited, suggestive/limited, no conclusion.	
Convincing evidence:	Evidence based on studies of determinants showing consistent associations between the variable and the behavioral outcome. The available evidence is based on a substantial number of studies including longitudinal observational studies and where relevant, experimental studies of sufficient size, duration and quality showing consistent effects. Specifically, the grading criteria include evidence from more than one study type and evidence from at least two independent cohort studies should be available, and strong and plausible experimental evidence.
Probable evidence:	Evidence based on studies of determinants showing fairly consistent associations between the variable and the behavioral outcome, but there are shortcomings in the available evidence or some evidence to the contrary, which precludes a more definite judgment. Shortcomings in the evidence may be any of the following: insufficient duration of studies, insufficient studies available (but evidence from at least two independent cohort studies or five case-control studies should be available), inadequate sample sizes, incomplete follow-up.
Limited, suggestive evidence:	Evidence based mainly on findings from cross- sectional studies. Insufficient longitudinal observational studies or experimental studies are available or results are inconsistent. More well- designed studies of determinants are required to support the tentative associations.
Limited, no conclusive evidence:	Evidence based on findings of a few studies which are suggestive, but are insufficient to establish an association between the variable and the behavioral outcome. No evidence is available from longitudinal observational or experimental studies. More well-designed studies of determinants are required to support the tentative associations.

TABLE 1.5 Characteristics of analyzed systematic reviews among youth

Author and date	Search range applied	Number of eligible studies included in the review/total number of studies included in the review	Designs of studies	Total sample size of eligible studies included in the review/Total sample size of all studies included in the review	Ages	Continent
Williams et al., 2014 [31]	Up to 2013	13/30	Cross-sectional n = 12, longitudinal n = 1	Total n = 570,403, range 610 to 529,367/ Total n = 1,550,415 (26 studies, NR: 4 studies), range 319 to 926,018	11 to 17y	North-America n = 6, Europe n = 5, Australasia n = 1, Asia n = 1
Gardner et al., 2011 [17]	No date limits were set.	4 studies (2 samples)/22 studies (21 samples)	Cross-sectional n = 4	Total n = 695, range 312 to 383/Total n = 6,121, range 93 to 876	High school students	Only Europe
Pearson & Biddle, 2011 [19]	NR	31 studies (240 samples (total), 33 samples (children), 207 samples (adolescents))/53 studies (111 samples)	Majority cross-sectional	NR/Children: mean n = 1,184, range 66 to 6,235, Adolescents: mean n = 8,356, range 60 to 14,407	<12, 12 to 18y	Children: majority North-America n = 13, Adolescents: half North-America n = 13
Adriaanse et al., 2011 [15]	Up to 2009	1 study/21 research articles describing 23 empirical studies	Healthy eating: cross-sectional n = 1, prospective n = 3, interventions n = 11; Unhealthy eating: longi-tudinal n = 1, interventions n = 8	NR/NR	11 to 16y	NR
McClain et al., 2009 [24]	From 1990 to 2009	50 studies/77 studies	Overall results: cross-sectional n = 64, prospective n = 11, interventions n = 2	NR/<50 n = 4, 51–99 n = 1, 100–499 n = 39, 500–999 n = 15, 1000–2999 n = 14, 3000–4999 n = 3, ≥5000 n = 3	<13, 13 to 18y	Overall results: North-America n = 48, Europe n = 32, Australasia n = 3, Africa n = 3, Asia n = 2, other n = 3
Van der Horst et al., 2007 [29]	From 1980 to 2004	36 studies (44 samples)/58 studies (77 samples)	Cross-sectional 95%, longitudinal 3%, case control 2%	NR/<100 n = 8, 100–199 n = 6, 200–299 n = 1, 300–499 n = 5, 500–999 n = 2, 1000–2999 n = 9; 3000–4999 n = 4, ≥5000 n = 2	<13, 13 to 18y	North-America 45 samples, Europe 26 samples, Asia 4 samples, Oceania 2 samples
Pearson et al., 2009 [25]	Up to 2008	24 studies (33 samples)/24 studies (33 samples)	Majority cross-sectional n = 23	Children: mean n = 1,534, range 136 to 4,314. Adolescents: mean n = 2,533, range 357 to 18,177	6 to 18y	Majority Europe n = 12 (papers)
De Craemer et al., 2012 [21]	From 1990 to 2010	6 studies/43 studies	Cross-sectional n = 35, longitudinal n = 6, cross-sectional and longitudinal n = 1, intervention n = 1	NR/<100 n = 3, 100–999 n = 28, >1000 n = 12. Study sample sizes ranged from 46 to 5,652	4 to 6y	North-America n = 21, Europe n = 9, Australasia n = 12, Asia n = 1

TABLE 1.5 *(Continued)*

Author and date	Search range applied	Number of eligible studies included in the review/total number of studies included in the review	Designs of studies	Total sample size of eligible studies included in the review/Total sample size of all studies included in the review	Ages	Continent
Pearson et al., 2009 [26]	Up to 2007	Total papers: n = 60. Children: 25 studies (33 samples). Adolescents: 38 studies (55 samples)/Total papers: n = 60. Children: 25 studies (33 samples). Adolescents: 38 studies (55 samples)	Majority cross-sectional n = 24. Children: cross-sectional n = 31, longitudinal n = 2; Adolescent: cross-sectional n = 55, ongitudinal n = 0	Mean n = 1,131, range 536 to 8,263. Children (6-11y): < 100 n = 8, 100–199 n = 2, 200–299 n = 1, 300–499 n = 1, 500–999 n = 6, 1000–2999 n = 10, 3000–4999 n = 3, unknown n = 2; Adolescent (12-18y): < 100 n = 2, 100–199 n = 3, 200–299 n = 3, 300–499 n = 11, 500–999 n = 4, 1000–2999 n = 12, 3000–4999 n = 8, >5000 n = 10	6 to 18y Children: 6-11y Adolescents: 12-18y	Children: North-America n = 15, Europe n = 15, Australasia n = 1, South-America n = 1, Asia n = 2; Adolescent: North-America n = 23, Europe n = 16, Australasia n = 9, South-America n = 2, Asia n = 5
Verloigne et al., 2012 [30]	From 1990 to 2010	17 studies/76 studies	Cross-sectional n = 16, longitudinal n = 1	100-199 n = 1, 300–499 n = 1, 500–999 n = 5, 1000–2999 n = 5, 3000–4999 n = 2, ≥5000 n = 3/< 100 n = 3, 100–199 n = 9, 200–299 n = 6, 300–499 n = 10, 500–999 n = 17, 1000–2999 n = 20, 3000–4999 n= 5, ≥5000 n = 6	10 to 12y	North-America n = 9, Europe n = 4, Australasia n = 4
Ford et al., 2012 [22]	NR	9 studies /12 studies	Cross-sectional n = 9	Total n = 13,280, range 240 to 4,983/ Total n = 13,386, range 106 to 4,983	2 to 6y	NR
Caspi et al., 2012 [16]	Up to 2011	5 studies /38 studies	Majority cross-sectional, intervention n = 3	NR/NR	Children5 to 6y, 10 to 12y, youth, boy scouts	North-America n = 4, Australasia n = 1
Moore & Cunningham, 2012 [18]	NR	2 studies /14 studies	Cross-sectional n = 2	Total n = 5,144, range 824 to 4,320/ Total n = 94,230, range 51 to 64,277	Preteens and 14 to 17y	NR
Lawman & Wilson, 2012 [23]	From 1995 to 2010	11 studies /38 studies	Cross-sectional n = 8, longitudinal n = 3.	Total n = 21,865, range 228 to 4,746/ Total n = 51,396, range 52 to 7,907	9 to 21y	North-America n = 32
Sleddens et al., 2011 [28]	Up to 2010	10 studies /36 studies	Cross-sectional: n = 9, longitudinal: n = 1	Total n = 14,567, range 74 to 4,555/ Total n = 35,146, range 48 to 4,983	NR	North-America n = 5, Europe n = 5

TABLE 1.5 *(Continued)*

Author and date	Search range applied	Number of eligible studies included in the review/total number of studies included in the review	Designs of studies	Total sample size of eligible studies included in the review/Total sample size of all studies included in the review	Ages	Continent
Berge, 2009 [20]	From 2000 onwards	48 studies /81 studies	Cross-sectional n = 39, longitudinal n = 8, intervention n = 11	Total n = 190,270, range 23 to 99,426/ Total n = 276,557, range 23 to 99,426	0 to 18y	NR
Rasmussen et al., 2006 [27]	Up to 2005	98 studies /98 studies	Cross-sectional n = 90, longitudinal n = 8	<500 n = 24, 500–1000 n = 20, >1000 n = 53, NR: n = 1/<500 n = 24, 500–1000 n = 20, >1000 n = 53, NR: n = 1	NR	North-America n = 50, Europe n = 31, Australasia n = 16, South-America n = 1

Note: Designs of studies: cross-sectional, longitudinal observational, case control, and intervention studies (experimental, behavioral laboratory, filed studies in which interventions were studied); NR: not reported; we were mainly interested to provide a more thorough description on the eligible studies of the included reviews (designs of studies, ages, continent).

Most of the studies included in the reviews used a cross-sectional study design. Six studies did not provide any information about sample sizes [15,16,19,21,24,29]. The remaining reviews included a total sample size of 695 to 570,403. The target groups of the eligible studies ranged in ages between the different reviews, although the focus was on primary school-aged children and adolescents. Most of the studies included in the reviews were conducted in North-America, followed by Europe.

1.3.2 Findings of the Reviews

Table 6 provides an overview of the correlates and outcomes (i.e. observable dietary behaviors) included in the reviews, and the overall findings, limitations and recommendations reported by the authors of these reviews. In the following two paragraphs we give an overview of the determinant-behavior relationships that have been studied so far, and give an overview of the importance and strength of evidence of potential determinants.

1.3.3 Determinant-behavior Relationship: Correlate and Outcome Measures

Potential determinants of a range of dietary behavior outcomes among youth were explored, and many studies included multiple dietary behavior outcomes.

Thirteen reviews explored associations between environmental factors and dietary behavior [16,18,20,21,23-31]. Within the environmental determinants, the social-cultural environment was most often studied (n=12) [16,18,20,21,23-30]. Thereafter, the physical environmental determinants (n=9) [16,21,23-26,29-31], the economic/financial environmental determinants (n=4) [16,21,29,30], and the political environment (n=1) [27]. Three reviews explored the associations between social-cognitive determinants and dietary behavior [15,24,27]. These social-cognitive determinants included attitude, self-efficacy/perceived behavioral control, and intention in the study of McClain et al. [24] and Rasmussen et al. [27], subjective norm in the study of Rasmussen et al. [27], and self-regulation in the study of Adriaanse et al. [15]. Two of these reviews also examined the influence between sensory determinants and dietary behavior [24,27]. One review addressed the relation between habit strength and dietary behavior [17]. And finally, three reviews looked at sedentary behavior in relation to dietary behavior [19,22,27].

TABLE 1.6 Results of the reviews about determinants of dietary behavior among youth

Author, date	Outcome measures	Correlate measures	Overall results of the reviews	Overall limitations of the review	Overall recommendations of the review
Williams et al., 2014 [31]	Sugar-sweetened beverages, fast food, fruit and vegetables	Food and retail outlets	Little evidence for an association between retail food environment surrounding schools and food consumption.	1) Meta-analysis not possible due to different conceptualizations and measures of the food environment surrounding schools. 2) Loss of detail; a review is dependent upon outcomes and analyses that individual papers reported.	1) Longitudinal studies needed. 2) Integrate validated classification systems of the retail food environment, explore the capacity of alternative methods for validating exposure data. 3) Specify individual-level measures of exposure to the food environment. 4) Collecting complementary measures of both qualitative and quantitative measures of food access. 5) Collect outcome measures that are appropriate relative to the exposures. 6) Take age and ethnicity differences into account
Gardner et al., 2011 [17]	Sugar-sweetened soft drinks	Habit strength	The weighted habit–behavior correlation effect estimate for nutritional habits was moderate to strong in size (fixed: r + =0.43; random: r + =0.41), and effects were of equal magnitude across healthful (fixed: r + =0.43; random: r + = 0.42) and unhealthful (fixed: r + =0.42; random: r + =0.41) dietary habits. The medium- to-large grand weighted mean habit– behavior correlation (r + ≈0.45) suggests that habit alone can explain around 20% of variation in nutrition related behaviors (i.e. R2 ≈ 0.20).	1) While it was not possible to meta-analyze interaction effects, habit often moderated the relationship between intention and behavior, such that intentions had reduced impact on behavior where habit was strong. This finding must be interpreted cautiously as it may reflect a bias towards publication of studies which find significant interaction, and so an overestimation of the robustness of this effect. 2) Many studies were cross-sectional, and so modeled habit as a predictor of past behavior. This fails to acknowledge the expected temporal sequence between habit and behavior, and is also conceptually problematic given that, at least in early stages of habit formation, repeated action strengthens habit. 3) Reliance on self-reports of behavior.	1) Explorations of the role of counter-intentional habits on the intention–be- havior relationship, such as the cap- acity for habitual snacking to obstruct intentions to eat a healthful diet, are needed. 2) Healthful behaviors can habituate. The formation of healthful ('good') habits, so as to aid maintenance of behavior change, thus represents a realistic goal for health promotion campaigns. 3) More methodologically rigorous research is required to provide more conceptually coherent and less biased observations of the influence of habit on action. 4) A more comprehensive understanding of nutrition behaviors, and how they might be changed, will be achieved by integrating habitual responses to contextual cues into theoretical accounts of behavior.

TABLE 1.6 *(Continued)*

Author, date	Outcome measures	Correlate measures	Overall results of the reviews	Overall limitations of the review	Overall recommendations of the review
Pearson & Biddle, 2011 [19]	Fruit, vegetables, fruit and vegetable intake combined, energy-dense snacks, fast foods, energy- dense drinks	Sedentary behavior: screen time (TV viewing, video/DVD, computer use, sitting while talking/reading/ homework)	Sedentary behavior, usually assessed as screen time and predominantly TV viewing, is associated with unhealthy dietary behaviors in children and adolescents. There appears no clear pattern for age acting as a moderator. There appears to be more consistent associations between sedentary behavior and diets for women/girls than for men/boys.	1) Many studies were cross-sectional. 2) Use of self-report measures of sedentary and dietary behaviors that lack strong validity. 3) Sedentary behavior is largely operationally defined as screen time, and this is mainly TV viewing, making it difficult to draw any conclusions regarding non-screen time and dietary intake. 4) Although "screen time" can include TV and computer use, this does not help in identifying whether it is TV, computer use, or both, that is associated with unhealthy diets.	1) More studies using objective measures of sedentary behaviors and more valid and reliable measures of dietary intake are required. 2) Examine the longitudinal association between sedentary behavior and dietary intake, and the tracking of the clustering of specific sedentary behaviors and specific dietary behaviors. For example, it appears from the mainly cross- sectional evidence presented that TV viewing is associated with unhealthy dietary patterns. Much less is known about diet and either computer use or sedentary motorized transport. It is likely that the main associations will be with TV, but this needs testing. 3) A focus on sedentary behaviors and dietary behaviors that "share" determinants as well as determinants of the clustering of sedentary and dietary behaviors will aid the development of targeted interventions to reduce sedentary behaviors and promote healthy eating.
Adriaanse et al., 2011 [15]	Fruit and vegetable consumption	Use of implementation intentions	Considerable support was found for the notion that implementation intentions can be effective in increasing healthy eating behaviors, with twelve studies showing an overall medium effect size of implementation intentions on increasing fruit and vegetable intake. However, when aiming to diminish unhealthy eating patterns by means of implementation intentions, the evidence is less convincing, with fewer studies reporting positive effects, and an overall effect size that is small.	NR	1) Although implementation intention instructions were not included as a moderator in the present meta- analysis due to the limited amount of studies, it seems prudent that future research takes into account the importance of using autonomy supportive instructions. 2) Stricter control conditions as well as better outcome measures are required. 3) Investigate efficacy of implementation intentions in diminishing unhealthy eating behaviors. In doing so, these studies should also compare the efficacy of different types of implementation intentions, as these may have differential effects on unhealthy food consumption.

TABLE 1.6 *(Continued)*

Author, date	Outcome measures	Correlate measures	Overall results of the reviews	Overall limitations of the review	Overall recommendations of the review
McClain et al., 2009 [24]	Fruit, juice and vegetable consumption, sugar, snacking, sweetened beverage consumption	Psychosocial correlates like: attitude, availability, intention, knowledge, norms, self-efficacy, preferences, parental factors, and more	Perceived modeling and dietary intentions to make healthy or less healthy dietary changes (such as intentions to decrease consumption of sugary beverages or intentions to increase consumption of medium fat milk) have the most consistent and positive associations with dietary behavior. Other psychosocial correlates such as liking, norms, and preferences were also consistently and positively associated with dietary behavior in children and adolescents. Availability, knowledge, outcome expectations, self-efficacy and social support did not show consistent relationships across dietary outcomes.	1) Many studies were cross-sectional. 2) Not possible to conduct meta-analysis. 3) Authors combined conceptually similar psychosocial determinants into one category, which may have introduced bias. 4) Most studies relied on self-report of dietary intake. 5) Bias might have been introduced due to possible lack of validity or reliability of both dietary and psychosocial measures. 6) Certain studies reported only significant findings and did not address non-significant findings. 7) Only studies included that were published in English in peer-reviewed journals (electronic databases). 8) This review did not separate children and adolescents into distinct categories, although research has suggested that children and adolescents exhibit different health behaviors.	1) Future intervention research may benefit from the incorporation of findings from this review to create more effective adolescent and childhood dietary interventions by targeting the variables shown in this review that are most consistently associated with the various eating behaviors such as intentions, modeling, norms, liking, and preferences. 2) Investigate variables that have been insufficiently examined to date, particularly the variables rooted in affective theories. It is quite plausible that affective factors, such as motivation, executive control, or meanings of behavior might drive the dietary behavior of children and adolescents. 3) Investigate psychosocial correlates of several dietary behaviors that are known to influence weight and metabolic health such as fat and fiber that have been understudied.
Van der Horst et al., 2007 [29]	Fruit intake, vegetable intake, juice intake, composite measure of fruit and vegetable intake, composite measure of fruit juice and vegetable intake, fast food consumption, snack food intake, pizza and snack, soft drink consumption.	Correlates are categorized under home/household, educational institutions, neighborhood, city/municipality.	Consistent evidence, for the relationship between parental intake and children's fruit and vegetable intake, and for parent educational level with adolescent's fruit and vegetable intake. A positive association was found for the relationship between availability and accessibility with children's fruit and vegetable intake. Further positive associations were found for modeling (fruit/vegetable), parental intake (soft drink), parenting style (fruit/vegetable), family connectedness	1) Many potential environmental determinants have been examined for a variety of dietary behaviors, but only few studies have been conducted on the same specific environmental factor—dietary behavior combination. 2) Many studies were cross-sectional. 3) Reliance on self-report measures. 4) Similar environmental determinants were collapsed conceptually into one category, although potential determinants in the same category were often dissimilar or measured in different ways.	1) Replication of studies on the same specific environmental factors is necessary, to generate more compelling evidence for associations between environmental factors and dietary intake. 2) The finding that parental behavior is associated with child and adolescent intakes implies that interventions should take the behavior of parents into account, or desensitize adolescents for the (unfavorable) behavior of their parents. Parents should be more strongly encouraged to give the right example, especially where fat and energy intakes are concerned.

TABLE 1.6 *(Continued)*

Author, date	Outcome measures	Correlate measures	Overall results of the reviews	Overall limitations of the review	Overall recommendations of the review
			(fruit/ vegetable) and encouragement to increase food intake (fruit/ vegetable).	5) Only studies included that were published in English in peer-reviewed journals (electronic databases). 6) Studies were heterogeneous in the conceptualization, measurement of the environmental determinant and/ or dietary intakes, samples and analyses used: not possible to assess the overall strength of associations. 7) Multiple environmental factors examined in one study were included in the review, so these associations are not independent.	3) Fruit and vegetable promotion should focus especially on adolescents from parents with lower levels of education. 4) Studies are needed that target the environmental levels and factors that have found to be (nearly) empty in the ANGELO framework, such as physical, socio-cultural, economic and political factors in the school (e.g. school food policy and food prices), neighborhood (e.g. availability and accessibility of foods in shops) and city/ municipality environment (e.g. food policy, food prices, marketing). Factors such as availability and accessibility at home, school and neighborhood should be studied in relation to energy, fat, soft drink, snacks and fast food intake. 5) Need for longitudinal studies with valid or objective measures.
Pearson et al., 2009 [25]	Breakfast consumption, breakfast skipping	Physical (availability and accessibility), food poverty, socio-cultural (e.g. two parent family, modeling, family communication, monitoring, food rules, parental presence), demographic (SES, parental education level and employment)	This review reported support for three family variables: Parental breakfast eating and living in two parent families were positively associated with adolescent breakfast consumption; and socio-economic deprivation was inversely associated with breakfast consumption.	1) Several studies may not have been powered to detect significant associations between family correlates and breakfast behaviors. 2) Diversity in the definition of breakfast across the literature.	1) Future studies should clearly define breakfast foods (e.g. breakfast cereal, breads, milk, snacks on the run) being measured as this will allow for an understanding of the healthfulness of this behavior and will provide scope for interventions to promote healthy breakfast consumption. 2) Importance of family structure should be considered when designing programs to promote breakfast consumption. 3) Future qualitative studies are needed to further explicate the mechanisms of the complex relationship between SES and adolescent breakfast behaviors.

TABLE 1.6 *(Continued)*

Author, date	Outcome measures	Correlate measures	Overall results of the reviews	Overall limitations of the review	Overall recommendations of the review
De Craemer et al., 2012 [21]	Sweet beverages, fruit and vegetable intake combined, snacks, milk intake	Demographic and biological variables, behavioral variables, physical environmental variables	TV viewing was positively associated with the intake of sweet beverages, snacks and inversely associated with fruit and vegetable intake. Parental modeling was associated with fruit and vegetable intake. No association with fruit and vegetable intake was found for restriction of eating, and an indeterminate result was found for pressuring the child to eat. Food availability was not associated with fruit and vegetable intake and snacking but had an indeterminate result for sweet beverages.	NR	1) Future research should investigate similar correlates of physical activity, sedentary behavior and eating behavior to develop more efficient interventions. 2) Future research should be on interventions to predict whether interventions targeting these correlates will have an impact. 3) Future research should focus on identifying the common correlates of physical activity, sedentary behavior and eating behavior in preschool- aged children so that better tailored interventions could be developed. 4) More longitudinal studies are needed.
Pearson et al., 2009 [26]	Fruit and vegetable consumption separately. fruit, fruit juice and vegetable consumption combined.	Physical (e.g. availability, accessibility), socio-cultural (parental modeling, parental intake, family rules), and demographic correlates (e.g. SES).	Children: home availability, family rules (demand/allow) and parental encouragement were positively associated with children's fruit and vegetable intake. Parental modeling and parental intake were positively associated with children's consumption of fruit and fruit juice and vegetable intake. Adolescents: parental intake and parental occupational status were found to be positively associated with adolescents' consumption of fruit. Parental intake was also positively associated with adolescents' vegetable consumption. There is also evidence for a positive association between parental education and adolescents' fruit juice and vegetable intake.	1) Diversity in character (e.g. measures used and correlates studied) 2) Difficult to assess overall consistency of associations. 3) Several studies may not have been powered to detect significant associations between family correlates and dietary behaviors. 4) Few studies have examined the same specific combination of family correlate and dietary behavior, thus limiting the possibilities of drawing strong or consistent conclusions. 5) Many studies were cross-sectional. 6) Reliance on self-report measures. 7) Little data on reliability and validity of measures of dietary outcomes and physical and socio-cultural family correlates. 8) Only studies included that were published in English	1) More longitudinal studies are needed. 2) More studies are needed to test understudied correlates to generate more convincing evidence for associations between correlates and dietary behaviors. 3) Studies should report the validity and reliability of measures used to assess predictor variables.

TABLE 1.6 *(Continued)*

Author, date	Outcome measures	Correlate measures	Overall results of the reviews	Overall limitations of the review	Overall recommendations of the review
Verloigne et al., 2012 [30]	Breakfast consumption, soft drink consumption.	Family and school environment: physical, socio-cultural, economic, political correlates.	Parental descriptive/ injunctive norms and control/supervision were positively related to breakfast. Parental catering on demands, avoidance of negative modeling behavior, permissiveness, and area deprivation were inversely related. School SES was negatively related and teacher injunctive norms was positively related to breakfast. Availability at home, parental soft drink, and permissive parenting style were positively related to soft drink. Having family dinners, household income, parental employment status, and limits were inversely related. Availability of soft drinks at school and intake at school were positively related with soft drink. Participation in healthy school lunches was inversely related.	1) Only studies included that were published in English 2) Did not take possible moderators and covariates into account. 3) Not all existing studies on this topic were covered. 4) Focused on the consistency of the association and not on the strength of the association. 5) Conceptually similar variables were combined into a single category, even if variables were measured in a different way. 6) Many studies were cross-sectional.	1) More longitudinal studies are needed. 2) Interventions could help parents to create a supportive environment for their children to promote healthy behavior. 3) More research is needed to focus on important school-environmental factors when developing an intervention program.
Ford et al., 2012 [22]	Vegetables, fruit and vegetable intake, (non)-fruit juice, high-energy/ sugar-sweetened drinks, whole or 2% milk, fast foods, breakfast	TV, video, and computer time in minutes.	Eleven of the 12 included studies reported significant associations between TV and adverse dietary behaviors in young children. Six studies reported significant inverse relationships between TV viewing and fruit and vegetable intake.	1) Reliance on parent-reported methods to assess child TV viewing. 2) Many studies were cross-sectional.	1) Guidelines for TV viewing use in young children should be further delimited. 2) More longitudinal studies are needed. 3) Direct measurement of TV use.
Caspi et al., 2012 [16]	Fruit and/or vegetables intake, 100% fruit juice consumption.	Food environment: 5 dimensions of food access (availability, accessibility, affordability, accommodation, acceptability).	Moderate evidence in support of the causal hypothesis that neighborhood food environments influence dietary health. Perceived measures of availability were consistently related to multiple healthy dietary outcomes.	NR	1) More standardized/validated measures for food environment assessment needed. 2) Develop/refine understudied measures. 3) Abandon purely distance-based measures of accessibility, and combine multiple environmental assessment techniques.

TABLE 1.6 *(Continued)*

Author, date	Outcome measures	Correlate measures	Overall results of the reviews	Overall limitations of the review	Overall recommendations of the review
					4) Researchers should continue to expound upon the conceptual definitions of food access as they develop and refine new combinations of measure for the food environment.
Moore & Cunningham, 2012 [18]	Daily fruit and vegetable consumption, snacking, breakfast consumption, soda consumption, meat intake.	Social status, stress.	Higher stress is related to less healthy dietary behaviors. The majority of studies reported that higher social position is related to healthier diet.	1) Only studies included that were published in English. 2) Many studies were cross-sectional. 3) Because obesity results from a prolonged period of positive energy imbalance, assessment of dietary behaviors at a single point in time makes inferences related to diet and obesity difficult. 4) Heterogeneity of measures.	1) More quantitative dietary assessment tools such as FFQ, repeated 24-hr recalls, and food diaries are needed. 2) More longitudinal studies are needed. 3) Important to acknowledge additional factors that influence energy intake, such as SES and stress levels. 4) Implementing appropriate monitoring and evaluation is essential to identifying successful, holistic strategies that can be used to improve quality of care.
Lawman & Wilson, 2012 [23]	Fruit, vegetables, fast food, soft drink, dairy, milk, breakfast.	Parenting (parental support for health behaviors, parenting style and parental monitoring surrounding health behaviors) and/or environmental factors (home availability/access, neighborhood availability/access and the built environment, neighborhood safety, neighborhood social factors).	The current review found support for some parenting and physical environmental factors for health behaviors, particularly parental monitoring and neighborhood social factors.	1) Many studies were cross-sectional. 2) Reliance on self-report measures.	1) More longitudinal studies are needed on at-risk youth. 2) More objective measures of health behaviors or multiple reporters, who may hold different perspectives are needed, when objective measures are not feasible. 3) Future research should be conscious of reporting results in a way that facilitates systematic review of the literature 4) Examine additional levels of the bio-ecological model such as interpersonal and other macro- or society and policy level factors. 5) Future research should explore the relation between home/environment and health behaviors, particularly neighborhood social contextual factors such as social cohesion, and how factors at multiple bio-ecological levels may be influencing them (e.g. moderators).

TABLE 1.6 *(Continued)*

Author, date	Outcome measures	Correlate measures	Overall results of the reviews	Overall limitations of the review	Overall recommendations of the review
					6) More research monitoring is needed. 7) Development of more valid measures of parenting, family, and home environment variables is warranted. 8) Examine how parenting style is related to health behavior outcomes.
Sleddens et al., 2011 [28]	Vegetables, fruit, sugar-sweetened beverages, soft drinks, breakfast, snacks/sweets	General parenting	In many studies significant associations with general parenting were found. Generally, children raised in authoritative homes were found to eat healthier.	1) Reliance on questionnaires and parental self-report measures. 2) Differences in conceptualization of parenting constructs across studies. 3) Different categorizations to classify parents into styles across studies. 4) Heterogeneity of measurements across studies and lacking information about distribution of independent and outcome variables. 5) Few studies examined the role of general parenting as a contextual factor that can influence the effectiveness of food-related parenting practices in predicting children's diet ary intake behaviors'(moderation analyses).	1) Additional research is needed to further study the influence of mediating and moderating factors influencing the general parenting - child weight relationship, preferably employing a longitudinal design with more extended follow-up periods. 2) More longitudinal studies are needed using diverse ethnic samples and age groups. 3) Larger samples of fathers should be included to allow for comparisons between mothers and fathers. 4) Intervention developers should increase their attention to the family context as it is an important factor influencing outcomes of overweight interventions for children.
Berge, 2009 [20]	Fruit and vegetable consumption, sugar sweetened beverages, dairy products, breakfast consumption, etc.	Parental domain (e.g. parenting style, parenting practices), family functioning domain (e.g. family meals, family emotional closeness/connection, family weight teasing).	Parental domain: authoritative parenting style is positively associated with dietary intake. Family functioning domain: from cross-sectional and longitudinal research there is convincing evidence that family meals have an enduring protective factor for children and adolescents, girls and boys, and across diverse ethnic groups related to healthy dietary intake.	1) Many studies were cross-sectional. 2) Many studies used single-group designs. 3) Reliance on self-report measures. 4) Many studies used single informant measures to measure family-level data 5) Many studies used single item measures. 6) Many studies adjusted for gender, SES and ethnicity as covariates, such as maternal MI and parental perception of child/adolescent weight.	1) More longitudinal, experimental and direct observational research in all family domains is needed. 2) Beneficial to incorporate mixed qualitative and quantitative designs. 3) There is a need for more within-in family measurements that utilize multi-level and multi-measurement approaches.

TABLE 1.6 *(Continued)*

Author, date	Outcome measures	Correlate measures	Overall results of the reviews	Overall limitations of the review	Overall recommendations of the review
					4) There is a need to use systemic outcome variables. More family system variables should be studies. 5) Examine possible mediator or moderator effects of the family domains. 6) Important to include covariates when studying familial correlates of child/adolescent obesity.
Rasmussen et al., 2006 [27]	Fruit and/or vegetable intake	Socio-demographic factors, personal factors, family- related, friends-related factors, school-related factors, meal patterns, TV watching, eating fast food.	The determinants supported by the greatest amount of evidence are social- economic position, preferences, parental intake, and home availability/accessibility. For nutritional knowledge, self-efficacy and shared family meals the evidence for positive associations is rather convincing.	1) Publications may have been missed due to the search strategy. 2) Within this review only significant associations are considered. 3) Many papers include analyses based on small study samples and samples that are non-representative or only representative of a restricted geographical area. 4) Often the validity of the applied instruments are only considered very superficially or not mentioned at all. 5) There is insufficient confounder control. 6) Large variety of approaches for conceptualizing, operationalizing, measuring and coding the outcome variable(s) exist.	1) More studies on the influence of the family setting for influencing fruit and vegetable intake among children and adolescents are needed to enable health promoters to make evidence based decisions. 2) Observational studies analyzing fruit and vegetable intake in a school setting are still lacking. 3) Future international comparative surveys should enable investigations of national level factors of importance e.g. price levels, policy, guidelines, supply, and exposure to mass media and commercials. 4) Future research should study the influence of e.g. local access to fruit and vegetables through grocery stores, local food policies, exposure to mass media and commercials, and fruit and vegetable availability in leisure time facilities for children and adolescents, like for instance local sport clubs. 5) Future research would benefit from improvements in design and methodology. 6) More longitudinal studies of children and adolescents' fruit and vegetable intake are needed.

TABLE 1.6 *(Continued)*

Author, date	Outcome measures	Correlate measures	Overall results of the reviews	Overall limitations of the review	Overall recommendations of the review
					7) Lack of knowledge about predictors of FVI among children and adolescents from non-western parts of the world. 8) Future studies should keep a very broad and comprehensive theoretical scope, in order not to exclude important etiological components of importance for child and adolescent FVI.

Note: The overall results/limitations/recommendations of the reviews that are reported are those reported by the review authors themselves.

In total, four reviews solely explored associations between determinants and fruit and/or vegetable consumption: self-regulation [15]; physical, social-cultural and economic environmental determinants [16]; physical and social-cultural determinants [26]; and social-cultural, political, and social-cognitive determinants, sensory processes, and sedentary behavior [27]. Additionally, one review solely explored associations between habit strength and sugar-sweetened beverage intake [17], and one review solely explored association between physical and social-cultural environmental determinants and breakfast consumption [25]. The other 11 reviews explored determinants of a variety of healthful and unhealthful dietary behaviors (e.g. snacks, fruit and vegetables, soft drinks, milk, breakfast) [18-24,28-31]. Dietary behaviors most often included as outcomes in the included reviews were fruit and/or vegetable consumption (n=14) [15,16,18-24,27-29,31], followed by sugar-sweetened beverage consumption (n=10) [17,18,20-24,28-30], snack consumption (n=9) [18,19,21-24,28,29,31] and breakfast consumption (n=7) [18,20,22,23,25,28,30] (see Table 5).

1.3.4 The Importance and Strength of Evidence of Potential Determinants

With regard to the importance of a determinant and its strength of evidence (Table 6), most determinant-behavior relationships were coded with a zero, indicating that the findings are mixed. The following categories of determinants were found to be significantly related to dietary behavior and/or reported a (non)-significant effect size larger than 0.30 in all identified eligible studies of the included reviews assessing these categories of determinants (++ in Table 3): some aspects of social-cognitive determinants (such as attitude, self-regulation, intention and self-efficacy) and dietary behavior [15,24,27]; habit strength and sugar-sweetened beverage intake [17]; sensory processes and snacking [24]; and sedentary behavior and sugar-sweetened beverage and breakfast consumption [22]. The following categories of determinants were found to be significantly related to dietary behavior and/or reported a (non)-significant effect size larger than 0.30 in more than 75% of the identified reviews assessing these categories of determinants (+ in Table 3): the physical environment and fruit intake [26]; the social-cultural environment and fruit and vegetable intake [16,18,21,24,27-29] and sugar-sweetened beverage consumption [18,20,21,23,24,28-30]; intention, sensory processes, and knowledge for fruit and vegetable intake [24,27];

and sedentary behavior and fruit intake [22], fruit and vegetable intake and snack intake [19,22]. The evidence is mostly limited (limited, suggestive: Ls), predominantly due to the abundance of studies with cross-sectional designs so that causal or predictive relations could not be established. Systematic review on the influence of political environments, self-regulation, subjective norm and automaticity were mostly lacking in the included reviews.

1.4 DISCUSSION

1.4.1 Main Results

The multitude of studies conducted on determinants of dietary behavior among youth provides mixed and sometimes quite convincing evidence regarding associations between potential determinants and a range of dietary behaviors. However, because of the general use of cross-sectional designs in the studies covered in the available reviews, the evidence for true determinants is suggestive at best.

In particular, environmental determinants (mainly the social-cultural environment) and social-cognitive determinants have been studied quite extensively for their association with different dietary behaviors, with somewhat mixed results. The included reviews suggest that in the past decade, environmental determinants have been studied most extensively. This is an important finding in itself, suggesting a paradigm shift in the field, i.e. from a focus on social-cognitive determinants to environmental factors. This shift towards more consideration of the social-ecological approach was also seen in our umbrella review on determinants of dietary behavior in adults [14]. Other potential determinants of dietary behavior, such as automaticity, self-regulation, and subjective norm, have been studied in relatively few studies, but study results are promising. With regard to the outcomes investigated, most reviews explored relations of potential determinants with fruit and/or vegetable intake.

In the reviewed papers we found evidence that the social-cultural environment, such as the familial influence (e.g. [21,24,27,28]) is a significant correlate of fruit and vegetable intake and snack consumption in youth in more than 75% of the available studies (see Table 7). Parents, as gatekeepers of the home food supply, can influence children's eating behavior either through the use of specific food parenting practices (i.e. context-specific acts of parenting on child eating including encouraging of food variety and controlling a child's intake of unhealthy products) or through the indirect influence of general parenting

TABLE 1.7 Summary of the results from reviews about determinants of dietary behavior among youth: Importance of a determinant and strength of evidence

Determinants	Dietary behavior					
	Fruit	Vegetable	Fruit & vegetable	Snack/fast food	Sugar-sweetened beverage	Breakfast
Physical environment	+, Ls [26]	0, Ls [26]	0, Ls [15,21,24,29,31]	0, Ls [21,23,24,29,31]	0, Ls [21,23,24,29,30]	0, Ls [23,25]
Social-cultural environment	0, Ls [20,23,26-28]	0, Ls [20,23,26-28]	+, Ls [16,18,21,24,27-29]	0, Ls [18,21,23,24,28,29]	+, Ls [18,20,21,23, 24,28-30]	0, Ls [18,20,23,25,28,30]
Economic/financial environment			0, Ls [16,21,29]	0, Ls [21,29]	-, Ls [21,29,30]	-, Lnc [30]
Political environment			0, Ls [27]			
Attitude	0, Lnc [24]	0, Lnc [24]	0, Ls [24,27]	++, Ls [24]	++, Lnc [24]	
Subjective norm			++, Lnc [27]			
Self-efficacy/perceived behavioral control	0, Ls [24]	0, Ls [24]	0, Ls [24,27]	0, Ls [24]	++, Lnc [24]	
Intention	++, Ls [24]	++, Lnc [24]	+, Ls [24,27]	++, Ls [24]	++, Lnc [24]	
Self-regulation			++, Ls [15] (implementation intentions)			
Habitual behavior, automaticity					++, Lnc [17]	
Sensory perceptions, perceived palatability foods			+, Ls [24,27]	++, Lnc [24]	–, Lnc [24]	
Other, knowledge	0, Ls [24]	0, Ls [24]	+, Ls [24,27]	0, Ls [24]	++, Lnc [24]	
Other, sedentary behavior	+, Ls [19,22,27]	0, Ls [19,22,27]	+, Ls [19,22,27]	+, Ls [19,22]	++, Ls [22]	++, Ls [22]

Note: Importance of a determinant: ++, +, 0, –, –- (see Table 3); strength of evidence (see Table 4): Co (Convincing evidence), Pr (Probable evidence), Ls (Limited, suggestive evidence), Lnc (Limited, no conclusion); studies including determinants such as stress and risks and dietary behavior such as milk and meat intake not included in this table.

[28]. Social-cognitive determinants have been studied often, but the evidence regarding their importance is limited (i.e. suggestive at best). Intention, a proximal indicator of actual behavior, was found to be a significant determinant of fruit and vegetable intake, snack intake, and sugar-sweetened beverage intake [24,27]. Socio-cognitive theories such as the Theory of Planned Behavior [6] are indicated to have limited value in predicting the translation of intention into action. This limitation is addressed in reviews on the constructs of habit [17] and implementation intentions [15]. The review on implementation intentions showed considerable support for the effect of implementation intentions on increasing fruit and vegetable intake (medium effect size) among youth. However, the effect of implementation intentions on the reduction of unhealthy eating patterns was less convincing. Habit strength was one of the factors to be significantly related to sugar-sweetened beverage intake with moderate to strong effect sizes in all identified eligible studies of the review of Gardner et al. [17]. Automatic processes, including habit strength appears to reduce the utility of cognitive factors for the prediction or association with dietary behavior [17]. Additionally, screen time was found to be consistently associated with dietary behavior [19,22,27]. The included reviews provide evidence that the amount of screen time was significantly related to dietary behavior; screen time was positively associated with snack and sugar-sweetened beverage intake [19-22] and inversely associated with fruit and vegetable intake [19-27]. An important mechanism linking screen time to unhealthy dietary behavior is exposure to marketing of unhealthy foods and beverages through screens [35,36]. The food and beverages depicted in these advertisements are predominantly unhealthy foods high in fat, salt and sugar [35,37]. Sedentary activities and unhealthy dietary behavior have repeatedly been found to cluster [38-40] and may also share similar environmental cues causing these behaviors to co-occur. Sedentary behavior offers a context for the consumption of energy-dense food products, disrupting the habituation to food cues.

Systematic reviews on the influence of political environments, self-regulation, subjective norm and habitual behavior were mostly lacking in the included reviews. In addition, some types or categories of potential determinants were not covered in the present umbrella review because we did not come across systematic reviews of such determinants. For instance, although we found two systematic reviews on sensory determinants of dietary behavior [24,27], most of the reviews were excluded as they did not comply to the quality standards of systematic reviews that we used as an inclusion criteria, e.g. [41]. This does not necessarily imply that such factors as taste and preferences are not important, but just that these have not been covered well at present in systematic reviews. Furthermore, it should be noted that lack of evidence for the importance of a possible determinant is not the same as evidence that the determinant is not important; since lack of well-designed studies is often the main reason for lack of evidence. We need to try to distinguish between well-researched determinants and still no evidence for importance, and determinants that have just not been studied (well enough) to make meaningful conclusions.

1.4.2 Limitations and Methodological Issues

Several limitations should be taken into consideration in reviewing these findings. These include the cross-sectional nature of many studies relying on self-report measures; heterogeneity of conceptualization, measurement, samples and analyses used, making it difficult to compare results between studies; inability to conduct a meta-analysis; lack of validity and reliability of dietary intake and correlate measures; and categorization of determinants into more global categories thereby losing important information. Additionally, the systematic reviews included a wide age range, i.e. respondents from birth to 18 years. During childhood many developmental transitions take place that may imply differential importance of distinct behavioral determinants. For instance, parents are highly responsible as gatekeepers of the home food supply for their children's dietary intake behavior. However, parental influence decreases with advancing age of the child as the child is increasingly exposed to other environments (e.g. school environment, peer influences).

In addition to the quality of the research design, the fact that some determinants have not been extensively studied yet, studies of some types of determinants have not been reviewed systematically, and the lack of robust results from this umbrella review may also be explained by the fact that groups or types of determinants are often studied in relative isolation. For instance, studies in which different categories of determinants—e.g. sensory determinants, self-regulation, and political environmental factors—were studied with integrative approaches are largely lacking. Such studies would allow for exploration and testing of mediating and moderating pathways between these determinants in influencing dietary behavior. Already some studies combining environmental and social-cognitive determinants have been reported in recent years and do support such mediating and moderating pathways, e.g. [42-45].

This is the first umbrella review that provides an overview of reviewed research regarding a broad range of potential determinants of dietary behavior in youth. Umbrella reviews in itself are, however, also prone to bias in various ways. Differences in reviewing methodology and reporting were apparent, as well as differences in for example categorizations of the determinants. By nature, umbrella reviews lead to loss of detail. In addition, some individual studies are included in multiple reviews which may have led to an overrepresentation of single studies in our results. Finally, we excluded reviews that primarily addressed biological determinants or papers with summative outcomes such as caloric intake, and we also did not include reviews that focused on qualitative data.

1.5 CONCLUSIONS AND RECOMMENDATIONS

The evidence gathered in our umbrella review suggests that intention and sedentary behavior have the strongest evidence base as determinants of healthy and unhealthy dietary behavior in youth. The influence of distinct determinants may, however, be stronger in interaction with other influences. We would advocate for studies that address combined, mediating and interactive influences on dietary behavior [46]. Such studies are advocated to include behaviors that have been found to cluster with dietary behavior, such as sedentary behavior. Other recommendations include the need for better designed studies, beyond mere cross-sectional research, –i.e. more longitudinal and experimental or intervention research, and research using natural experiments-, larger samples among specific age groups, and more valid and reliable measures (dietary behavior and correlates). Our results underline the importance of embracing theories and factors additional to determinants derived from socio-cognitive theories that are often used to inform interventions to promote healthy dietary behaviors. Theories that are promising of further research for determinants of dietary behavior research include habit theory and (social-) ecological models of health behavior.

REFERENCES

1. Craigie AM, Lake AA, Kelly SA, Adamson AJ, Mathers JC. Tracking of obesity-related behaviours from childhood to adulthood: A systematic review. Maturitas. 2011;70:266–84.
2. Astrup A, Dyerberg J, Selleck M, Stender S. Nutrition transition and its relationship to the development of obesity and related chronic diseases. Obes Rev. 2008;9(s1):48–52.

3. Brug J, Oenema A, Ferreira I. Theory, evidence and Intervention Mapping to improve behavior nutrition and physical activity interventions. Int J Behav Nutr Phys Act. 2005;2:2.
4. Azjen I. Attitudes, personality and behavior. Milton Keynes: Open University Press; 1988. p. 2005.
5. Bandura A. Social foundations of thought and action: a social cognitive theory. Englewood Cliffs: Erlbaum; 1986.
6. Rosenstock IM. Historical origins of the health belief model. Health Educ Monogr. 1974;2:1–8.
7. Eertmans A, Baeyens F, Van den Bergh O. Food likes and their relative importance in human eating behavior: Review and preliminary suggestions for health promotion. Health Educ Res. 2001;16:443–56.
8. Brug J, Van Lenthe F. Environmental determinants and interventions for physical activity, nutrition and smoking: a review. Zoetermeer: Speed-print; 2005.
9. Kremers S, Martens M, Reubsaet A, De Weerdt I, De Vries N, Jonkers R. Programmeringstudie overgewicht. Rescon: Universiteit Maastricht; 2008.
10. Swinburn B, Egger G, Raza F. Dissecting obesogenic environments: The development and application of a framework for identifying and prioritizing environmental interventions for obesity. Prev Med. 1999;29:563–70.
11. Booth SL, Sallis JF, Ritenbaugh C, Hill JO, Birch LL, Frank LD, et al. Environmental and societal factors affect food choice and physical activity: Rationale, influences and leverage-points. Nutr Rev. 2001;59:S21–39.
12. Davison KK, Birch LL. Childhood overweight: A contextual model and recommendations for future research. Obes Rev. 2001;2:159–71.
13. Kremers SPJ, De Bruijn G-J, Visscher TLS, Van Mechelen W, De Vries NK, Brug J. Environmental influences on energy balance-related behaviors: a dual-process view. Int J Behav Nutr Phys Act. 2006;3:9.
14. Sleddens EFC, Kroeze W, Kohl LFM, Bolten LM, Velema E, Kaspers P, et al. Determinants of dietary behavior amoung adults: An umbrella review. Nutr Rev. 2015; accepted 22 Jan 2015, in press.
15. Adriaanse MA, Vinkers CDW, De Ridder DTD, Hox JJ, De Wit JBF. Do implementation intentions help to eat a healthy diet? A systematic review and meta-analysis of the empirical evidence. Appetite. 2011;56:183–93.
16. Caspi CE, Sorensen G, Subramanian SV, Kawachi I. The local food environment and diet: A systematic review. Health Place. 2012;18:1172–87.
17. Gardner B, De Bruijn G-J, Lally P. A systematic review and meta-analysis of applications of the self-report habit index to nutrition and physical activity behaviours. Ann Behav Med. 2011;42:174–87.
18. Moore CJ, Cunningham SA. Social position, psychological stress, and obesity: A systematic review. J Acad Nutr Diet. 2012;112:518–26.
19. Pearson N, Biddle SJ. Sedentary behavior and dietary intake in children, adolescents, and adults: A systematic review. Am J Prev Med. 2011;41:178–88.
20. Berge JM. A review of familial correlates of child and adolescent obesity: What has the 21st century taught us so far? Int J Adolesc Med Health. 2009;21:457–84.
21. De Craemer M, De Decker E, De Bourdeaudhuij I, Vereecken C, Deforche B, Manios Y, et al. Correlates of energy balance-related behaviours in preschool children: a systematic review. Obes Rev. 2012;13(s1):13–28.

22. Ford C, Ward D, White M. Television viewing associated with adverse dietary outcomes in children ages 2–6. Obes Rev. 2012;13:1139–47.
23. Lawman HG, Wilson DK. A review of family and environmental correlates of health behaviors in high-risk youth. Obesity (Silver Spring). 2012;20:1142–57.
24. McClain AD, Chappuis C, Nguyen-Rodriguez ST, Yaroch AL, Spruijt-Metz D. Psychosocial correlates of eating behavior in children and adolescents: A review. Int J Behav Nutr Phys Act. 2009;6:54.
25. Pearson N, Biddle SJH, Gorely T. Family correlates of breakfast consumption among children and adolescents. A systematic review. Appetite. 2009;52:1–7.
26. Pearson N, Biddle SJH, Gorely T. Family correlates of fruit and vegetable consumption in children and adolescents: A systematic review. Public Health Nutr. 2009;12:267–83.
27. Rasmussen M, Krølner R, Klepp K-I, Lytle L, Brug J, Bere E, et al. Determinants of fruit and vegetable consumption among children and adolescents: a review of the literature. Part I: Quantitative studies. Int J Behav Nutr Phys Act. 2006;3:22.
28. Sleddens EFC, Gerards SMPL, Thijs C, De Vries NK, Kremers SPJ. General parenting, childhood overweight and obesity-inducing behaviors: A review. Int J Pediatr Obes. 2011;6:e12–27.
29. Van der Horst K, Oenema A, Ferreira I, Wendel-Vos W, Giskes K, Van Lenthe F, et al. A systematic review of environmental correlates of obesity-related dietary behaviors in youth. Health Educ Res. 2007;22:203–26.
30. Verloigne M, Van Lippevelde W, Maes L, Brug J, De Bourdeaudhuij I. Family-and school-based correlates of energy balance-related behaviours in 10–12-year-old children: A systematic review within the ENERGY (EuropeaN Energy balance Research to prevent excessive weight Gain among Youth) project. Public Health Nutr. 2012;15:1380–95.
31. Williams J, Scarborough P, Matthews A, Cowburn G, Foster C, Roberts N, et al. A systematic review of the influence of the retail food environment around schools on obesity-related outcomes. Obes Rev. 2014;15:359–74.
32. De Vet E, De Ridder DTD, De Wit JBF. Environmental correlates of physical activity and dietary behaviours among young people: A systematic review of reviews. Obes Rev. 2011;12:e130–42.
33. Thomas H, Miccuci S, Ciliska D, Mirza M. Effectiveness of school-based interventions in reducing adolescent risk behaviours: a systematic review of reviews. City of Hamilton: Effective Public Health Practice Project (EPHPP), Epidemiology and Evaluation, Public Health Services; 2005.
34. World Cancer Research Fund. Food, nutrition, physical activity, and the prevention of cancer: a global perspective. Washington DC: American Institute for Cancer Research; 2007.
35. Boyland EJ, Halford JC. Television advertising and branding. Effects on eating behaviour and food preferences in children. Appetite. 2013;62:236–41.
36. Chamberlain LJ, Wang Y, Robinson TN. Does children's screen time predict requests for advertised products? Cross-sectional and prospective analyses. Arch Pediatr Adolesc Med. 2006;160:363–8.
37. Scully P, Macken A, Leddin D, Cullen W, Dunne C, Gorman CO: Food and beverage advertising during children's television programming. Ir J Med Sci 2014. [Epub ahead of print]
38. Gubbels JS, Kremers SPJ, Stafleu A, Dagnelie PC, De Vries SI, De Vries NK, et al. Clustering of dietary intake and sedentary behavior in 2-year-old children. J Pediatr. 2009;155:194–8.

39. Gubbels JS, Kremers SPJ, Stafleu A, Goldbohm RA, De Vries NK, Thijs C. Clustering of energy balance-related behaviors in 5-year-old children: Lifestyle patterns and their longitudinal association with weight status development in early childhood. Int J Behav Nutr Phys Act. 2012;9:77.
40. Leech RM, McNaughton SA, Timperio A. The clustering of diet, physical activity and sedentary behavior in children and adolescents: A review. Int J Behav Nutr Phys Act. 2014;11:4.
41. Schwartz C, Scholtens PA, Lalanne A, Weenen H, Nicklaus S. Development of healthy eating habits early in life. Review of recent evidence and selected guidelines. Appetite. 2011;57:796–807.
42. Cameron AJ, Van Stralen MM, Brug J, Salmon J, Bere E, Chin A, et al. Television in the bedroom and increased body weight: potential explanations for their relationship among European schoolchildren. Pediatr Obes. 2013;8:130–41.
43. Ray C, Roos E, Brug J, Behrendt I, Ehrenblad B, Yngve A, et al. Role of free school lunch in the associations between family-environmental factors and children's fruit and vegetable intake in four European countries. Public Health Nutr. 2013;16:1109–17.
44. Tak NI, Te Velde SJ, Kamphuis CBM, Ball K, Crawford D, Brug J, et al. Associations between neighbourhood and household environmental variables and fruit consumption: exploration of mediation by individual cognitions and habit strength in the GLOBE study. Public Health Nutr. 2013;16:505–14.
45. Tak NI, Te Velde SJ, Oenema A, Van der Horst K, Timperio A, Crawford D, et al. The association between home environmental variables and soft drink consumption among adolescents. Exploration of mediation by individual cognitions and habit strength. Appetite. 2011;56:503–10.
46. Gubbels JS, Van Kann DHH, De Vries NK, Thijs C, Kremers SPJ. The next step in health behavior research: the need for ecological moderation analyses—an application to diet and physical activity at childcare. Int J Behav Nutr Phys Act. 2014;11:52.

CHAPTER 2

Dietary Intake of Children Participating in the USDA Summer Food Service Program

Betty Del Rio-Rodriguez and Karen W. Cullen

2.1 INTRODUCTION

Food insecurity is defined as "*the limited or uncertain availability of nutritionally adequate and safe foods or limited or uncertain ability to acquire acceptable foods in socially acceptable ways*" [1,2]. In 2012, about 14.5% of US households were food insecure at least some time during the year, including 5.7% with very low food security [3,4]. Food insecurity is usually higher during the summer months, especially among households with children [5]. Families with school-age children may struggle to provide nutritious food for their children who receive free breakfast and lunch during the school year. The Summer Food Service Program (SFSP) provides free meals during the summer months to all children up to the age of 18 years old living in low-income areas where at least 50% of children qualify for free and reduced school meals [6]. The SFSP was created as a 3-year pilot in 1968 and made permanent in 1975 [7]. State agencies administer the program and sponsors such as school food authorities, government agencies, summer camps, and non-profit organizations run the program in various sites including schools, parks, community centers, and churches.

All meals served to the children must follow the National School Lunch Program (NSLP) guidelines. Prior to the 2012-2013 school year, NSLP lunches had to meet the applicable recommendations of the Dietary Guidelines for Americans: no more than 30% of calories from fat, and less than 10% from saturated fat. School lunches also had to provide one-third of the Recommended Dietary Allowances of protein, Vitamin A, Vitamin C, iron, calcium, and calories. The food pattern offered to children had to include one serving of protein food, 2 servings of fruit and/or vegetables, 1 grain serving, and 8 ounces of milk. A recent study reported that the SFSP has the potential to reduce food insecurity among those with very low food security by as much as 33% [8].

Unfortunately, poor participation from children and sponsors has been a major obstacle for the program to reach its mission [9]. During the summer of 2012, only 14.3 children received summer meals for every 100 low-income students who received lunch in the 2011-2012 school year [9]. In recent years, efforts have concentrated on increasing program participation; but little research has been published on the nutrition provided by these meals.

Therefore, the objective of this paper is to examine the quality of the SFSP meals selected and consumed by children participating in the program. It was hypothesized that the meals selected and consumed by children participating in the SFSP would meet the NSLP standards.

2.2 METHODS AND MATERIALS

This was a cross-sectional study of children participating in a SFSP sponsored one school district during the summer of 2011. This school district is located in the Houston area. At the time of this study, 81% of the students were Hispanic and 82% of the students were eligible for free or reduced price meals. Fourteen schools were selected for observation (10 elementary, 2 middle, and 2 intermediate) by the Food Service Director. The study protocol was approved by the Baylor College of Medicine Institutional Review Board. Informed consent was not required for the anonymous observations.

The school cafeterias were open for breakfast and lunch to every child up to 18 years old. For this study, children were observed only during the lunch period. Participating children were enrolled in summer school, summer camp at the school, or walked in from the surrounding community with a parent or by themselves. Selection of children for observation was based on table seating and order, and no more than 4children were observed at the same time by the observer.

The lunch was prepared at the schools by the cafeteria staff. Table 1 illustrates the menu items offered by day. The school utilized the offer versus serve (OVS) option, whereby children only had to select three of the five menu components for the meal to qualify as reimbursable [10]. Prior to the observation, a checklist was created using the lunch menu items as planned by the school district. Observers were trained during one lunch period and used the checklist to note what menu items the child selected in the cafeteria line. During the observation period, the portion (0, ¼, ½, ¾, all) of food items consumed, exchanged and wasted was recorded. The quarter waste method (0, ¼, ½, ¾, all) has high inter-rater and inter-method reliability [11]. No demographic information was collected from the children other than sex and grade level (elementary or intermediate school), and there was no interaction with the children before or during lunch. Children were not aware of the reason of for the presence of the observers in the cafeteria and only the school administration knew the purpose of the visit.

TABLE 2.1 One-Week Four-Day Cycle Menu and Lunch Meal Pattern for the SFSP

	Milk (1 serving)	**Fruits/Vegetables (2 serving)**	**Grains (1 serving)**	**Meat/ Meat Alternate (1 serving)**
Monday	White 1% Fat or Chocolate Fat-free	Chilled Peaches Beans (lowfat refried w cheese)	Soft whole wheat tortilla Spanish Rice	Beef taco meat with cheese
Tuesday	White 1% Fat or Chocolate Fat-free	Mashed Potatoes Green Beans Spiced Apples	Dinner roll	Chicken Nuggets or Roasted Chicken
Wednesday	White 1% Fat or Chocolate Fat-free	Peas or Corn Pear Cup	Whole Wheat bread Cookie	Grilled Cheese Sandwich
Thursday	White 1% Fat or Chocolate Fat-free	Baked French Fries Pickle Spears Rosy Applesauce	Whole wheat buns	Cheeseburger or Hamburger patty

Note: Serving sizes consist of: 1 cup of fluid milk; ¾ cup of fruits/vegetables; 1 slice of bread or 1 serving of roll or ½ cup of grains; 2 oz. of lean meat or poultry or alternate protein product or cheese; ½ cup of cooked dry beans or peas; 4 Tbsp. peanut butter.

For each lunch observation form, the foods selected and consumed for each student were entered into separate Nutrition Data System for Research files (version 2010, Nutrition Coordinating Center, University of Minnesota, MN) by trained dietitians to obtain lunch intake of selected and consumed nutrients and food groups. The mean amounts of nutrients and food groups selected and consumed by grade level were calculated. The percentage of the food groups consumed was calculated by dividing the amount consumed by the total amount selected. The percentage of food groups wasted was calculated by subtracting the percent consumed from 100%. Differences in the percentage of food groups consumed by grade level were assessed with independent t tests or Mann-Whitney tests (for non-normal distribution) depending on distribution. SPSS (IBM SPSS Statistics for Windows, Version 19.0. Armonk, NY: IBM Corp) was used for all calculations.

2.3 RESULTS

Three hundred and two (N=302) children were observed during a four-week period in the 14 schools. 50% were male and 75% were in elementary grades. Parents attended with 62 elementary school students (26%). Most of the students eating lunch attended summer school (73% elementary and 86% intermediate).

The mean amounts of nutrients in the meals selected by the elementary school students (n=240) met the USDA NSLP standards for all nutrients except energy and vitamin C (Table 2). The mean amount of fruit and vegetables selected by the students was 1.1 servings per meal, not the two servings that were allowable for the meal. Only 53% selected at least one fruit and 76% selected at least one vegetable. The elementary school students did not consume adequate energy, iron, vitamins A and C, or the various food groups to meet the NSLP standards (Table 2). Elementary school students consumed only 64% of energy in the meals they selected, reflecting a wasting of almost one third of the kcals selected (Table 4). The percentages of fruit and vegetables consumed were 61% and 44%, respectively, which reflects wastes of 39% of fruit and 56% of vegetables selected.

The intermediate school students (n=62) did not select foods that met the USDA NSLP energy or vitamin C standards, nor did they select two servings of total fruit and vegetables or 2 ounces of protein foods as per the NSLP meal pattern (Table 3). Only 55% and 46% selected at least one fruit or vegetable for lunch, respectively. Three intermediate school students did not consume their lunch. Those records were deleted from the consumption analyses. Intermediate school students did not consume enough energy, iron, or vitamins A and C to meet the NSLP standards (Table 3). They only consumed only 73% of energy selected fruit and vegetables selected, respectively (Table 4). These values represent wasting 25% of energy selected, 35% of fruit and 67% of vegetables. There were no significant differences in percentage of food groups consumed by grade level.

TABLE 2.2 Mean Amounts of Calories and Foods Selected and Consumed at Lunch by 240 Elementary School Students in the 10 Schools Participating in the Summer Food Service Program, Summer, 2011

	USDA Lunch Standard	Nutrients and Foods Selected		Nutrients and Foods Consumed	
		Mean	SD[1]	Mean	SD
Energy	633	611	90	387	152
Protein (gram)	9	40	10	26	13
% Energy from Fat	<30%	25	4	24	7
% Energy from Saturated Fat	<10%	9.2	2.1	8.7	3.3
Calcium (milligram)	267	578	273	400	252
Iron (milligram)	3.3	4.3	1.5	2.6	1.5
Vitamin A (Retinol Equivalent)	200	273	90	190	88
Vitamin C (milligram) Sodium	15 none	10.4	8.4	5.5	6.9
(milligram)	set none	1500	371	936	460
Total Dietary Fiber (gram)	set	6.5	2.8	3.7	2.1
Fruit (serving)	2 total fruit	0.28	0.26	0.17	0.23
Total Vegetables (serving)	and vegetables	0.83	0.67	0.40	0.65
Grains (serving)	1 none	2.20	1.12	1.20	0.90
Whole grains (serving)	set	0.88	1.07	0.44	0.65
Protein Foods (ounce)	2	2.2	2.1	1.4	1.7
Milk (ounce)	8	7.6	1.8	6.0	2.7

TABLE 2.3 Mean Amounts of Calories and Foods Selected and Consumed at Lunch by 62 Intermediate School Students in the 10 Schools Participating in the Summer Food Service Program, Summer, 2011

	NSLP lunch Standard	Nutrients and Foods Selected[a]		Nutrients and Foods Consumed[b]	
		Mean	SD	Mean	SD
Energy	785	628	85	450	231
Protein (gram)	15	38	7	28	17
% Energy from Fat	<30%	25	5	24	9
% Energy from Saturated Fat	<10%	9.00	1.80	8.40	3.20
Calcium (milligram)	370	639	251	493	361
Iron (milligram)	4.20	4.20	1.30	2.80	1.70
Vitamin A (Retinol Equivalent)	285	299	84	222	141
Vitamin C (milligram) Sodium	17 none	4.90	5.30	3.20	6.00

TABLE 2.3 *(Continued)*

	NSLP lunch Standard	Nutrients and Foods Selected[a]		Nutrients and Foods Consumed[b]	
(milligram)	set none	1678	416	1168	695
Total Dietary Fiber (gram)	set	8.00	2.80	5.20	3.10
Fruit (serving)	2 total fruit	0.29	0.28	0.21	0.28
Total Vegetables (serving)	and vegetables	0.31	0.49	0.18	0.56
Grains (serving)	1 none	2.90	0.80	1.96	1.20
Whole grains (serving)	set	1.96	1.05	1.20	1.10
Protein Foods (ounce)	2	1.50	1.67	1.20	1.80
Milk (ounce)	8	7.10	2.60	5.70	1.96

[a]n=62 [b]n=59 (3 students did not eat their selected meals.)

TABLE 2.4 Percent of Energy and Food Groups Consumed at Lunch by 240 Elementary and 62 Intermediate School Students in the 14 Schools Participating in the Summer Food Service Program, Summer, 2011

	Mean percent consumed	
	Elementary	**Intermediate**
Energy	64	73
Fruit (serving)	61	65
Total Vegetables (serving)	44	33
Grains (serving)	59	69
Whole grains (serving)	54	64
Protein Foods (ounce)	66	66
Milk (ounce)	78	77

No significant differences in percentage of food groups consumed by grade level.

2.4 DISCUSSION

This study assessed the nutrients and food groups selected and consumed by elementary and intermediate school students participating in the SFSP. The SFSP meals as offered to the students in this study met the NSLP meal patterns. Only two previous studies were found that assessed SFSP lunches. In a 2001 study, observers recorded the foods selected and leftover for SFSP lunches [6]. The meals served to the students met all the nutrient and food group standards, except for fat and saturated fat. Similar findings were reported with a plate waste study on SFSP meals consumed by youth in Delaware [12].

Neither the elementary or intermediate school students in this current study selected foods with enough energy or vitamin C; the intermediate students also did not select enough protein foods. The greatest proportion of food waste by elementary and intermediate school students was for fruit (39-35%), vegetables (56-67%), and s (41-31%) (Tables 2 and 3). This waste contributed to the inadequate lunch consumption of kilocalories, iron, vitamins A and C, compared to the NSLP meal standards. The student plate waste results are very similar to a national study where about 32% of calories, 36% of meat, 37% of fruit, 39% of bread, and 48% of vegetables were wasted [6]. In Delaware, the mean amount of calories selected was 668; the mean amounts consumed ranged from 375-440 for the 4-13 year old children; and the authors estimated that 38% of kilocalories were wasted [12].

In 2002, 203 interviews and two focus groups about the SFSP menus were conducted with Delaware SFSP participants [12]. The major reason reported for wasting foods was dislike of the items served. Perceptions of food quality were also important. Items that were smashed, soggy, or frozen were rejected, as was warm milk [12]. The involvement and support of the SFSP vendor, school, and parents are needed. Promising strategies to promote consumption of new foods include taste testing, signage promoting the foods being served and marketing [13-15].

Other reasons for the food waste include whether the foods were culturally acceptable to this predominately Hispanic population. Children also prefer energy dense high fat foods [16]. Perhaps the children were not used to the fruit, vegetables, and low fat milk on the menu. This is an important area for future research. Sodium intake was high for both grade levels, something not discussed in previous SFSP studies. New NSLP standards include sodium limits with a target implementation date of 2023 [Lunch meals ≤640mg (grades K-5); ≤710mg (grades 6-8); ≤740mg (grades 9-12)] [17]. These values are substantially lower than the 936 and 1168 mg consumed in this study. Because most sodium (75%) in school meals comes from processed foods like combination entrees and accompaniments, new lower sodium products and recipes that are acceptable to students will be needed [18], creating a need for a very important area for future research.

Plate waste and not selecting fruit and vegetables are also issues for lunches served during the school year. In a Texas study with middle school students who completed lunch records in the cafeteria, 40.2% consumed fruit and 66.9% consumed vegetables [19]. Actual lunch consumption was 0.89 serving of total vegetables (0.45 cup) (excluding high-fat vegetables), 0.45 serving fruit and juice (0.23 cup), and 6.5 ounces of milk during the 2005-2006 school year [20]. These results identify the need for nutrition education and marketing efforts both during the school year and during the summer programming.

There are several limitations that should be noted. The study took place in one school district in South Texas, limiting generalizability. Only gender and grade level were recorded; information on ethnicity and parent demographics were not collected, reducing the outcomes that could be reported. Diet for the entire day was not recorded, so the impact of this meal on total day's intake was not assessed. Future studies should include dietary intake for the entire day. However, the observation method used to record intake is an important strength of the study, as it reduces error from remembering foods consumed in previous meals. Finally, new school meal guidelines were implemented in the fall of 2012,that aligned the meal patterns to the 2010 US Dietary Guidelines [21,22]. These changes increased to three (1 fruit and 2 vegetables) that are allowed for a reimbursable lunch meal, as well as increase the number of whole foods on the menu. The level of sodium must be decreased over a ten year period. These changes may impact food selection and consumption for the SFSP; further research is warranted.

2.5 CONCLUSION

The SFSP is an important program that should improve child food security and nutrition during the summer months when school is not in session. However, not all children have the opportunity to receive summer meals because of low participation by sponsors during the summer months. Also food waste is a concern. Further research is needed to increase SFSP program availability and to improve consumption of the meal.

REFERENCES

1. United States (2014) Department of Agriculture - Economic Research Service. Food security in the U.S: Key statistics & graphics.
2. Hamilton WL, Cook JT, Thompson WW, Buron LF, Frongillo EA, et al. (1997) Household food security in the United States in 1995: Summary report of the Food Security Measurement Project. Alexandria, VA: Food and Consumer Service, U.S. Department of Agriculture.
3. Coleman-Jensen A, Nord M, Andrews M, Carlson S (2012) Household food security in the United States in 2011. United States Department of Agriculture - Economic Research Service.
4. Coleman-Jensen A, Nord M, Singh A (2013) Household food security in the United States in 2012. United States Department of Agriculture - Economic Research Service.

5. Nord M, Romig K (2006) Hunger in the summer: Seasonal food insecurity and the National School Lunch and Summer Food Service programs. J Child Poverty 12: 141-58.
6. Gordon A, Briefel R (2003) Feeding low-income children when school is out-The Summer Food Service Program: Executive summary.
7. Department of Agriculture -Food and Nutrition Service (2013) Program History-Summer Food Service Program. United States.
8. Department of Agriculture - Economic Research Service (2013) SummerFood Service Program distribution sites and average daily attendance in July, fiscal 1989-2013. United States.
9. Burke M, Sims K, Anderson S, FitzSimons C, Hewins J (2013) Hunger doesn't take a vacation: Summer nutrition status report 2013. Food Research and Action Cente.
10. Food and Nutrition Service – US (2000) Department of Agriculture. Menu planning in the National School Lunch Program.
11. Hanks AS, Wansink B, Just DR (2014) Reliability and accuracy of real-time visualization techniques for measuring school cafeteria tray waste: Validating the quarter-waste method. J Acad Nutr Diet 114: 470-4.
12. Cotugna N, Vickery CE (2004) Children rate the Summer Food Service Program. Fam Econ Nutr Rev 16: 3-12.
13. Fulkerson JA, French SA, Story M, Nelson H, Hannan PJ (2004) Promotions to increase lower-fat food choices among students in secondary schools: Description and outcomes of TACOS (Trying Alternative Cafeteria Options in Schools). Public Health Nutr 7: 665-74.
14. Snyder P, Anliker J, Cunningham-Sabo L, Dixon LB, Altaha J, et al. (1999) The Pathways study: a model for lowering the fat in school meals. Am J Clin Nutr 69: 810S-5S.
15. Wechsler H, Basch CE, Zybert P, Shea S (1998) Promoting the selection of low-fat milk in elementary school cafeterias in an inner-city Latino community: Evaluation of an intervention. Am J Public Health 88: 427-33.
16. Birch LL (1992) Children's preferences for high-fat foods. Nutr Rev 50: 249-55.
17. Food and Nutrition Service - U.S (2012) Department of Agriculture. Nutrition standards in the National School Lunch and School Breakfast Programs. Final rule. Fed Regist 77: 4088-167.
18. Gordon A, Crepinsek MK, Nogales R, Condon E (2007) School nutrition dietary assessment study III: Volume I: School foodservice, school food environment, and meals offered and served. Washington, D.C, United States Department of Agriculture - Food and Nutrition Service.
19. Cullen KW, Watson KB, Dave JM (2011) Middle-school students' school lunch consumption does not meet the new Institute of Medicine's National School Lunch Program recommendations. Public Health Nutr 14:1876-81.
20. Cullen KW, Watson K, Zakeri I (2008) Improvements in middle school student dietary intake after implementation of the Texas Public School Nutrition Policy. Am J Public Health 98:111-7.
21. Stallings VA, Suitor CW, Taylor CL (2009) School Meals: Building Blocks for Healthy Children. Institute of Medicine/The National Academies Press. Washington, D.C, USA.
22. Food and Nutrition Service - U.S (2010) Department of Agriculture. Healthy, Hunger- Free Kids Act of 2010.

PART II

Family Environment and Socioeconomic Status

CHAPTER 3

Parental Feeding Practices and Child Weight Status in Mexican American Families: A Longitudinal Analysis

Jeanne M. Tschann, Suzanna M. Martinez, Carlos Penilla, Steven E. Gregorich, Lauri A. Pasch, Cynthia L. De Groat, Elena Flores, Julianna Deardorff, Louise C. Greenspan, and Nancy F. Butte

3.1 INTRODUCTION

The high prevalence of obesity among children is of great concern. Obese children are likely to be obese as adults; and obesity is a risk factor for type 2 diabetes, cardiovascular disease, and sleep apnea [1–4]. Mexican American children have an elevated prevalence of obesity, compared to non-Hispanic white children. Among children 6–11 years old, 22.4% of Mexican American girls and 21.8% of Mexican American boys were obese in 2009–2010, compared with 10.7% of non-Hispanic white girls and 16.8% of non-Hispanic white boys [5].

There is a critical need to identify modifiable risk factors for obesity among Mexican American children. One important influence on children's weight, for which interventions could be developed, is parental feeding practices. Parental feeding practices are thought to influence children's weight gain, through children's eating behavior and nutritional intake. Controlling feeding practices, such as restriction of food, pressure to eat, and use of food to control behavior, may cause children to focus on external cues and impede their ability to self-regulate their food intake [6, 7]. In general, restricting foods appears to increase their desirability, while pressure to eat may reduce foods' desirability [7]. Consistent with this conceptualization, most cross-sectional studies have reported that parents' restriction of food is linked to children's higher weight status [8–13], and pressure to eat is associated with children's lower weight status [9–15]. In contrast, positive feeding practices, often conceptualized as a child-centered and including behaviors such as encouraging healthy eating and new foods, may allow children to develop self-regulation using their internal cues of hunger and satiety [16].

Longitudinal research can provide guidance for obesity prevention interventions. If parental feeding practices influence child weight status, such information could be incorporated into obesity prevention interventions; but if parental feeding practices are largely a response to child weight, then interventions could focus more on addressing parents' concerns about their children's weight. However, because most studies have been cross-sectional, the direction of influence between parental feeding practices and child weight status is unclear [12]. Moreover, the few existing longitudinal studies have reported inconsistent findings. In young children, two studies have reported that mothers' pressure to eat predicted lower weight status [17, 18], one study found that restriction of food predicted lower weight status in contrast to cross-sectional studies [17], and one found that use of food as a reward predicted higher weight status [19]. Other longitudinal studies have found effects of parental feeding practices only among certain subgroups, such as children of overweight mothers [20, 21], younger children (ages 5–6) but not older children (ages 10–12) [22], or among boys but not girls [23]. Several longitudinal studies have found no effects of parental feeding practices on children's subsequent weight [24–27].

Parents may also modify their feeding practices in response to children's weight status, and this possibility has been examined in three longitudinal studies. Rhee and colleagues [23] found that for girls (but not boys) who had greater weight gain, mothers subsequently used more controlling feeding. Webber and colleagues [27] found that higher baseline child weight predicted increased maternal monitoring and reduced pressure to eat over a 3-year period. Finally, Jansen and colleagues [18] reported that higher baseline child weight predicted greater maternal restriction and less pressure to eat 2 years later.

Relatively few studies of parental feeding practices and children's weight have focused specifically on Latino families [10, 14, 28–32]. Despite the fact that Latinos are the largest ethnic minority group in the U.S., and 63% of Latinos are Mexican Americans [33], no previous longitudinal study of parental feeding practices and child weight status has focused on Mexican Americans or any Latino group.

The major purpose of this study was to examine the mutual influences between parental feeding practices and child weight over a 2-year period, in Mexican American families with children 8–10 years old. Both mothers and fathers participated in the research. Most previous cross-sectional studies of parental feeding practices have focused only on maternal feeding practices. To date, no longitudinal research has reported on whether fathers' feeding practices influence children's weight status, although evidence is beginning to emerge that fathers' feeding practices are also associated with their children's weight [34–39].

The current study examined four types of parental feeding practices: restriction of amount of food, pressure to eat, use of food to control behavior, and positive involvement in child eating. There is evidence that Latino parents use all of these feeding practices [10, 40]. Restriction of food and pressure to eat have been examined in numerous studies [12]. Use of food to control behavior has been studied less often, but a recent longitudinal study reported that using food as a reward—one aspect of using food to control behavior—predicted children's weight gain one year later [19]. Finally, positive involvement in child eating was conceptualized as a child-centered feeding practice, encompassing monitoring of high-calorie foods, encouraging healthy eating and new foods, and providing small servings [10]. Among Mexican American children, greater maternal positive involvement in child eating has been linked to children's lower weight status [10].

In this study, we examined whether parental feeding practices and child weight status influenced each other at three points over a 2-year period, in Mexican American families with children who were 8–10 years old at baseline. We hypothesized that parental feeding practices would predict child weight status: specifically, that restriction of food and using food to control behavior would predict increased child weight status, and that pressure to eat and positive involvement in child eating would predict lower child weight status. We also examined whether child weight status would predict parental feeding practices; specifically, whether greater child weight status would predict more restriction of food, less pressure to eat, and less use of food as a reward. We examined these relationships for both mothers' and fathers' feeding practices. We also assessed these relationships separately by child gender, because previous research suggests that parental feeding practices may influence boys and girls differently [23].

3.2 METHODS

3.2.1 Participants

Parents of 322 Mexican American children ages 8–10 were enrolled in the research. Eligibility criteria for participation included: a mother of Mexican descent (Mexican or U.S. born), and a child between 8 and 10 years old, who had no major illnesses. Families were eligible whether or not fathers participated, but every effort was made to recruit fathers. If the father did not reside in the same household as the mother and child, the primary father figure (biological father living apart or residential parental figure) was recruited to participate. Of the 322 families participating in the study, 57% (n = 182) of fathers participated.

3.2.2 Procedure

We recruited families to participate in a 24-month longitudinal cohort study to understand parental influences on obesity in Mexican American children. Parents were members of Kaiser Permanente Northern California, an integrated health delivery system, between 2007 and 2009. Kaiser Permanente is one of the largest health care providers in California, with membership occurring through employer-provided insurance coverage, individual enrollment, or state-funded (Medi-Cal) programs. A computer program was used to select potential participants from a Kaiser Permanente membership list. Selection criteria were members with a Spanish surname and a child in the eligible age range. These parents were sent letters introducing the research, were telephoned by research assistants, were screened for eligibility, and if eligible, were invited to participate in the study. 37% of eligible families participated in the research.

If the mother or both parents agreed to participate, a baseline assessment home visit was scheduled. At home visits, bilingual research assistants first obtained written parental informed consent and verbal child assent. Families were assessed at baseline (BL), 1-year follow-up (Yr1), and 2-year follow-up (Yr2). All study materials were developed in both Spanish and English, and interviews were conducted in the language of participants' choice. Most parents chose to be interviewed in Spanish (71% of mothers, 69% of fathers). Research assistants interviewed family members individually in their homes, and recorded responses to the questionnaires in laptop computers. Research assistants also measured family members' height, weight, and waist circumference. The in-home interview and assessment lasted about 5 hours per time point. The study was approved by the university and Kaiser Permanente Northern California institutional review boards.

3.2.3 Measures

3.2.3.1 Parental Feeding Practices

At each assessment, parents completed the 55-item Parental Feeding Practices (PFP) Questionnaire [10] about the study child. The PFP was developed for use with Latino parents, and has good validity and reliability [10]. It includes items based on focus group discussions, as well as items adapted from previous measures, and contains four subscales: restriction of amount of food (12 items, e.g., "How often do you tell your child he/she has eaten enough?"; $\alpha_{mothers} = 0.77$, $\alpha_{fathers} = 0.70$), pressure to eat (10 items, e.g., "How often do you tell your child to eat everything on the plate?"; $\alpha_{mothers} = 0.86$, $\alpha_{fathers} = 0.84$), use of food to control behavior (9 items, e.g., "How often do you give your child something to eat or drink to make him/her happy, even if you think he/she isn't hungry?"; $\alpha_{mothers} = 0.78$, $\alpha_{fathers} = 0.75$), and positive involvement in child eating (24 items, e.g., "How often do you find out how much your child ate during the day?"; $\alpha_{mothers} = 0.88$, $\alpha_{fathers} = 0.91$). All questions were worded in terms of frequency of behavior, and response options ranged from never (=1) to always (=5). For each subscale, mean scores were calculated; higher scores represented more use of that feeding practice. In previous research, mothers' and fathers' feeding practices scores were modestly to moderately correlated (rs = 0.19 - 0.46) [10]. In addition, most feeding practices subscales were related to children's weight status for both parents (rs = 0.18–0.35). Exceptions were mothers' use of food to control behavior and fathers' positive involvement in child eating [10].

3.2.3.2 Children's Weight Status: Waist-height Ratio (WHtR) and Body Mass Index (BMI)

At each assessment, child height, weight and waist circumference were obtained using standard procedures; and in duplicate while the participants were wearing light indoor clothing and no shoes [41, 42]. Waist-height ratio (WHtR) was used as a measure of the distribution of central adiposity. This sensitive and specific marker of upper body fat is a good predictor of cardiovascular disease risk factors in children [43, 44]. WHtR was obtained by dividing the child's waist circumference by their height. As a clinical measure, WHtR should be less than 0.5, reflecting the standard that an individual's waist circumference should be less than half their height [45]. Children's body mass index (BMI) was also calculated (weight[kg]/height[m]^2). Raw BMI scores were used in analyses, because these allow for variability in extreme scores to be more accurately assessed over time, compared to BMI z-scores [46, 47].

3.2.3.3 Covariates: Parent and Child Characteristics

We included several parental characteristics as possible covariates: family-level socioeconomic status (SES), acculturation, and parental BMI at BL. Family-level SES was a standardized score based on each parent's years of education and occupational status. Occupational status could range from unskilled (=1) to major professional (=9) [48]. Acculturation was assessed using the Spanish Language Use and English Language Use subscales of the Bidimensional Acculturation Scale for Hispanics [49]. An example item is "How often do you speak English with your friends?" Items are scored from never (=1) to always (=5), and have good reliabilities (α for mothers and fathers = 0.88–0.94). Parents' BMI was calculated (weight[kg]/height[m]^2).

We also included child gender, age, and pubertal status at BL as potential covariates. Pubertal status has been associated with obesity in previous studies [50]. We used the 5-item Pubertal Development Scale [51], which was completed by mothers at BL. This measure, with versions for males and females, asks about physical development on characteristics associated with physical maturation, with response options ranging from no (=1) to yes, a lot (=3). Separate mean scores were calculated by gender.

3.2.4 Statistical Analyses

Pearson correlations were used to examine the relationships between covariates and child weight status (WHtR and BMI) at BL. Covariates that were significantly related to child weight status were included in multivariate analyses. We fit cross-lagged panel models to estimate the effects of parental feeding practices and child weight status on one another over time. Cross-lagged panel models are widely used with longitudinal data to examine the direction of influence between two variables that are measured repeatedly over time. Cross-lagged models provide estimates of regression coefficients between each variable measured at one wave and the other variable at the next wave. In the current study, there were three time points (BL, Yr1, Yr2), and the two variables measured at each time were parental feeding practices and child weight status (general model shown in Fig 1). Each cross-lagged model controlled for covariates at BL. Separate models were estimated for mothers' and fathers' four feeding practices, and for WHtR and BMI (16 models). Satorra-Bentler scaled Chi-square test statistics assessed goodness-of-fit of each model, and approximate model fit was examined using the recommendations of Hu and Bentler [52]; i.e., root mean square error of approximation [RMSEA] ≤ 0.06, and standardized root mean square residual [SRMR] ≤ 0.08. Modeling was performed using Mplus 7, with full information maximum likelihood to accommodate missing values [53].

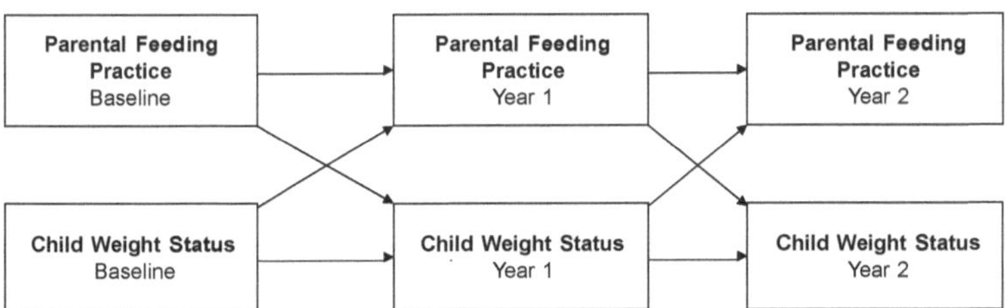

FIGURE 3.1 General cross-lagged panel model, showing mutual influences of parental feeding practices and child weight status across three time points.

We also tested whether child gender modified the cross-lagged effects between each parental feeding practice and child weight status variable. This was accomplished by comparing the fit of a model that allowed cross-lagged effects to freely vary across child gender, to a model that constrained corresponding cross-lagged effects to be equal across child gender. A significant χ^2 difference test would indicate significantly improved fit for the freely-estimated model—an omnibus test of the moderating effect of child gender. For freely-estimated models that showed significantly improved fit, we fit cross-lagged panel models separately by child gender.

A total of 246 mothers had complete data at all three time points, 44 were missing data at one time point, and 32 were missing data at two time points. A total of 98 fathers had complete data at all three time points, 67 were missing data at one time point, and 17 were missing data at two time points. All 322 mothers were included in the analyses of mothers' feeding practices and all 182 fathers were included in the analyses of fathers' feeding practices.

3.3 RESULTS

3.3.1 Participant Characteristics

Demographic characteristics of mothers, fathers and children are shown in Table 1. Additional demographic information included the following: most participating fathers were biological fathers living with the mothers (90%); the remainder were stepfathers (7%), or biological fathers living apart from the mothers (3%). Most parents were born in Mexico (78% mothers; 74% fathers), while most participating children (95%) had been born in the U.S. By design, all mothers were of Mexican heritage. Most fathers were also of Mexican heritage (83%); the rest were other Latino heritage (9%), or other/mixed ethnicities (8%). Most parents were employed (75% of mothers, 93% of fathers). Parents' average occupational status was skilled worker (=3). Descriptive statistics for parental feeding practices are shown in Table 1.

TABLE 3.1 Demographic characteristics and parental feeding practices in Mexican American families at baseline

	Mean (SD) or%		
	Mother	**Father**	**Child**
Variable (range)	(*n* = 322)	(*n* = 182)	(*n* = 322)
Parent characteristics			
Education (0–19 years)	10.77 (3.69)	11.02 (3.67)	
Occupational status (1–9)	3.25 (2.09)	3.53 (1.84)	
Acculturation (1–5)			
Spanish language	4.23 (1.10)	4.01 (1.10)	
English language	2.64 (1.27)	2.94 (1.11)	
BMI (18–72)	30.29 (6.69)	29.81 (4.33)	
Child characteristics			
Gender (% female)			53%
Age (8–10 years)			9.29 (0.92)
Pubertal status (1–3)			1.10 (0.32)

TABLE 3.1 *(Continued)*

	Mean (SD) or%		
	Mother	**Father**	**Child**
Waist-height ratio (WHtR) (0.37–0.79)			0.50 (0.08)
BMI(14–48)			20.35 (4.75)
Parental feeding practices (1–5)			
Restriction of amount of food	2.28 (0.44)	2.29 (0.47)	
Pressure to eat	2.30 (0.86)	2.43 (0.85)	
Use of food to control behavior	1.50 (0.44)	1.62 (0.50)	
Positive involvement in meals	3.35 (0.69)	3.11 (0.70	

Most parents were overweight (BMI ≥ 25 and <30; 33% of mothers, 47% of fathers) or obese (BMI ≥30; 48% of mothers, 45% of fathers). Based on age- and gender-specific BMI percentiles [54], 20% of the children were overweight (≥85th%ile, <95th%ile) and 31% were obese (≥95th%ile) at BL (baseline). 42 percent of children had a WHtR > 0.50.

3.3.2 Correlations between study variables

Correlations between covariates and BL child weight status are shown in Table 2. Based on significant correlations with child WHtR or BMI, covariates included in subsequent multivariate analyses were SES, Spanish language acculturation, parental BMI, child age, and child pubertal status. As shown in Table 3, most parental feeding practices were significantly related to child WHtR and/or BMI at BL, with the exception of positive involvement in child meals. Child WHtR and BMI were significantly related at BL, Yr1, and Yr2 (rs = 0.58, 0.84, 0.53, ps < 0.001, respectively).

TABLE 3.2 Correlations between demographics and child weight status in Mexican American families at baseline

Demographics	Child WHtR1	Child BMI
Family SES	−0.12*	−0.12*
Mother acculturation (Spanish)	0.14*	0.08
Mother acculturation (English)	−0.08	−0.03
Father acculturation (Spanish)	0.10	0.18*
Father acculturation (English)	−0.07	0.12

TABLE 3.2 *(Continued)*

Demographics	Child WHtR1	Child BMI
Mother BMI	0.21***	0.36***
Father BMI	0.30***	0.23***
Child gender	−0.01	0.00
Child age	0.14*	0.28***
Child pubertal status	0.22***	0.33***

*p < 0.05; **p < 0.01; ***p < 0.001

1. WHtR waist-height ratio

TABLE 3.3 Correlations between parental feeding practices and child weight status in Mexican American families at baseline

	Child waist-height ratio		Child BMI	
	Girls	Boys	Girls	Boys
Mothers' feeding practices (n = 322)				
Restriction	0.38***	0.24**	0.51***	0.45***
Pressure	−0.18*	−0.27***	−0.34***	−40***
Use food to control	−0.09	−0.15	−0.24**	−0.22**
Positive involvement	−0.04	−0.11	−0.03	−0.05
Fathers' feeding practices (n = 182)				
Restriction	0.37***	0.13	0.39***	0.47***
Pressure	−0.23*	−0.29**	−0.19	−43***
Use food to control	−0.11	−0.24*	−0.13	−0.25*
Positive involvement	−0.03	−0.09	0.05	0.01

*p < 0.05; **p < 0.01; ***p < 0.001

3.3.3 Longitudinal Relationships between Parental Feeding Practices and Child WHtR

Fig 1 illustrates the general model used to assess the relationships between parental feeding practices and child weight status over time, using cross-lagged panel models. For child WHtR, tests for interactions found that child gender significantly modified the cross-lagged effects between feeding practices and child WHtR in most models, including mothers' restriction, pressure to eat, and use of food to control behavior; and fathers' restriction, pressure to eat, and positive involvement in child eating. For these models, comparisons between freely estimated models and constrained models all showed that the freely estimated models had significantly improved fit (Table 4). All freely estimated models met the fit criteria (see Additional file 1). Therefore, cross-lagged panel model results for these models are reported separately by child gender. The models without significant interactions involving child gender—mothers' positive involvement in child eating and fathers' use of food to control behavior—also had no significant cross-lagged effects between feeding practices and child WHtR (data not shown).

TABLE 3.4 Comparisons of models with cross-lagged effects freely estimated across child gender and models with constrained cross-lagged effects, for waist-height ratio

Model	S-Bχ^2	df	p	ΔS-Bχ^2	Δdf	Δp
Mothers						
Restriction $_{Free}$	39.56	36	0.31			
Restriction $_{Constrained}$	92.43	49	<0.001	54.57	13	<0.001
Pressure $_{Free}$	20.89	36	0.98			
Pressure $_{Constrained}$	102.103	49	<0.001	67.20	13	<0.001
Control $_{Free}$	24.21	36	0.93			
Control $_{Constrained}$	82.31	49	<0.01	59.40	13	<0.001
Fathers						
Restriction $_{Free}$	47.06	36	0.10			
Restriction $_{Constrained}$	82.90	49	<0.01	36.06	13	<0.001
Pressure $_{Free}$	38.85	36	0.34			
Pressure $_{Constrained}$	97.07	49	<0.001	46.44	13	<0.001
Involvement $_{Free}$	42.65	36	0.21			
Involvement $_{Constrained}$	113.24	49	<0.001	58.64	13	<0.001

Note: S-Bχ^2: Satorra-Bentler χ^2 for ΔS-Bχ^2: Satorra-Bentler difference χ^2
Δdf: difference in degrees of freedom between nested models
Δp: p-value for ΔS-Bχ^2.

Cross-lagged panel model results for girls' and boys' WHtR, showing standardized regression coefficients, are summarized in Tables 5 and 6. (See Additional file 1 for figures.) All models included parental BMI, SES, Spanish language acculturation, and child pubertal status as covariates (covariates not shown in tables).

TABLE 3.5 Cross-lagged panel models: parental feeding practices predicting girls' and boys' weight-height ratio (WHtR)

Cross-lagged effects	Mothers' feeding practices		Fathers' feeding practices	
	Girls' WHtR β	Boys' WHtR β	Girls' WHtR β	Boys' WHtR β
Baseline feeding practices → Year 1 child WHtR				
Restriction	0.23**	0.22**	0.21**	0.40***
Pressure	−0.12	−0.23**	−0.07	−0.29**
Use food to control	−0.10	−0.11	na	na
Positive involvement	na	na	0.10	0.08
Year 1 feeding practices → Year 2 child WHtR				
Restriction	−0.02	0.02	−0.11*	0.18*
Pressure	−0.01	−0.05	−0.04	−0.03
Use food to control	−0.03	0.02	na	na
Positive involvement	na	na	−0.07	0.15*

*$p < 0.05$; **$p < 0.01$; ***$p < 0.001$
na: not applicable because the interaction between child gender and feeding practice was not significant

TABLE 3.6 Cross-lagged panel models: girls' and boys' weight-height ratio (WHtR) predicting parental feeding practices

Cross-lagged effects	Mothers' feeding practices		Fathers' feeding practices	
	Girls' WHtR β	Boys' WHtR β	Girls' WHtR β	Boys' WHtR β
Baseline child WHtR → Year 1 feeding practices				
Restriction	0.06	−0.00	0.07	−0.02
Pressure	−0.04	−0.20**	−0.02	0.01
Use food to control	−0.04	−0.03	na	na
Positive involvement	na	na	−0.04	-0.03
Year 1 child WHtR → Year 2 feeding practices				
Restriction	0.00	0.19*	0.07	0.03
Pressure	−0.10	−0.06	−0.20*	−0.07
Use food to control	−0.05	−0.31***	na	na
Positive involvement	na	na	−0.23**	0.09

*p < 0.05; **p < 0.01; ***p < 0.001
na: not applicable because the interaction between child gender and child WHtR was not significant.

3.3.4 Parental Feeding Practices Predicting Child WHtR

3.3.4.1 Mothers' Feeding Practices

Mothers' restriction at BL predicted girls' higher WHtR at Yr1 ($\beta = 0.23$; Table 5). Mothers' restriction at BL predicted boys' higher WHtR at Yr1 ($\beta = 0.22$). Mothers' pressure to eat at BL predicted boys' lower WHtR at Yr1 ($\beta = -0.23$).

3.3.4.2 Fathers' Feeding Practices

Fathers' restriction at BL predicted girls' higher WHtR at Yr1 ($\beta = 0.21$), but fathers' restriction at Yr1 predicted girls' lower WHtR at Yr2 ($\beta = -0.11$). Fathers' restriction at BL and Yr1 predicted boys' higher WHtR at subsequent years (βs = 0.40, 0.18, respectively). Fathers' pressure to eat at BL predicted boys' lower WHtR at Yr1 ($\beta = -0.29$). Fathers' positive involvement in boys' eating at Yr1 predicted boys' higher WHtR at Yr 2 ($\beta = 0.15$).

3.3.5 Child WHtR Predicting Parental Feeding Practices

3.3.5.1 Mothers' Feeding Practices

Girls' WHtR did not significantly predict mothers' feeding practices. Boys' higher WHtR at Yr1 predicted mothers' greater restriction at Year 2 ($\beta = 0.19$; Table 6). Boys' lower WHtR at BL predicted mothers' less pressure to eat at Yr1 ($\beta = -0.20$). Boys' lower WHtR at Yr1 predicted mothers' less use of food to control behavior at Yr2 ($\beta = -0.31$).

3.3.5.2 Fathers' Feeding Practices

Girls' higher WHtR at Yr1 predicted fathers' less pressure to eat at Yr2 ($\beta = -0.20$), as well as fathers' less positive involvement in girls' eating at Yr2 ($\beta = -0.23$). Boys' WHtR did not significantly predict fathers' feeding practices.

3.3.5.3 *Parental Feeding Practices and Child BMI*

For child BMI, tests for interactions showed that child gender did not significantly modify the cross-lagged effects between feeding practices and child BMI in any model. Therefore, the constrained models for data pooled across child gender are reported. All models included parental BMI, SES, Spanish language acculturation, child pubertal status, and child age as covariates.

Models for mothers' restriction, mothers' use of food to control behavior, and fathers' pressure revealed significant cross-lagged effects between feeding practices and child BMI, and had adequate fit. (See Additional file 1 for figures and fit statistics.) Parental feeding practices did not significantly predict child BMI in any of these models. However, child BMI predicted several parental feeding practices. Child greater BMI at BL predicted mothers' greater restriction at Yr1 ($\beta = 0.18$). Child greater BMI at Yr1 predicted mothers' less use of food to control behavior ($\beta = -0.14$) and fathers' less pressure to eat ($\beta = -0.21$) at Yr2.

3.4 DISCUSSION

This research addresses the urgent need to identify modifiable risk factors for childhood obesity among Mexican American children. This longitudinal family-based study included both mothers and fathers in the research, examined the mutual influences of parental feeding practices and children's weight status over time, and utilized the Parental Feeding Practices Questionnaire [10], which was validated for use with this population. Hypotheses were partially supported. Both mothers' and fathers' feeding practices, particularly restriction of amount of food and pressure to eat, predicted children's subsequent weight status. However, parents' positive involvement in child feeding and use of food to control child behavior had minimal or no influence on children's subsequent weight status. Child weight status also predicted several parental feeding practices, with gender-specific findings: mothers altered some feeding practices in response to their sons' weight status, and fathers altered some feeding practices in response to their daughters' weight status.

A consistent pattern of findings was that parents' use of food restriction predicted subsequent higher weight status in both girls and boys at Year 1. For fathers, this effect was also seen at Year 2, suggesting that fathers' restriction in particular may have a continuing effect on child weight status. These findings are consistent with previous cross-sectional research [8–13], although most previous longitudinal studies found this link only among certain subgroups [20–22], or reported no significant effects [19, 24, 26, 27].

Parents' use of pressure to eat predicted lower weight status at Year 1, among boys but not girls. Previous cross-sectional studies [9–15] and two longitudinal studies [17, 18] have reported that pressure to eat was related to children's lower weight status, although several other longitudinal studies were unable to confirm this link [24, 26, 27]. However, none of the previous studies reported the effects of parental feeding practices on boys and girls separately, as we did in the present study.

Our findings regarding parental restriction and pressure to eat are longitudinal evidence that parents' controlling feeding practices may have unintended influences on child weight status in Mexican American families. When parents attempt to restrict their children's dietary intake, children subsequently tend to weigh more, and when parents urge their children to increase their food intake, boys tend to subsequently weigh less over time. Consistent with current theorizing [7], controlling feeding practices appear to increase Mexican American children's reliance on external cues when eating.

There are several possible explanations for this study's findings that parental restriction and pressure to eat influenced children's weight status, in contrast to the nonsignificant findings of some previous longitudinal studies. First, we used waist-height ratio (WHtR), a measure of central adiposity, as well as body mass index (BMI) to assess children's weight status, rather than the commonly used BMI z-scores [e.g., 19–20; 22–24]. Most of this study's significant findings regarding parental influences on child weight status were those using WHtR. Because nearly a third of the study children were obese at baseline (i.e., above the 95% percentile of BMI scores), the WHtR measure may have yielded significant results due to its sensitivity to extreme scores [45]. Second, our sample of 322 mothers and 182 fathers was larger than those of most previous longitudinal studies; other larger studies also reported some significant findings [19, 21–23]. Third, we used an elaborated, culturally-based measure of parental feeding practices, developed and validated for use with this population [10]. Finally, some of our results were due to the inclusion of fathers and separate analyses by child gender. Overall, our findings suggest that some feeding practices likely do predict child weight status over time. More longitudinal research is needed in this area, particularly research using sensitive measures and large samples that include both mothers and fathers.

It is worth noting the particular effect of fathers' feeding practices on boys' weight status. When fathers engaged in more restriction, used less pressure to eat, and were more positively involved in their sons' eating, their sons tended to have a higher weigh status a year later. These findings are intriguing, given that little is known about the feeding practices utilized by fathers, regardless of ethnicity [37]. Our results suggest that Mexican American fathers are involved in their children's eating, and that future research including both parents in Mexican American families could illuminate the ways in which fathers and mothers interact with their sons and daughters regarding dietary intake. Moreover, future obesity interventions could be designed to include fathers as well as mothers as participants.

This is one of few longitudinal studies to examine the effects of child weight status on parental feeding practices. Parents appeared to alter some feeding practices in response to their children's weight, in gender-specific ways. In particular, boys' weight status predicted maternal feeding practices, while girls' weight predicted fathers' feeding practices. Mothers of boys with higher weight status subsequently used less pressure to eat at Year 1, more restriction of food at Year 2, and less use of food to control their sons' behavior at Year 2. Fathers of girls with higher weight status at Year 1 subsequently engaged in less pressure to eat and were less positively involved in their daughters' eating at Year 2. Our findings appear to be consistent with some previous longitudinal research with mothers and children, although those previous studies did not report results separately by child gender [18, 27]. However, our results contrast with those of Rhee and colleagues [23], who found that mothers of girls (but not boys) who gained more weight subsequently used more controlling feeding practices. Overall, our findings hint at the possibility that mothers and fathers have distinct parental roles regarding feeding practices, a topic that is beginning to receive some attention [37, 55, 56]. These cross-gender findings also underscore the importance of examining parental feeding practices separately by parents' and children's gender.

Our finding that children's weight status predicts some parental feeding practices also suggests that parents who alter their feeding practices in response to their child's weight may be experiencing concerns about their child's weight. This notion is consistent with several cross-sectional studies reporting that maternal concerns about child weight are related to parental feeding practices (e.g., [27, 57, 58]). Parents may welcome interventions that could address these concerns and provide guidance for utilizing constructive feeding practices, such as recognizing children's hunger and satiety cues while setting appropriate limits [59, 60].

This longitudinal study sheds light on the question of whether parental feeding practices influence children's subsequent weight, or whether children's weight influences parents' subsequent feeding practices. We found some evidence for both directions of influence. Because this was not a randomized controlled trial, causal inferences cannot be drawn. Moreover, the sample was a convenience sample drawn from a large health care provider. However, a strength of this study was the fact that we assessed participants at three points in time, allowing for the mutual influences of parental feeding practices and child weight to be examined. Another limitation of this research is that results cannot be generalized beyond Mexican American families with mostly immigrant parents. The generalizability of the findings is also limited because only about one-third of eligible families participated in the research, possibly partially because of the considerable time commitment required. It would be of interest to investigate whether our findings also apply to other Latino subgroups, such as those who are more acculturated, as well as other cultural, ethnic, or economic groups; and whether the same findings would apply if research participation was less time-consuming. Moreover, because the PFP Questionnaire is relatively new, further investigation of its reliability and validity is needed. Finally, we studied only children ages 8–10 at baseline, and followed them for 2 years to ages 10–12. We speculate that the influence of parental feeding practices may be stronger at younger ages, as hinted by the findings of some previous research [17, 19, 22]. A valuable contribution to the literature would be to assess the ages at which the influence of parental feeding practices on child weight begins to diminish, as well as when parental responses to child weight begin to occur. Such information could be of use in designing future obesity prevention interventions.

3.5 CONCLUSIONS

This study provides longitudinal evidence that parental feeding practices influence children's weight status in Mexican American families, and that children's weight status also influences parental feeding practices. Both mothers' and fathers' feeding practices appear to influence children's weight status, underscoring the importance of including fathers in research on parental feeding practices and child obesity. Our findings suggest that both mothers and fathers should be included in obesity prevention interventions focusing on parental feeding practices in Latino populations. Finally, this longitudinal research adds to accumulating evidence regarding the undesirable effects of controlling feeding practices. Obesity prevention interventions may benefit from educating parents to avoid using controlling feeding practices—such as restriction of food and pressure to eat—from an early age, regardless of children's weight. Toward this aim, interventions could address parents' concerns about their children's weight, by helping them to understand and be responsive to children's hunger and satiety cues [60]. Interventions should also focus on healthy behaviors for the entire family, such as improved diet and physical activity, which help prevent childhood obesity [60, 61].

REFERENCES

1. Freedman DS, Mei Z, Srinivasan SR, Berenson GS, Dietz WH. Cardiovascular risk factors and excess adiposity among overweight children and adolescents: the Bogalusa Heart Study. J Pediatr. 2007;150(1):12–7. e12.
2. L'Allemand-Jander D. Clinical diagnosis of metabolic and cardiovascular risks in overweight children: early development of chronic diseases in the obese child. Int J Obes (Lond). 2010;34(2):S32–6.
3. Singh AS, Mulder C, Twisk JW, van Mechelen W, Chinapaw MJ. Tracking of childhood overweight into adulthood: a systematic review of the literature. Obes Rev. 2008;9(5):474–88.
4. Skinner AC, Steiner MJ, Henderson FW, Perrin EM. Multiple markers of inflammation and weight status: cross-sectional analyses throughout childhood. Pediatrics. 2010;125(4):e801–9.
5. Ogden CL, Carroll MD, Kit BK, Flegal KM. Prevalence of obesity and trends in body mass index among US children and adolescents, 1999–2010. JAMA. 2012;307(5):483–90.
6. Fisher JO, Birch LL. Restricting access to foods and children's eating. Appetite. 1999;32:405–19.
7. Mitchell GL, Farrow C, Haycraft E, Meyer C. Parental influences on children's eating behaviour and characteristics of successful parent-focussed interventions. Appetite. 2013;60(1):85–94.
8. Gray WN, Janicke DM, Wistedt KM, Dumont-Driscoll MC. Factors associated with parental use of restrictive feeding practices to control their children's food intake. Appetite. 2010;55(2):332–7.
9. Jansen PW, Roza SJ, Jaddoe VW, et al. Children's eating behavior, feeding practices of parents and weight problems in early childhood: results from the population-based generation R study. Int J Behav Nutr Phys Act. 2012;9:130.
10. Tschann JM, Gregorich SE, Penilla C, et al. Parental feeding practices in Mexican American families: initial test of an expanded measure. Int J Behav Nutr Phys Act. 2013;10:6.
11. Wehrly SE, Bonilla C, Perez M, Liew J. Controlling parental feeding practices and child body composition in ethnically and economically diverse preschool children. Appetite. 2014;73:163–71.
12. Ventura AK, Birch LL. Does parenting affect children's eating and weight status? Int J Behav Nutr Phy. 2008;5:15.
13. Hurley KM, Cross MB, Hughes SO. A systematic review of responsive feeding and child obesity in high-income countries. J Nutr. 2011;141(3):495–501.
14. Matheson DM, Robinson TN, Varady A, Killen JD. Do Mexican-American mothers' food-related parenting practices influence their children's weight and dietary intake? J Am Diet Assoc. 2006;106:1861–5.

15. Birch LL, Fisher JO, Grimm-Thomas K, Markey CN, Sawyer R, Johnson SL. Confirmatory factor analysis of the child feeding questionnaire: a measure of parental attitudes, beliefs and practices about child feeding and obesity proneness. Appetite. 2001;36(3):201–10.
16. Hughes SO, Power TG, Orlet Fisher J, Mueller S, Nicklas TA. Revisiting a neglected construct: parenting styles in a child feeding context. Appetite. 2005;44:83–92.
17. Farrow CV, Blissett J. Controlling feeding practices: cause or consequence of early child weight? Pediatrics. 2008;121(1):e164–9.
18. Jansen PW, Tharner A, van der Ende J, et al. Feeding practices and child weight: is the association bidirectional in preschool children? Am J Clin Nutr. 2014;100(5):1329–36.
19. Rodgers RF, Paxton SJ, Massey R, et al. Maternal feeding practices predict weight gain and obesogenic eating behaviors in young children: a prospective study. Int J Behav Nutr Phys Act. 2013;10:24.
20. Faith MS, Berkowitz RI, Stallings VA, Kerns J, Storey M, Stunkard AJ. Parental feeding attitudes and styles and child body mass index: prospective analysis of a gene-environment interaction. Pediatrics. 2004;114:e429–36.
21. Francis LA, Birch LL. Maternal weight status modulates the effects of restriction on daughters' eating and weight. Int J Obes (Lond). 2005;29(8):942–9.
22. Campbell K, Andrianopoulos N, Hesketh K, Ball K, Crawford D, Brennan L, et al. Parental use of restrictive feeding practices and child BMI z-score. A 3-year prospective cohort study. Appetite. 2010;55:84–8.
23. Rhee KE, Coleman SM, Appugliese DP, Kaciroti NA, Corwyn RF, Davidson NS, et al. Maternal feeding practices become more controlling after and not before excessive rates of weight gain. Obesity. 2009;17:1724–9.
24. Gregory JE, Paxton SJ, Brozovic AM. Maternal feeding practices, child eating behaviour and body mass index in preschool-aged children: a prospective analysis. Int J Behav Nutr Phys Act. 2010;7:55.
25. Gregory JE, Paxton SJ, Brozovic AM. Maternal feeding practices predict fruit and vegetable consumption in young children. Results of a 12-month longitudinal study. Appetite. 2011;57(1):167–72.
26. Spruijt-Metz D, Li C, Cohen E, Birch L, Goran M. Longitudinal influence of mother's child-feeding practices on adiposity in children. J Pediatr. 2006;148(3):314–20.
27. Webber L, Cooke L, Hill C, Wardle J. Child adiposity and maternal feeding practices a longitudinal analysis. American J Clin Nut. 2010;92:1423–8.
28. Anderson CB, Hughes SO, Fisher JO, Nicklas TA. Cross-cultural equivalence of feeding beliefs and practices: the psychometric properties of the child feeding questionnaire among Blacks and Hispanics. Prev Med. 2005;41:521–31.
29. Cardel M, Willig AL, Dulin-Keita A, Casazza K, Beasley TM, FernSndez JR. Parental feeding practices and socioeconomic status are associated with child adiposity in a multi-ethnic sample of children. Appetite. 2012;58:347–53.
30. Hughes SO, Anderson CB, Power TG, Micheli N, Jaramillo S, Nicklas TA. Measuring feeding in low-income African-American and Hispanic parents. Appetite. 2006;46:215–23.
31. Melgar-Quinonez HR, Kaiser LL. Relationship of child-feeding practices to overweight in low-income Mexican-American preschool-aged children. J Am Diet Assoc. 2004;104:1110–9.
32. Robinson TN, Kiernan M, Matheson DM, Haydel KF. Is parental control over children's eating associated with childhood obesity? Results from a population-based sample of third graders. Obes Res. 2001;9:306–12.

33. The Hispanic population: 2010 Census briefs [http://www.census.gov/prod/cen2010/briefs/c2010br-04.pdf]
34. Blissett J, Meyer C, Haycraft E. Maternal and paternal controlling feeding practices with male and female children. Appetite. 2006;47:212–9.
35. Brann LS, Skinner JD. More controlling child-feeding practices are found among parents of boys with an average body mass index compared with parents of boys with a high body mass index. J Am Diet Assoc. 2005;105:1411–6.
36. Johannsen DL, Johannsen NM, Specker BL. Influence of parents' eating behaviors and child feeding practices on children's weight status. Obesity (Silver Spring). 2006;14:431–9.
37. Khandpur N, Blaine RE, Fisher JO, Davison KK. Fathers' child feeding practices: a review of the evidence. Appetite. 2014;78:110–21.
38. Musher-Eizenman DR, de Lauzon-Guillain B, Holub SC, Leporc E, Charles MA. Child and parent characteristics related to parental feeding practices. A cross-cultural examination in the US and France. Appetite. 2009;52:89–95.
39. Zhang L, McIntosh WA. Children's weight status and maternal and paternal feeding practices. J Child Health Care. 2011;15(4):389–400.
40. Martinez SM, Blanco E, Rhee K, Boutelle K. Latina mothers' attitudes and behaviors around feeding their children: the impact of the cultural maternal role. J Acad Nutr Diet. 2014;114(2):230–7.
41. Lohman TG, Roche AF, Martorell R. Anthropometric Standardization Reference Manual. Champaign, IL: Human Kinetics Books; 1989.
42. Stallings VA, Fung EB. Clinical nutritional assessment of infants and children. In: Shils ME, Olson JA, Shike M, Ross AC, editors. Modern Nutrition in Health and Disease. 9th ed. Philadelphia: Lippincott, Williams & Wilkins; 1999. p. 885–93.
43. Savva SC, Tornaritis M, Savva ME, et al. Waist circumference and waist-to-height ratio are better predictors of cardiovascular disease risk factors in children than body mass index. Int J Obes Relat Metab Disor. 2000;24(11):1453–8.
44. Taylor RW, Jones IE, Williams SM, Goulding A. Evaluation of waist circumference, waist-to-hip ratio, and the conicity index as screening tools for high trunk fat mass, as measured by dual-energy X-ray absorptiometry, in children aged 3–19 y. Am J Clin Nutr. 2000;72(2):490–5.
45. McCarthy HD, Ashwell M. A study of central fatness using waist-to-height ratios in UK children and adolescents over two decades supports the simple message - /'keep your waist circumference to less than half your height/'. Int J Obes. 2006;30(6):988–92.
46. Cole TJ, Faith MS, Pietrobelli A, Heo M. What is the best measure of adiposity change in growing children: BMI, BMI%, BMI z-score or BMI centile? Eur J Clin Nutr. 2005;59(3):419–25.
47. Field AE, Laird N, Steinberg E, Fallon E, Semega-Janneh M, Yanovski JA. Which metric of relative weight best captures body fatness in children? Obes Res. 2003;11(11):1345–52.
48. Hollingshead AB. Four-factor index of social status: Department of Sociology, Yale University. 1975.
49. Marin G, Gamba RJ. A new measurement of acculturation for Hispanics: The bidimensional acculturation scale for Hispanics (BAS). Hispanic J Behav Sci. 1996;18:297–316.
50. Biro FM, Khoury P, Morrison JA. Influence of obesity on timing of puberty. Int J Androl. 2006;29(1):272–7.

51. Petersen AC, Crockett L, Tobin-Richards M, Boxer A. Measuring Pubertal Status: Reliability and Validity of a Self-Report Measure. Pennsylvania State University: University Park; 1985.
52. Hu LT, Bentler PM. Cutoff criteria for fit indexes in covariance structure analysis: conventional criteria versus new alternatives. Struct Equ Modeling. 1999;6:1–55.
53. Muthen LK, Muthen BO. How to use a Monte Carlo study to decide on sample size and determine power. Struct Equ Modeling. 2002;9(4):599–620.
54. Kuczmarski RJ, Ogden CL, Grummer-Strawn LM, Flegal KM, Guo SS, Wei R, et al.: CDC growth charts: United States. Adv Data 2000:1-27.
55. Cabrera NJ, Bradley RH. Latino fathers and their children. Child Dev Perspect. 2012;6(3):232–8.
56. Freeman E, Fletcher R, Collins CE, Morgan PJ, Burrows T, Callister R. Preventing and treating childhood obesity: time to target fathers. Int J Obes (Lond). 2012;36(1):12–5.
57. Gregory JE, Paxton SJ, Brozovic AM. Pressure to eat and restriction are associated with child eating behaviours and maternal concern about child weight, but not child body mass index, in 2- to 4-year-old children. Appetite. 2010;54(3):550–6.
58. May AL, Donohue M, Scanlon KS, et al. Child-feeding strategies are associated with maternal concern about children becoming overweight, but not children's weight status. J Am Diet Assoc. 2007;107(7):1167–75.
59. Rollins BY, Loken E, Savage JS, Birch LL. Maternal controlling feeding practices and girls' inhibitory control interact to predict changes in BMI and eating in the absence of hunger from 5 to 7 year. Am J Clin Nutr. 2014;99(2):249–57.
60. Birch LL, Ventura AK. Preventing childhood obesity: what works? Int J Obes (Lond). 2009;33 Suppl 1:S74–81.
61. Crawford PB, Gosliner W, Anderson C, et al. Counseling Latina mothers of preschool children about weight issues: suggestions for a new framework. J Am Diet Assoc. 2004;104(3):387–94.

CHAPTER 4

Development of the General Parenting Observational Scale to Assess Parenting During Family Meals

Kyung E Rhee, Susan Dickstein, Elissa Jelalian, Kerri Boutelle, Ronald Seifer, and Rena Wing

4.1 BACKGROUND

There has been long-standing interest in the influence of general parenting on many aspects of child development. In more recent years, there has been particular interest in its relationship to childhood obesity [1]. However, measuring general parenting styles can be difficult, partly due to differences between measures regarding underlying constructs, level of parenting behavior being measured, psychometric properties of the measures, and participants' understanding of individual assessment items [2,3]. This variability has resulted in inconsistencies regarding the relationship between parenting and childhood obesity [4-7]. As a result, the American Heart Association and the International Society for Behavioral Nutrition and Physical Activity have called for better measures of parenting to help inform the impact of general parenting on weight related behaviors and ultimately childhood obesity [2,8].

Within the domain of parent feeding and child nutrition, there are three different levels of parenting that have been reported on in the literature: specific parenting practices, parent feeding style, and general parenting (Figure 1) [9]. General parenting is the broadest concept of parenting and is traditionally thought of as the underlying attitude and socialization goal parents have towards their children [10]. It often provides the backdrop or emotional context in which specific parenting behaviors are delivered and interpreted by the child. As such, it should not be viewed as what parents do (which is better defined as specific parenting practices), but how they do it. Because it represents an underlying attitude and approach towards parenting however, it can be difficult to measure. For example, a question that is often asked in obesity-related research is whether or not parents limit the amount of food their child eats. This is generally thought of as a question that assesses a specific parenting practice. However, parents may do this by discussing what the appropriate amount is to eat and encouraging children to slow down and not take seconds (authoritative style), or by abruptly telling the child s/he should stop eating and taking the food away after it has been partially consumed (authoritarian style). Depending on how the parent limits food intake (i.e., which general parenting style is used), the impact of the specific parent behavior (in this case, limiting food consumption) on child eating behavior or weight may be altered. This moderating effect of general parenting on specific parenting practices has been demonstrated in a few studies [11-13]. For example, van der Horst and colleagues found that parents were more effective at limiting their child's consumption of sugar-sweetened beverages when they used an authoritative parenting style compared to when they used an authoritarian parenting style [11]. These studies therefore indicate that higher-order general parenting is an important construct to consider when examining the impact of parent behaviors on child outcomes.

Parent feeding styles reflect the specific attitudes and socialization goals parents have around feeding their child [14], and is another level of parenting that has been examined in relation to pediatric obesity-related outcomes. While the terminology used to describe parent feeding styles are derived from the general parenting literature, this type of parenting is typically thought of as a domain-specific form of parenting (around food) that is nested within the broader concept of general parenting. Because these different levels of parenting have not always been clearly differentiated in the literature, there appear to be inconsistent findings around "parenting" and child obesity-related outcomes [9]. For example, the indulgent/permissive *parent feeding style* has been associated with greater child weight status [15,16] while in other studies, the authoritarian *parenting style* (general parenting) has been associated with greater child weight status [4,17]. As a result, it can be confusing to delineate how parenting relates to child obesity-related outcomes. Nevertheless, because parent feeding styles pertain to a different level of parenting and reflect domain specific goals around child eating, this level of analysis has its own merit and should be considered separately from the higher-order dimension of general parenting.

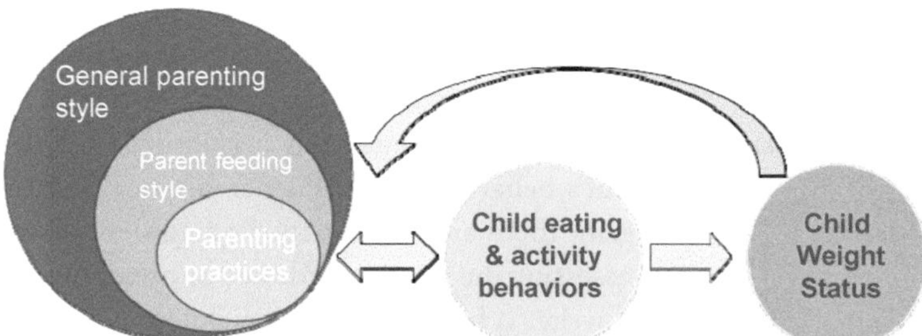

FIGURE 4.1 Parent levels of influence on child behaviors and weight. There are three levels of parenting that have been identified as impacting child eating and activity behaviors and weight status. The broadest is general parenting style, which is thought to moderate the effect of specific parenting practices and possibly parent feeding style. Each of these levels of parenting can influence child eating and activity behaviors and ultimately child weight status, either individually or in conjunction with each other. Child eating and activity behaviors directly affect child weight status. This relationship however seems to be bi-directional, and child weight status and eating and activity behaviors influence parenting behaviors.

While specific parenting practices or feeding behaviors often have a stronger relationship with child eating behaviors and weight status than general parenting [18,19], there are several studies to suggest that general parenting style alone is also related to these outcomes [4,20,21]. This is best demonstrated in a recent study that involved a general parenting intervention for children with behavioral problems [22]. The goal of the original intervention was to improve parents' ability to interact with their children and manage their behavioral problems. While weight loss was not a goal of the original study and nutrition and physical activity counseling was not a component of the intervention, they were still able to demonstrate an effect on obesity rates, with children from the intervention group having lower rates of obesity three to five years later compared to children who did not receive this intervention [22]. Thus it appears that general parenting can have a significant impact on broader aspects of child health and well-being. Understanding the effect of general parenting on these outcomes will help us determine how to incorporate parenting training, specifically which aspect of general parenting training, into obesity prevention and treatment efforts. However, in order to assess this dimension, better measures of general parenting need to be developed.

Because general parenting taps into more abstract parenting concepts like socialization goals and emotional climate, there is an added complexity to assessing it. Contemporary parenting measures have typically relied on self-report or survey items and focus on specific parenting behaviors [1]. Unfortunately, these types of assessments can lead to recall bias and have the added problem of social desirability. Parents may also lack awareness of their own parenting style and behaviors [23]. Others have suggested that using child reports of parenting behavior can result in more relevant accounts since it is ultimately the child's perspective of his/her parent's behaviors that influence his/her development [24,25]. However, here again, there are issues with finding developmentally appropriate measures and assessing the views of toddlers or preschool children who are unable to read and write. While there are several newer methods that have the ability to improve the reliability of self-report measures (e.g., using implicit measures, ecological momentary assessment, or computerized adaptive testing [26]), observational methods are a traditional method of assessment that allow for more objective evaluation free from recall bias. Observational methods have their own limitations, such as social desirability, coder biases, and time and labor intensity to analyze. Nevertheless, as interest in the relationship between general parenting and childhood obesity-related behaviors grows, additional methods of assessing general parenting are needed and a return to direct observational methods may be warranted.

4.1.1 Defining General Parenting Styles and Dimensions

The classic general parenting dimensions include: 1) warmth, support and responsiveness, and 2) behavioral control and demands for maturity [27-29]. The dimension of "warmth, support and responsiveness" is defined by displays of support and emotional connection with the child to foster autonomy and self-efficacy. "Behavioral control/demands for maturity" is characterized by the setting of expectations for the child to display certain levels of maturity and compliance with behavioral norms. Crossing these dimensions result in the four classic parenting styles of authoritative parenting (high in warmth/support and behavioral control/maturity demands), authoritarian parenting (low in warmth/support, high in behavioral control/maturity demands), permissive parenting (high in warmth/support, low in behavioral control/maturity demands) and neglectful parenting (low in warmth/support and behavioral control/maturity demands) [30]. While much of the literature focuses on these four parenting styles, growing attention has been paid to the specific dimensions encompassing these parenting styles. For coding purposes, it may also be simpler and more accurate to assess each of the general parenting dimensions separately. This will allow us to determine specifically which aspects of general parenting are affecting child weight-related outcomes.

4.1.2 Creation of General Parenting Observational Scale

Based on work by Baumrind [27], Maccoby and Martin [30], Barber [31], and Slater and Power [32], several dimensions of parenting were selected for this direct observational scale. These included traditional dimensions of warmth and support, behavioral control, and demands for maturity, but also included newer concepts like psychological control and structure (Table 1). Similar to how Maccoby and Martin operationalized parenting [30], these were then divided into two categories of parenting, one that characterizes the emotional climate of the parent–child interaction and one that characterizes the behavioral aspects of parenting.

TABLE 4.1 Parenting dimensions of the General Parenting Observational Scale

GPOS Dimension	Definition
Emotional Dimensions:	
Warmth and affection	Parent expresses warmth and affection towards the child by saying "I love you" or other words of affection, praising the child, or showing that they care about the child. This affection can be reflected in the parent's tone of voice, facial expressions, physical signs (like hugging, patting on the back, or gentle touching), or other affectionate acts. Parent may also provide positive reinforcement for child behaviors. Overall, parent shows genuine affection, care and attachment towards their child.
Support and sensitivity	Parent provides support and helps the child in some manner. Parent can listen to the child's ideas; shows physical, emotional, or intellectual support and understanding of the child's behaviors, thoughts, or emotions; appreciates the child's ideas and behaviors; helps child to problem solve; and helps child through difficulties. Parent is sensitive to the child's needs and goals. Ultimately, parent is aware of what the child is doing and adjusting his/her own behavior to take the child's behaviors and needs into consideration.

TABLE 4.1 *(Continued)*

GPOS Dimension	Definition
Negative Affect	Parent shows anger, hostility, disdain, or disappointment towards the child. Parent may criticize, yell, make fun of child (mocking), belittle, make sarcastic comments towards child, or be frustrated by what the child is saying or doing. This attitude can be reflected in the tone of voice, facial expressions, or hostile acts.
Detachment	Parent is uninvolved or unresponsive towards the child. For example, the child may do something nice for the parent, but the parent does not acknowledge it. Parent can be distant or is "going through the motions", but displays no feeling of attachment with the child. There is an overall lack of connection with child. Parent may be actively ignoring the child (e.g. child is trying to interact or get the parent's attention but is not getting a response, or the child is being "boxed" out of conversation/interaction).
Behavioral Dimensions:	
Firm discipline and structure	This dimension captures how parents structure the environment to control or manage the child's behaviors. Parents have a defined set of rules, guidelines, and boundaries for behaviors that are somehow expressed on the recording. For example, parent may enforce or remind the child about a rule or expectation, explain reasons for a rule, allow discussion around a rule, provide warnings, or carry through with some disciplinary action or consequence. Parent may demonstrate flexibility around certain rules but usually has a limit which is not negotiable. Parent tries to be consistent when disciplining and carry through with the discipline or consequence. He/she expects the child to follow rules and structures the environment to support these behaviors. (Parents can be calm or angry when disciplining, but if they are angry, using threats, raising their voice, or bullying, then also code for negative affect.)
Demands for maturity	Parent expects certain behaviors from the child that demonstrate maturity and respect for others, like not interrupting, saying please and thank you, using a napkin or silverware appropriately, etc. Parent also expects self-control of behaviors, emotions, and attitudes. Parents may remind the child of these expectations verbally or refer to these expectations through physical acts, gestures, or facial expressions.
Psychological control	This type of control intrudes into the psychological and emotional development of the child, and typically includes guilt or coercion to influence the child's behaviors (guilt induction). Parents can show disappointment in the child behaviors or tell the child about all the sacrifices that were made for the child with the intention of guilting or persuading him/her to execute or complete the desired

TABLE 4.1 *(Continued)*

GPOS Dimension	Definition
	behavior. Parent may bring up previous bad behavior as a reminder to influence a new behavior. Parent may also withdraw affection if the child does something bad (love withdrawal), invalidate the child's feelings, make a personal attack on the child, and demonstrate erratic emotional behavior (change their emotional reaction to suit their needs and goals). Parent can also be intrusive and push his/her goals and agenda on the child without regard for what the child is doing. Parent typically wants to control all of the child's behaviors and wants to tell the child what to do. Child has no autonomy in this situation.
Physical control	Parent uses physical force to control the child's behavior. Parent may physically hurt the child, push or grab the child, or spank the child when he/she disobeys.
Permissive	In this situation, the child usually decides what to do and controls his/her behaviors, actions, and daily schedule. The child can also determine the rules, e.g. what to eat, how much to eat. There are typically no rules. Parents are more laissez-faire. They may label the child's misbehavior, but provide no follow-through with discipline. Parents may be more concerned with the child liking them and are therefore not as concerned about the discipline. These parents usually cannot say no to the child.
Neglectful	Parent does not provide support or respond to the child's physical needs. For example, if the child hurts him- or herself, parent does not respond or show concern; or the parent does not provide more food or drink if the child asks for it or looks hungry. This is different from detachment in that it does not address the emotional needs of the child.

Dimensions were based on classic parenting concepts introduced by Baumrind, Maccoby and Martin, Barber, and Slater and Power.

Videotapes are divided into 2 minute time-periods and each dimension is scored on a scale from 1 (not at all present) to 5 (present a great deal). Composite scores are calculated for each dimension based on a 20 minute videotape of a family meal.

4.1.2.1 Emotional Dimensions of Parenting

The emotional dimensions of parenting included warmth and affection, support and sensitivity, negative affect, and detachment. *Warmth and affection* was rated on how often the index parent demonstrated love, caring and affection for the index child, either verbally, physically, or through facial expressions. *Support and sensitivity* was rated on how engaged the parent was with what the child was saying or doing, demonstrating sensitivity to his/her needs and providing understanding and support for the child's behaviors, thoughts, and emotional expressions. *Negative affect* was scored when parents demonstrated hostility and anger towards the child. Sarcastic remarks were also included in this category. Parents were scored for *detachment* if they were unresponsive towards the child and displayed any behavioral expression to suggest a lack of feeling of attachment or interest in what the child was feeling, saying or doing.

4.1.2.2 Behavioral Dimensions of Parenting

The behavioral dimensions of parenting included firm discipline and structure, demands for maturity, psychological control, physical control, permissiveness, and neglect. *Firm discipline and structure* was rated on how often parents limited behaviors and enforced rules. Consistency in enforcing these rules contributed to scoring in this dimension. Because structure complements the concept of firm discipline, it was coded together. *Structure* is defined as having clear rules and routines, consistent boundaries, and an organized environment in which the child can exist [32]. Parenting that does not include structure does not provide an organized environment in which the child can learn what their parent's behavioral expectations are. The organized home environment and consistent parenting provided by structure ultimately provides the child with stable expectations and an ability to develop and learn new skills successfully [33]. Recently, this dimension of general parenting has appeared in a comprehensive self-report measure of parenting [34] and is garnering more interest in the field. The use of routines, reference to rules that had previously been set, or the discussion of new rules were included when scoring for firm discipline and structure. *Demands for maturity* is a behavioral dimension that compliments that of firm discipline and structure, and refers to the behavioral expectation that parents have for their child to demonstrate self-control and maturity. Parents who remind their children of these behavioral expectations were coded as displaying demands for maturity. If any of these demands were delivered with negative affect, coders would include that rating in the appropriate emotional dimension of parenting.

In addition to these dimensions, *psychological control* was included. Psychological control is different from behavioral control in that it uses more coercive and emotionally-laden parenting behaviors (e.g., guilt induction, withdrawal of love, disappointment, shame) as well as excessive use of personal control (e.g., possessiveness and protection) to manage a child's behaviors [31].

Parents who use this more intrusive type of parenting often impose their agenda onto the child, reflecting a more domineering type of control over the child's autonomy. This type of parenting can have a negative impact on child social and emotional growth and development into an autonomous, independent, and self-efficacious person. It has also been shown to have a negative impact on adolescent substance abuse [35], internalizing problems, and self-efficacy [19]. More recently, it was found to be associated with higher child BMI z-scores [36] and was therefore included in this scale. Psychological control was rated on whether the parent used coercive behaviors like guilt induction or withdrawal of love and attention to control or shape the child's behaviors. Parents who were intrusive, or showed little regard for their child's interests or agenda, were rated highly on this dimension.

Other aspects of behavioral parenting included *physical control, permissiveness,* and *neglect. Physical control* was intended to capture any physical actions that the parent used to control the child's behavior. *Permissiveness* was scored when parents showed little control over their child's behaviors and allowed the child to determine the rules. Parents were also rated as being permissive if they did not follow through with any suggestion of discipline or had a hard time placing limits on the child's behaviors. *Neglect* was included to capture parents who were not responsive to the child's physical needs. This was meant to be different from detachment in that detachment pertained to whether or not the parent addressed the child's emotional needs and displayed a level of emotional attachment with the child. A parent could be detached emotionally, but still meet the child's physical needs, and therefore not be neglectful.

With this new observational schema, we set out to assess general parenting dimensions during a family meal. While other parenting coding schemas use the play-situation [37,38], this setting may not be developmentally appropriate for older children. Mealtimes offer a naturalistic setting where parents are often managing child behaviors, imposing rules and expectations, and interacting with their children. Furthermore, it allows one to assess other parent level behaviors, like feeding style and feeding practices, as well as family functioning that may be associated with obesity-related outcomes. Several behavioral observational measures of parent/caregiver-child interactions during mealtime exist [39-44]. While one of these measures claims to assess maternal parenting style, closer examination of this tool reveals that it measures feeding specific behaviors instead (e.g., prompts to eat and number of times food is offered) [39]. Several of the other tools also report on feeding-specific parenting behaviors or prompts that occur prior to eating [40,42,43]. Finally, one tool characterizes caregiver feeding behaviors into the four classic parenting styles, thus capturing parent feeding styles and not general parenting per se [44]. As such, very few observational tools truly assess the higher-order level of general parenting. The purpose of this study was to develop and test a tool to assess general parenting as it pertains to obesity-related outcomes. The Mealtime Family Interaction Coding System (MICS) has been used in previous studies to assess family functioning in homes with overweight children [45,46] and several of its dimensions capture similar emotional and behavioral control aspects of parenting, albeit at a different level of interaction. Therefore, we used the MICS and several self-report measures of parenting to examine the correlation between their constructs of parenting to those from our newly developed General Parenting Observational Scale (GPOS).

4.2 METHODS

4.2.1 Subjects

Families were recruited through advertisements in physicians' offices and schools in Providence, Rhode Island and San Diego, California. Families with overweight (body mass index (BMI) ≥ 85th percentile but < 95th percentile) or obese (BMI ≥ 95th percentile) children were recruited to participate in a family-based weight control intervention for children between the ages of 8 and 12 years old. Eligible families had a child with a BMI ≥ 85th percentile but were less than 100% overweight, and were willing to participate in the 16-week program. Families were excluded if the child was taking medication that affected his/her weight or growth, was severely developmentally delayed, had a major psychiatric illness that prevented him/her from participating in the group sessions, or they were moving outside the area during the timeframe of the study. Families were provided with informed consent and IRB approval was obtained from relevant institutions in both cities.

4.2.2 Procedure

Families who contacted the research center completed a brief phone screen. Those who were eligible were invited to the center for an orientation session where they learned more about the weight control intervention. Families with overweight children were invited to participate in a 16-week family-based weight control program based on the Traffic Light Diet [47,48]. Children and parents met in separate 1-hour weekly group sessions and learned about behavioral strategies that would help them make changes to their eating and physical activity behaviors. A total of 226 parents contacted the research center. However, 182 families were excluded because of failure to meet eligibility criteria (19%), lack of interest or time commitment (54%), did not respond to phone calls or attend orientation (21%), or failure to complete pre-intervention assessments (6%). As a result, only 44 families entered the study. Pre- and post-intervention assessments were completed by both children and parents. Only pre-intervention assessment data from families were used in this study.

Each family participated in a video-taped family meal before and after the intervention. Research assistants (RA) scheduled a time to go to the family's home during one of their regular dinner hours (times ranged from 3:30 to 7:30 P.M.). The RA set up a video camera in their dining area and turned the camera on when they were ready to eat. She then left the house and returned in 30 minutes. Since previous studies have demonstrated that parent–child behaviors during a meal are similar across three different tapings [49-51], only one taping was performed for each family. However, to ensure the validity of this taping, after the meal parents were asked to rate: 1) how similar the meal was to their typical meal, and 2) how similar the parent–child interaction was to their typical interactions. Scores were rated on a scale of 1 (not very typical) to 4 (very typical). Parents who scored the meal or the interaction as a 1 or 2 were told that an additional meal would have to be taped to ensure the validity of the data being collected. Only 2 families required an additional taping.

4.2.3 Measures

4.2.3.1 General Parenting Observational Scale (GPOS)

Based on the Home Observation Coding System [52], a 5-point global rating scale was used to determine the prevalence of these general parenting dimensions during the meal. Coding began when all family members were at the table. Meals averaged 18.1 minutes (S.D. 3.2 minutes) in length (median = 20 minutes, interquartile range = 4 minutes). Therefore tapes were coded for 20 minutes. Each 20-minute videotaped family meal was divided into 10, two-minute time-periods. At the end of each 2 minute segment, the tape was stopped and coders scored the index parent (i.e., the parent who enrolled and came to the intervention) and child interaction for each of the 10 parenting dimensions.

Scores ranged from 1 (not present at all) to 5 (present a great deal). Scores were summed for each dimension with a possible range of 10 to 50. Meals less than 20 minutes long were coded and summary scores standardized to fit a 20 minute coding period.

Two coders were trained on the Global Parenting Observational Scale. Coders were educated on the different parenting dimensions included in the scale. Education included coding of ten training tapes in a group setting so that coders could learn to differentiate between the different dimensions. Coders then individually coded "gold-standard" training tapes until they reached at least 70% reliability on these tapes. When they reached this goal, they began coding study tapes. Coders met weekly with the trainer and coded 2 training tapes together to prevent observer drift. All tapes were reviewed by both coders and reliability checked. Inter-rater reliability was determined by performing intraclass correlations between the summary scores for each of the 10 parenting dimensions. Intraclass correlations for each dimension were: warmth/affection = 0.87, support/sensitivity = 0.89, negative affect = 0.91, detachment = 0.81, firm discipline/structure = 0.87, demands for maturity = 0.91, psychological control = 0.95, physical control = 0.96, permissiveness = 0.85, and neglect = 0.74. Coders reached consensus on any discrepant scores and these scores were used for analysis.

4.2.4 Mealtime Family Interaction Coding System (MICS)

The MICS is an observational coding system based on the McMaster Model of Family Functioning [53,54] and was adapted from the McMaster Structured Interview of Family Functioning. The MICS demonstrates moderate to high correlation with other measures of parent and family functioning [55] and codes six dimensions of family functioning: Task accomplishment, Communication, Affect management, Interpersonal involvement, Behavioral control, and Roles. Overall Family Functioning is the seventh and final dimension that is rated and is not an average of the other six dimensions. Instead, it provides an overall assessment of the quality of the family's interactions and functioning at the meal. Given the similarity of some of these dimensions with the GPOS parenting dimensions of warmth/affection, support/sensitivity, firm discipline/structure, and demands for maturity, we compared constructs between both measures.

Affect management and *interpersonal involvement* assess the emotional aspects of the family meal. *Affect management* addresses the appropriateness and intensity of the emotions expressed at the meal as well as the responsiveness and sensitivity of these emotional responses towards other family members. *Interpersonal involvement* captures the degree to which family members show respect, interest, and value in each other's activities and thoughts (similar to support and sensitivity in the GPOS). *Behavior control* assesses the way in which the family maintains rules around physical expectations at the table and social behaviors. It categorizes the behaviors as chaotic, laissez-faire, rigid, and flexible, and is similar in part to the parenting styles of permissive, authoritarian, and authoritative. Families who shift between different control styles and use more chaotic, rigid, or laissez-faire methods score lower in this domain. *Task accomplishment* also assesses the structure and organization of the meal and reflects on the parent's ability to have control over the meal. Families who display smooth transitions between tasks and can adequately handle disruptions score higher in this domain. *Communication* rates the verbal interaction of the family, particularly the rate of exchange of information, the quality of the communication, and the appropriateness between different age groups. Finally, *roles* reflect on the patterns of behavior of each family member and whether or not they are able to fulfill expected tasks. Each dimension is rated on a Likert scale from 1 to 7, with scores of 5 or greater being considered categorically different (healthy) from those with scores less than 5 (unhealthy).

Coding for the MICS was performed by independent trained coders who were blind to study hypotheses.

4.2.5 Child Measures

Child's Report of Parental Behavior Inventory (CRPBI) [56] asks children to assess their parent's parenting behaviors [57], and can be completed by children aged eight years and older [58]. It has been used in pediatric weight control studies [59], as well as adapted to assess parent involvement and strictness in relation to dietary [20,21] and smoking behavior [60]. The inventory assesses three dimensions of parenting: acceptance vs. rejection, psychological control vs. autonomy, and firm vs. lax control. The 30 item version (CRPBI-30 [61]), which is a shortened version of the 108-item scale [62], was used in this study and includes the top ten items with the highest correlation within each dimension. Children rated each item on a 3-point Likert scale ranging from "like", "somewhat like", or "not like" their parent's behavior. Children completed this measure for their mother and father's parenting behaviors separately. Factor analysis demonstrated that each of the items loaded significantly on a single principle axis with 96%, 94%, and 87% of the variance respectively. The alpha values for Acceptance, Psychological control, and Firm control have been previously reported as 0.75-0.73, 0.72-0.63, and 0.65-0.63 respectively [61]. The test-retest correlations ranged from 0.79-0.89. This inventory has been reported to have strong discriminative validity [63].

"Getting Along with My Parent" [64] is a 38-item questionnaire (19 items relating to the mother and 19 items for the father) that assesses the child's ratings of the caregiver's behaviors. The items map onto 2 dimensions, warmth/support and hostility. Examples of the warmth/support items include: "When you and your mother spend time talking or doing things together, how often does your mother: let you know she really cares about you; listens carefully to your point of view; acts supportive and understanding towards you; helps you do something that is important to you?" Examples of the hostility items include: "When you and your mother spend time talking or doing things together, how often does your mother: get angry at you; criticize your ideas; shout or yell because she is mad at you; insult or swear at you?" Four-point scales were used to assess parent behaviors from "a lot" to "not at all". The items have been previously reported to have an internal consistency of 0.78 for the warmth scale and 0.79 for the hostility scale [65].

4.2.6 Parent Measures

Parent Report of Parental Behavior Inventory (PRPBI) is a 30-item measure that parallels the CRPBI-30 and was used to assess parent's views of their own parenting behaviors towards the index child. This measure assesses the same three dimensions of parenting as the CRPBI, has the same scoring system, and has been used successfully in previous studies [66,67].

Raising Children Checklist (RCC) [68] is a simplified revision of Greenberger's Raising Children Checklist [69], a standardized measure of parenting strategies that was based on Baumrind's concepts of responsiveness and disciplinary control. This measure has been used in NICHD's Study of Early Child Care and Youth Development [70] and was chosen for its brevity and apparent face validity with Baumrind's dimensions of parenting. Three dimensions of parenting are obtained with this survey—firm (authoritative), harsh (authoritarian), and lax (permissive) parenting. These dimensions have been found to differentiate children based on school adjustment, academic achievement, and behavioral problems [69]. Cronbach's alpha for each of these dimensions were reported as 0.67, 0.75, and 0.73 respectively.

4.2.6.1 Anthropometrics

Child height and weight were obtained to determine BMI percentile and BMI z-scores. Weight was measured in kilograms to the nearest 0.1 kg on a Tanita Digital Scale (model WB-110A). Weight was measured twice and the average of the values was used for analysis. Height was measured using a portable Tanita stadiometer. Height was recorded to the nearest 0.1 cm for both trials, and the average of the 2 values used for analysis. Body mass index (BMI = [kg/m^2]) was calculated and translated to BMI percentiles for age and sex using the CDC growth charts [71] and to standardized BMI z-scores (BMI-Z) [72].

Several sociodemographic variables were included in this study: parent and child age and gender, parent race/ethnicity, marital status and educational level. In this sample, the primary racial/ethnic groups were Caucasian, Hispanic, and other. Maternal education was dichotomized into "some college or less" and "college degree or higher". Marital status was dichotomized into "married or living with significant other" and "widowed, divorced, separated or never married".

4.2.6.2 Analysis

Descriptive statistics and correlations were completed using SAS, version 9.3. Distributions of the GPOS dimensions were not normally distributed for all dimensions except warmth/affection and support/sensitivity. As a result, medians and interquartile ranges were presented. Spearman's correlations were used to determine correlations between the GPOS parenting dimensions and the MICS family functioning dimensions, child reports of parenting behaviors, and parent reports of parenting behaviors. Correlations between parenting dimensions and parent demographics were also explored. Alpha level of 0.05 was used to determine significance.

4.3 RESULTS

The sample included 44 parent–child dyads. Mean child age was 10.0 years and two-thirds were female. Mean child BMI percentile was 98.2. The majority of parents were mothers with a mean age of 41.4 years. Most children lived in two parent households and about half of parents had a college degree or higher (Table 2). There were no significant differences in demographic characteristics between those families recruited in Rhode Island and California.

TABLE 4.2 Child and parent demographics

Variable	Percent or Means (S.D.) (n = 44)
Child characteristics	
Sex	
Male	34%
Female	66%
Age (years)	10.0 (1.3)
BMI percentile	98.2 (1.3)
BMI z-score	2.2 (0.3)
Parent characteristics	
Sex	
Male	5%
Female	95%
Race/ethnicity	
White	52%
Hispanic	36%
Other	11%
Education	
No degree	47%
Bachelor's degree or higher	53%
Marital status	
Married/living with significant other	77%
Widowed/divorced/Separated/never married	23%
Age (years)	41.4 (6.9)
BMI (kg/m^2)	30.1 (5.8)

S.D. = Standard deviation.

Scores for the observed parenting dimensions ranged between 10 and 34 (Table 3). Only five dimensions had a wide range of scores: warmth/affection, support/sensitivity, negative affect, detachment, and firm discipline/structure. Of these dimensions, the most commonly observed behaviors were warmth/affection, support/sensitivity, and firm discipline/structure. All other parenting dimensions were not commonly observed during the videotaped family meals.

TABLE 4.3 Range of observed parenting dimensions in the General Parenting Observational Scale

	Mean (S.D.)	Median (IQR)	Range
Emotional Dimensions			
Warmth and Affection	23.70 (6.49)	24.0 (9.5)	10-34
Support and Sensitivity	23.37 (5.28)	24.44 (6.43)	10-33
Negative Affect	10.99 (3.18)	10.0 (1.0)	10-30
Detachment	10.99 (3.42)	10.0 (0)	10-30
Behavioral Dimensions			
Firm discipline/structure	12.95 (3.64)	12.0 (4.44)	10-29
Demands for maturity	10.52 (0.73)	10.0 (1.0)	10-13
Psychological control	10.09 (0.59)	10.0 (0)	10-14
Physical Control	10.05 (0.34)	10.0 (0)	10-12
Permissive	10.38 (1.14)	10.0 (0)	10-16
Neglect	10.13 (0.63)	10.0 (0)	10-14

Tapes were coded for 20 minutes. Tapes were divided into 10 two-minute intervals and coded for all 10 parenting dimensions. Summary scores for each dimension ranged from 10–50.

S.D. = Standard deviation.

IQR = Inter-Quartile Range.

Several parenting dimensions were highly correlated with the family functioning dimensions of the MICS (Table 4). Families who scored highly in warmth/affection (GPOS) scored highly in affect management, interpersonal involvement, and communication (MICS) ($r = 0.39$, 0.56, and 0.44, respectively). Support/sensitivity (GPOS) was also highly correlated with affect management, interpersonal involvement, and communication (MICS) ($r = 0.38$, 0.55, and 0.45, respectively). High scores in negative affect (GPOS) were inversely correlated with affect management, interpersonal involvement, communication, behavior control and overall family functioning (MICS). In the behavioral dimensions, there was an inverse relationship between firm discipline/structure (GPOS) and the family functioning dimensions of affect management, behavior control, task accomplishment, and roles. Higher permissive scores in the GPOS were also negatively correlated with these dimensions.

When comparing observed parenting dimensions with self-report measures of parenting by children, there were fewer significant correlations. Only child report of warmth ("Getting along with my parent" survey) was inversely correlated with detachment ($r = -0.41$, $p < 0.01$). Parent reports of psychological

TABLE 4.4 Correlation between General Parenting Observational Scale and other measures of parenting and family functioning

	Warmth/ Affection	Support/ Sensitivity	Negative Affect	Detach-ment	Firm Discipline/ Structure	Maturity Demands	Psycholo-gical Control	Physical Control	Permis-siveness	Neglect
MICS:										
Task Accomplishment	0.19	0.15	−0.20	−0.09	−0.31	−0.07	−0.28	−0.28	−0.36	−0.15
	0.23	0.34	0.20	0.59	0.04	0.66	0.06	0.06	0.04	0.32
Communication	0.44	0.45	−0.40	−0.13	−0.23	0.16	−0.27	−0.27	−0.20	−0.31
	<0.01	<0.01	<0.01	0.39	0.13	0.31	0.08	0.08	0.19	0.05
Affect Management	0.39	0.38	−0.44	−0.31	−0.32	0.04	−0.28	−0.28	−0.41	−0.39
	0.01	0.01	<0.01	0.04	<0.03	0.81	0.07	0.07	<0.01	0.01
Interpersonal Involvement	0.56	0.55	−0.42	−0.14	−0.25	0.03	−0.27	−0.27	−0.38	−0.30
	<0.001	<0.001	<0.01	0.36	0.11	0.84	0.08	0.08	0.01	0.05
Behavior Control	0.31	0.27	−0.30	−0.24	−0.35	0.07	−0.29	−0.29	−0.47	−0.38
	0.05	0.08	0.05	0.12	0.02	0.64	0.07	0.07	0.001	0.01
Roles	0.50	0.56	−0.37	−0.32	−0.24	0.15	−0.29	−0.29	−0.37	−0.22
	<0.001	<0.001	0.01	.04	0.12	0.34	0.06	0.06	0.01	0.17
Family Functioning	0.48	0.51	−0.40	−0.26	−0.34	−0.03	−0.27	−0.27	−0.38	−0.30
	<0.01	<0.001	<0.01	0.09	0.02	0.85	0.08	0.08	0.01	0.05
Getting along with my parent:										
Warmth	−0.25	−0.29	−0.06	−0.41	−0.12	−0.19	−0.21	−0.21	0.09	−0.05
	0.12	0.06	0.70	<0.01	0.46	0.24	0.18	0.18	0.58	0.75
Hostility	0.05	0.11	−0.19	−0.26	0.00	0.06	0.01	0.01	−0.002	−0.18
	0.75	0.49	0.22	0.10	0.99	0.70	0.93	0.93	0.99	0.27
CRPBI:										
Acceptance	0.19	0.05	−0.22	0.13	−0.14	0.08	−0.19	−0.19	−0.23	−0.25
	0.24	0.77	0.17	0.41	0.39	0.61	0.24	0.24	0.14	0.12

TABLE 4.4 *(Continued)*

	Warmth/ Affection	Support/ Sensitivity	Negative Affect	Detachment	Firm Discipline/ Structure	Maturity Demands	Psychological Control	Physical Control	Permissiveness	Neglect
Psychological Control	−0.15	0.06	−0.11	−0.15	−0.01	−0.22	−0.24	−0.24	−0.04	−0.30
	0.35	0.73	0.50	0.37	0.94	0.16	0.13	0.13	0.79	0.06
Firm Control	−0.08	−0.00	0.08	−0.09	0.12	−0.14	0.04	0.04	−0.05	0.17
	0.62	0.99	0.61	0.57	0.44	0.38	0.83	0.83	0.77	0.30
PRPBI:										
Acceptance	−0.18	−0.21	0.04	−0.01	0.06	−0.06	−0.20	−0.20	0.06	−0.11
	0.26	0.18	0.80	0.96	0.70	0.73	0.21	0.21	0.71	0.49
Psychological Control	−0.45	−0.38	0.25	0.28	0.32	0.00	0.27	0.27	0.36	0.16
	<0.01	0.01	0.11	0.08	0.04	0.98	0.09	0.09	0.02	0.31
Firm Control	−0.52	−0.48	0.19	0.25	0.25	−0.18	0.07	0.07	0.34	0.10
	<0.001	0.001	0.22	0.11	0.11	0.27	0.65	0.65	0.03	0.52
Raising Children Checklist										
Harsh	−0.30	−0.22	0.02	−0.11	0.05	−0.20	−0.04	−0.04	−0.05	−0.20
	0.05	0.16	0.88	0.49	0.73	0.21	0.81	0.81	0.77	0.20
Firm	0.05	0.09	−0.27	−0.15	−0.30	−0.09	−0.24	−0.24	−0.29	−0.29
	0.75	0.56	0.09	0.33	0.05	0.56	0.13	0.13	0.07	0.06
Lax	0.11	0.11	0.08	0.27	0.36	0.29	0.01	0.01	0.27	0.18
	0.48	0.48	0.60	0.09	0.02	0.07	0.94	0.94	0.08	0.25

Spearman's correlation was used to examine the correlation between the 10 dimensions of the GPOS and the MICS and several other child- or self-report measures of parenting. "Getting along with my parent" and the CRPBI are child reports of parenting. The PRPBI and Raising Children Checklist ask parents to report on their parenting. Correlation coefficients (r) and p-values are presented.
MICS = Mealtime Family Interaction Coding System.
CRPBI = Child's Report of Parental Behavior Inventory.
PRPBI = Parent Report of Parental Behavior Inventory.

control and firm control (PRPBI) and harsh parenting (Raising Children Checklist) were inversely correlated with observed measures of warmth/affection and support/sensitivity (GPOS). Interestingly, parents self-reporting higher firm (authoritative) parenting (Raising Children Checklist) were viewed as using less firm discipline on the GPOS ($r = -0.30$). However self-report of lax behaviors was positively correlated with firm discipline on the GPOS ($r = 0.36$). Similarly, psychological control and firm control (PRPBI) were both positively correlated with permissive behaviors on the GPOS.

Parent demographics were correlated with certain parenting dimensions. Parents with higher BMIs had lower warmth/affection ($r = -0.38$, $p = 0.02$) and support/sensitivity scores ($r = -0.32$, $p = 0.05$). Older parents had higher warmth/affection ($r = 0.33$, $p = 0.04$) and support/sensitivity scores ($r = 0.42$, $p = 0.01$). Parents with higher education also had higher warmth/affection scores ($r = 0.33$, $p = 0.04$).

4.4 DISCUSSION

The goal of this study was to develop a General Parenting Observational Scale that could be used to assess general parenting dimensions in the context of family meals, and compare these dimensions to those captured in other observational and self-report measures of parenting and family functioning. Parenting dimensions were based on the four classic parenting styles [27,30] and more recent dimensions of interest, i.e., psychological control and structure. The most robust dimensions in the GPOS were warmth/affection, support/sensitivity, and firm discipline/structure. The emotional dimensions of warmth/affection and support/sensitivity were positively associated with the family functioning dimensions assessing interpersonal involvement, affect management, and communication. Thus parents displaying high warmth, affection, and support for their child on the GPOS were also viewed as having good communication, effective and appropriate emotional displays, and being involved with or expressing empathy and concern for their child. Warmth/affection and support/sensitivity were also inversely correlated with parent self-report measures of harsher parenting behaviors. Thus it appears that the emotional dimensions of parenting were captured well in the GPOS.

With regards to the behavioral dimensions, firm discipline/structure in the GPOS was inversely correlated with affect management as well as behavior control and task accomplishment in the MICS. While on the surface this may seem contradictory and questions the validity of this GPOS parenting dimension, these results may actually complement each other and provide us with a more complete picture of what is happening during the family meal. Parents who have to frequently make comments to remind children of the rules and provide a structure for their children so that they comply with these rules (coded as high discipline and structure on the GPOS) may appear to have low behavioral control of the situation on the MICS because of this constant reminding. Furthermore, they may have had to shift between several types of control styles to maintain this order (e.g., chaotic or laissez-faire as defined by the MICS), thus causing them to score low on the MICS. In a similar vein, the frequent reminders about rules may have caused parents to appear as if they were unable to maintain an organized meal with minimal disruptions, resulting in low scores for task accomplishment. The complexity of these family interactions may also explain the results for the GPOS dimension of permissiveness. Parents who were permissive on the GPOS could have had poor behavioral control of the mealtime situation and be unsuccessful at completing the task of eating a meal with minimal disruptions. Thus parents who were permissive would have been categorized as having poor family functioning on the MICS, as was seen in this analysis. These results suggest that the parenting dimensions in the GPOS are related to the concepts captured by the MICS, but not completely overlapping. Overall, the GPOS focuses more on parent behaviors while the MICS takes the whole family and the child's response to parent behaviors into account. As a result, the GPOS views the behavioral aspect of parenting from another angle, which may potentially complement the results of the MICS. A previous study noted no significant relationship between task accomplishment, behavior control and child BMI z-score [46]. Whether or not the dimensions of firm discipline/structure and permissiveness from the GPOS are related to child BMI remains to be seen. This type of analysis could highlight whether or not the behavioral aspects of parenting captured by the GPOS are providing us with additional information that is not captured in the MICS, thereby providing us with a more complete picture of the parenting and family dynamics during mealtimes.

It is interesting to note that the self-report measures were not as well correlated with the observed parenting behaviors of the GPOS. It was not surprising to see that parents who were viewed as warm/affectionate as well as supportive/sensitive to their child's needs self-report that they did not engage in psychologically controlling or harsh parenting behaviors. However, observed behaviors of firm discipline, behavioral control, and structure on the GPOS were not self-reported as such. Instead, these parents self-reported more lax parenting behaviors (as measured by the Raising Children's Checklist). In addition, observed permissive parenting behaviors were self-reported by parents as being more psychologically controlling and firm (PRPBI). When children reported on their parent's behaviors, only detachment was inversely correlated with parent displays of warmth. There was no correlation between the behavioral dimensions of parenting as assessed by the GPOS or self-report measures. Thus, overall it appears that the emotional dimensions of parenting may be more accurately reported while behavioral dimensions may be subject to personal biases or social desirability. While a few studies have found poor correlations between parent and child reports of parenting behaviors [66,73], we are unaware of any study to date that has compared direct observation of parenting behaviors with parent or child self-report measures of parenting. The results of our study highlight the potential difficulty in using self-report measures of parenting, and suggest that the emotional dimensions of parenting may be more accurately captured in these self-report measures than the behavioral dimensions of parenting.

In our analyses, we also found that parents with higher education, lower BMI scores, and older age scored higher on warmth/affection and support/sensitivity. A few studies using self-report measures of parenting have found that authoritative parenting is associated with higher parental SES [17], and parents with higher levels of education were less likely to use controlling behaviors like coercion or overprotection [34]. Studies have reported that both demographic factors (like higher income and educational attainment [74]) and authoritative or supportive parenting [4] are associated with lower risk for obesity. Whether parenting mediates the relationship between demographic factors and child weight status has not been investigated. Given the correlation between certain parenting behaviors and SES/educational level, this relationship should be clarified and may provide further evidence for targeting general parenting in future interventions.

While several of the dimensions captured in the General Parenting Observational Scale appear to be robust, there were a few limitations. First, the sample was relatively small and only conducted on overweight children and their parents, who were also primarily overweight. Many children also came from two parent families, where general parenting behaviors may be different than in single parent families. Validity of this measure should be tested in larger samples that include a broader range of marital statuses, weight categories, racial/ethnic and cultural groups, and educational backgrounds. Our ability to only record one family meal per subject may have also limited the generalizability of our findings. However other groups have reported that one video recording may be sufficient [49-51], and meals were re-recorded if the parent indicated that the interactions or the meal itself was not typical. Finally, several dimensions were relatively unobserved in this mealtime setting (psychological control, physical control, permissiveness, neglect), and it begs the question as to whether a different parent–child interaction setting should be used to assess a broader range of these general parenting behaviors. Other observational systems, like the Home Observation for Measurement of the Environment (HOME) [37] and Dyadic Parent Child Interaction Coding Scheme (DPICS) [38], have typically been used in play situations. But as children grow older and we assess parenting behaviors at this later time, play situations may not be developmentally appropriate. Given that we are interested in using this scale to determine the relationship between general parenting and childhood obesity and other weight-related behaviors, the mealtime interaction seems to be an appropriate setting. However, we did not videotape and code other eating or activity related situations, like snack time, and the interactions found here may only be relevant to the meal time situation. Examination of this tools' efficacy in other settings should be explored.

4.5 CONCLUSION

There is growing interest in the role of general parenting behaviors in the development and potential treatment of childhood obesity. At this time several studies report that authoritative or supportive parenting behaviors are associated with lower risk of obesity [4,5] and improved eating behaviors [20,21]. However, there are still discrepancies reported in these relationships [6,19] and the use of self-report measures of parenting may be contributing to this discrepancy. While there is a role for self-report measures of parenting, particularly when a child reports on his/her parent's behaviors and this is correlated with his/her developmental outcomes, these measures may still be limited by difficulties with understanding the selected concepts or recall bias. Many people also find it difficult to recognize how their own behaviors impact and are viewed by others. Therefore, an observational tool may provide a more objective or standardized means of measuring parenting. Since there are few observational assessments of general parenting, we developed the General Parenting Observational Scale to assess parent behaviors in a mealtime situation. It appears that the primary dimensions of warmth/affection, support/sensitivity, and firm discipline/structure were robustly captured in this tool. Continued use of this tool among families with a wider age range of child weights and demographic variability will help to determine the versatility of this tool. While observational methods may be more labor and time-intensive, it offers another standardized and possibly more objective means of assessing general parenting. This may result in more homogeneity in research results, allowing one to determine the true relationship between general parenting and obesity-related behaviors.

REFERENCES

1. Sleddens EF, Gerards SM, Thijs C, de Vries NK, Kremers SP. General parenting, childhood overweight and obesity-inducing behaviors: a review. Int J Pediatr Obes. 2011;6(2–2):e12–27.
2. Faith MS, Van Horn L, Appel LJ, Burke LE, Carson JA, Franch HA, et al. Evaluating parents and adult caregivers as "agents of change" for treating obese children: evidence for parent behavior change strategies and research gaps: a scientific statement from the American Heart Association. Circulation. 2012;125(9):1186–207.
3. Pritchett R, Kemp J, Wilson P, Minnis H, Bryce G, Gillberg C. Quick, simple measures of family relationships for use in clinical practice and research. A systematic review Fam Pract. 2011;28(2):172–87.
4. Rhee KE, Lumeng JC, Appugliese DP, Kaciroti N, Bradley RH. Parenting styles and overweight status in first grade. Pediatrics. 2006;117(6):2047–54.
5. Wake M, Nicholson JM, Hardy P, Smith K. Preschooler obesity and parenting styles of mothers and fathers: Australian national population study. Pediatrics. 2007;120(6):e1520–7.
6. Agras WS, Hammer LD, McNicholas F, Kraemer HC. Risk factors for childhood overweight: a prospective study from birth to 9.5 years. J Pediatr. 2004;145(1):20–5.
7. Chen JL, Kennedy C. Factors associated with obesity in Chinese-American children. Pediatr Nurs. 2005;31(2):110–5.
8. Baranowski T, O'Connor T, Hughes S, Sleddens E, Beltran A, Frankel L, et al. Houston... We have a problem! Measurement of parenting. Child Obes. 2013;9(Suppl):S1–4.
9. Kremers S, Sleddens E, Gerards S, Gubbels J, Rodenburg G, Gevers D, et al. General and food-specific parenting: measures and interplay. Child Obes. 2013;9(Suppl):S22–31.
10. Darling N, Steinberg L. Parenting Style as Context: An Integrative Model. Psychol Bull. 1993;113(3):487–96.
11. van der Horst K, Kremers S, Ferreira I, Singh A, Oenema A, Brug J. Perceived parenting style and practices and the consumption of sugar-sweetened beverages by adolescents. Health Educ Res. 2007;22(2):295–304.
12. Hennessy E, Hughes SO, Goldberg JP, Hyatt RR, Economos CD. Parent behavior and child weight status among a diverse group of underserved rural families. Appetite. 2010;54(2):369–77.
13. Musher-Eizenman DR, Holub SC. Children's eating in the absence of hunger: the role of restrictive feeding practices. In: Flamenbaum R, editor. Childhood obesity and health research. Hauppauge, NY, USA: Nova Science Publishers; 2006. p. 135–56.
14. Hughes SO, Power TG, Orlet FJ, Mueller S, Nicklas TA. Revisiting a neglected construct: parenting styles in a child-feeding context. Appetite. 2005;44(1):83–92.

15. Hughes SO, Shewchuk RM, Baskin ML, Nicklas TA, Qu H. Indulgent feeding style and children's weight status in preschool. J Dev Behav Pediatr. 2008;29(5):403–10.
16. Tovar A, Hennessy E, Pirie A, Must A, Gute DM, Hyatt RR, et al. Feeding styles and child weight status among recent immigrant mother-child dyads. Int J Behav Nutr Phys Act. 2012;9:62.
17. Berge JM, Wall M, Bauer KW, Neumark-Sztainer D. Parenting characteristics in the home environment and adolescent overweight: a latent class analysis. Obesity (Silver Spring). 2010;18(4):818–25.
18. Vereecken C, Legiest E, De Bourdeaudhuij I, Maes L. Associations between general parenting styles and specific food-related parenting practices and children's food consumption. Am J Health Promot. 2009;23(4):233–40.
19. De Bourdeaudhuij I, Te Velde SJ, Maes L, Perez-Rodrigo C, de Almeida MD, Brug J. General parenting styles are not strongly associated with fruit and vegetable intake and social-environmental correlates among 11-year-old children in four countries in Europe. Public Health Nutr. 2009;12(2):259–66.
20. Kremers SP, Brug J, de Vries H, Engels RC. Parenting style and adolescent fruit consumption. Appetite. 2003;41(1):43–50.
21. Pearson N, Atkin AJ, Biddle SJ, Gorely T, Edwardson C. Parenting styles, family structure and adolescent dietary behaviour. Public Health Nutr. 2010;13(8):1245–53.
22. Brotman LM, Dawson-McClure S, Huang KY, Theise R, Kamboukos D, Wang J, et al. Early childhood family intervention and long-term obesity prevention among high-risk minority youth. Pediatrics. 2012;129(3):e621–8.
23. Power TG, Sleddens EF, Berge J, Connell L, Govig B, Hennessy E, et al. Contemporary research on parenting: conceptual, methodological, and translational issues. Child Obes. 2013;9(Suppl):S87–94.
24. Taylor A, Wilson C, Slater A, Mohr P. Parent- and child-reported parenting. Associations with child weight-related outcomes Appetite. 2011;57(3):700–6.
25. Haines J, Neumark-Sztainer D, Hannan P, Robinson-O'Brien R. Child versus parent report of parental influences on children's weight-related attitudes and behaviors. J Pediatr Psychol. 2008;33(7):783–8.
26. Masse LC, Watts AW. Stimulating innovations in the measurement of parenting constructs. Child Obes. 2013;9(Suppl):S5–13.
27. Baumrind D. Child care practices anteceding three patterns of preschool behavior. Genet Psychol Monogr. 1967;75(1):43–88.
28. Becker WC, Peterson DR, Luria Z, Shoemaker DJ, Hellmer LA. Relations of factors derived from parent-interview ratings to behavior problems of five-year-olds. Child Dev. 1962;33:509–35.
29. Shaefer ES. A circumplex model for maternal behavior. J Abnormal Soc Psychol. 1959;59: 226–35.
30. Maccoby E, Martin J. Socialization in the Context of the Family: Parent–child Interaction. In: Hetherington E, editor. Handbook of Child Psychology: Socialization, Personality and Social Development. New York: Wiley; 1983. p. 1–101.
31. Barber BK. Parental psychological control: revisiting a neglected construct. Child Dev. 1996;67(6):3296–319.

32. Slater MA, Power TG. Multidimensional assessment of parenting in single-parent families. In: Vincent JP, editor. Advances in Family Intervention, Assessment and Theory. Greenwich, CT, USA: JAI Press; 1987. p. 197–228.
33. Carr A, Pike A. Maternal scaffolding behavior: links with parenting style and maternal education. Dev Psychol. 2012;48(2):543–51.
34. Sleddens EF, O'Connor TM, Watson KB, Hughes SO, Power TG, Thijs C, et al. Development of the Comprehensive General Parenting Questionnaire for caregivers of 5–13 year olds. Int J Behav Nutr Phys Act. 2014;11:15.
35. Otten R, Harakeh Z, Vermulst AA, Van den Eijnden RJ, Engels RC. Frequency and quality of parental communication as antecedents of adolescent smoking cognitions and smoking onset. Psychol Addict Behav. 2007;21(1):1–12.
36. Rodenburg G, Kremers SP, Oenema A, van de Mheen D. Psychological control by parents is associated with a higher child weight. Int J Pediatr Obes. 2011;6(5–6):442–9.
37. Caldwell BM, Bradley RH. Home Observation for Measurement of the Environment (HOME) - Revised Edition. Little Rock, Arkansas: University of Arkansas; 1984.
38. Eyberg S.M., Bessmer J., Newcomb K., Edwards D., and Robinson E.A. Dyadic Parent–child Interaction Coding Scheme II:A manual. April, 2009 [http://pcit.phhp.ufl.edu/measures/dpics%20%283rd%20edition%29%20manual%20version%203.07.pdf]
39. Drucker RR, Hammer LD, Agras WS, Bryson S. Can mothers influence their child's eating behavior? J Dev Behav Pediatr. 1999;20(2):88–92.
40. Klesges RC, Coates TJ, Brown G, Sturgeon-Tillisch J, Moldenhauer-Klesges LM, Holzer B, et al. Parental influences on children's eating behavior and relative weight. J Appl Behav Anal. 1983;16(4):371–8.
41. Koivisto UK, Fellenius J, Sjoden PO. Relations between parental mealtime practices and children's food intake. Appetite. 1994;22(3):245–57.
42. McKenzie TL, Sallis JF, Nader PR, Patterson TL, Elder JP, Berry CC, et al. BEACHES: an observational system for assessing children's eating and physical activity behaviors and associated events. J Appl Behav Anal. 1991;24(1):141–51.
43. Orrell-Valente JK, Hill LG, Brechwald WA, Dodge KA, Pettit GS, Bates JE. "Just three more bites": an observational analysis of parents' socialization of children's eating at mealtime. Appetite. 2007;48(1):37–45.
44. Hughes SO, Patrick H, Power TG, Fisher JO, Anderson CB, Nicklas TA. The impact of child care providers' feeding on children's food consumption. J Dev Behav Pediatr. 2007;28(2):100–7.
45. Moens E, Braet C, Soetens B. Observation of family functioning at mealtime: a comparison between families of children with and without overweight. J Pediatr Psychol. 2007;32(1):52–63.
46. Berge JM, Jin SW, Hannan P, Neumark-Sztainer D. Structural and interpersonal characteristics of family meals: associations with adolescent body mass index and dietary patterns. J Acad Nutr Diet. 2013;113(6):816–22.
47. Epstein LH, Valoski A, Koeske R, Wing RR. Family-based behavioral weight control in obese young children. J Am Diet Assoc. 1986;86(4):481–4.
48. Epstein LH, Wing RR. Behavioral treatment of childhood obesity. Psychol Bull. 1987;101(3):331–42.

49. Stark LJ, Jelalian E, Powers SW, Mulvihill MM, Opipari LC, Bowen A, et al. Parent and child mealtime behavior in families of children with cystic fibrosis. J Pediatr. 2000;136(2):195–200.
50. Powers SW, Patton SR, Byars KC, Mitchell MJ, Jelalian E, Mulvihill MM, et al. Caloric intake and eating behavior in infants and toddlers with cystic fibrosis. Pediatrics. 2002;109(5):E75–5.
51. Stark LJ, Jelalian E, Mulvihill MM, Powers SW, Bowen AM, Spieth LE, et al. Eating in preschool children with cystic fibrosis and healthy peers: behavioral analysis. Pediatrics. 1995;95(2):210–5.
52. Belsky J, Crnic K, Woodworth S. Personality and parenting: exploring the mediating role of transient mood and daily hassles. J Pers. 1995;63(4):905–29.
53. Epstein NB, Bishop DS, Levin S. The McMaster Model of family functioning. Journal of Marriage and Family Counseling. 1978;4:19–31.
54. Dickstein S, Hayden L, Schiller M, Seifer R, San Antonio W. Providence Family Study. Family Mealtime Interaction coding system. Unpublished coding manual. Brown University School of Medicine. Providence, RI, USA: Bradley Hospital; 1994.
55. Hayden L, Schiller M, Dickstein S, Seifer R, Sameroff A, Miller I, et al. Levels of family assessment I: Family, marital and parent–child interaction. J Fam Psychol. 1998;12:7–22.
56. Schaefer E. Children's reports of parental behavior: an inventory. Child Dev. 1965;36:413–24.
57. Armentrout J, Burger G. Children's reports of parental child-rearing behavior at five grade levels. Dev Psychol. 1972;7:44–8.
58. Mann BJ, Sanders S. Child dissociation and the family context. J Abnorm Child Psychol. 1994;22(3):373–88.
59. Stein RI, Epstein LH, Raynor HA, Kilanowski CK, Paluch RA. The influence of parenting change on pediatric weight control. Obes Res. 2005;13(10):1749–55.
60. den Exter Blokland EA, Hale 3rd WW, Meeus W, Engels RC. Parental support and control and early adolescent smoking: a longitudinal study. Subst Use Misuse. 2007;42(14):2223–32.
61. Schludermann S, Schludermann E. Questionnaire for Children and Youth (CRPBI-30). Winnipeg: University of Manitoba; 1988.
62. Schludermann E, Schludermann S. Replicability of factors in Children's Report of Parent Behavior (CRPBI). J Psychol. 1970;76:239–49.
63. Locke LM, Prinz RJ. Measurement of parental discipline and nurturance. Clin Psychol Rev. 2002;22(6):895–929.
64. Conger RD, Ge X. Conflict and cohesion in parent-adolescent relations: Changes in emotional expression from early to mid-adolescence. In: Cox M, Brooks-Gunn J, editors. Conflict and cohesion in families: Causes and consequences. Mahwah, NJ: Erlbaum; 1999. p. 185–206.
65. Conger RD, Wallace LE, Sun Y, Simons RL, McLoyd VC, Brody GH. Economic pressure in African American families: a replication and extension of the family stress model. Dev Psychol. 2002;38(2):179–93.
66. Schwarz JC, Barton-Henry ML, Pruzinsky T. Assessing child-rearing behaviors: a comparison of ratings made by mother, father, child, and sibling on the CRPBI. Child Dev. 1985;56(2):462–79.
67. Tien JY, Roosa M, Michaels M. Agreement between parent and child reports of parental behaviors. J Marriage Fam. 1994;56(2):341–55.

68. Shumow L, Vendell D, Posner J. Harsh, firm, and permissive parenting in low-income families: Relations to children's academic achievement and behavioral adjustments. J Fam Issues. 1998;19:483–507.
69. Greenberger E, Goldberg W. Work, Parenting, and the Socialization of Children. Dev Psychol. 1989;25:22–35.
70. NICHD Study of Early Child Care and Youth Development https://www.nichd.nih.gov/research/supported/seccyd/Pages/overview.aspx#instruments
71. Ogden CL, Kuczmarski RJ, Flegal KM, Mei Z, Guo S, Wei R, et al. Centers for Disease Control and Prevention 2000 growth charts for the United States: improvements to the 1977 National Center for Health Statistics version. Pediatrics. 2002;109(1):45–60.
72. Kuczmarski RJ, Ogden CL, Grummer-Strawn LM, Flegal KM, Guo SS, Wei R, et al. CDC growth charts: United States. Adv Data. 2000;314:1–27.
73. Huver RM, Engels RC, Vermulst AA, de Vries H. Bi-directional relations between anti-smoking parenting practices and adolescent smoking in a Dutch sample. Health Psychol. 2007;26(6):762–8.
74. Ogden CL, Lamb MM, Carroll MD, Flegal KM. Obesity and socioeconomic status in children and adolescents: United States, 2005–2008. NCHS Data Brief. 2010;51:1–8.

CHAPTER 5

Mealtime Behavior Among Siblings and Body Mass Index of 4–8 Year Olds: A Videotaped Observational Study

Rana H. Mosli, Alison L. Miller, Niko Kaciroti, Karen E. Peterson, Katherine Rosenblum, Ana Baylin, and Julie C. Lumeng

5.1 INTRODUCTION

Childhood obesity continues to be a public health concern [1]. Family-based interventions have shown promise for childhood obesity prevention, though as with other obesity intervention strategies, effects tend to be modest [2]. Careful examination of interaction patterns between family members that may contribute to childhood obesity risk could provide novel targets for refining and strengthening the effectiveness of family-based interventions. The family mealtime is often used as a venue for studying family interaction patterns and has also been a key focus of childhood obesity prevention programs [3–5]. Most studies examining features of family mealtimes and childhood obesity have focused on mother-child interactions or the mealtime environment [5–11]. There is a lack of understanding of how siblings interact during mealtimes and how different interaction patterns relate to child body mass index (BMI).

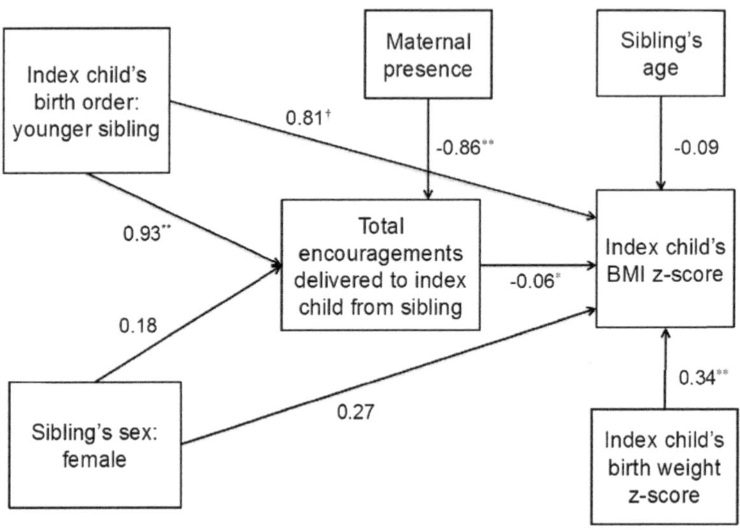

FIGURE 5.1 Path model showing path coefficients for associations between index child's birth order, sibling's sex, total encouragements delivered to index child from sibling, and index child's BMI z-score. * $p \leq 0.05$ ** $p \leq 0.01$ † $p \leq 0.1$

Interactions between siblings during childhood can influence development and behavior [12] through caregiving and role modeling interactions [12–14]. During mealtimes, sibling caregiving or role modeling behaviors may be observed as encouragements to eat. Although some studies found that mothers encourage their children to eat as a response to lower child BMI [15], others suggest that maternal encouragement to eat is a predictor of child weight status, such that encouragements to eat may override the child's ability to respond to internal satiety cues and lead to increased risk of obesity or obesity-promoting eating behaviors [10, 16, 17]. Mothers encouraging children to eat has been a frequent target for obesity prevention efforts. However, we have been unable to identify any published studies examining the potential role of siblings encouraging a child to eat in shaping children's eating behavior and obesity risk.

The child's birth order and sex of siblings shape the nature of interactions between the siblings [12]. Older siblings and sisters more often act as caregivers and role models for their siblings than do younger siblings and brothers and thus may be more likely to encourage their siblings to eat [12, 14, 18]. We and others have previously reported that children who are the youngest in a sibship are more likely to be obese [19–22] and that having a sister, compared with a brother, is associated with greater likelihood of being overweight [23, 24]. Prior work has not yet identified a mechanism for this association [19, 20, 24]. The objective of this study was therefore to test the hypothesis that encouragement to eat initiated by older siblings and sisters is an underlying process for the association of being a younger sibling and having a sister with higher BMI.

5.2 METHODS

5.2.1 Participants and Procedures

The study sample includes 301 child-mother dyads recruited through Head Start programs in South Central Michigan. Head Start is a federally funded preschool program for low-income, high-risk families in the United States (US). Participants were drawn from a longitudinal cohort initiated in 2009 to investigate associations between stress and eating among low-income children. Children described in this study were between the ages of 4 and 8 years at the time of data collection. Inclusion criteria were: caregiver is fluent in English and does not have a college degree; and child is not in foster care, has no serious medical problems or history of food allergies and was born at ≥ 35 weeks gestation without significant perinatal or neonatal complications. For this analysis we only included children who were living with their biological mothers (as this represents the majority of this sample), who were living with only one sibling, and who had complete data on all variables (n = 102). Of those 102 children, we only included index children whose siblings were at least a year old (n = 86) on the premise that the processes via which infants may influence eating behavior of siblings could be fundamentally different. Mothers provided written informed consent for themselves and for their children. The University of Michigan Institutional Review Board approved this study.

During two study visits, mothers completed questionnaires, and trained staff members obtained child anthropometry. Three videotaped home mealtime observations were completed for each family. Each mother was asked to record three routine evening meals within a single week. Research assistants called each mother after the meal to obtain information regarding individuals present. These family mealtime observations (FMOs) followed standard procedures that have been previously described [25].

For the present study, inclusion criteria for the FMO videotape included that the index child (IC) was eating with his/her sibling, and that the IC was not eating with other children in addition to the sibling. We systematically selected one of the three FMO videos for each IC. We started video selection with the second

FMO video on the premise that we would expect families to be more acclimated to the camera by the second home observation. If the second FMO video did not meet the inclusion criteria, we then assessed the third FMO video; if the third FMO video did not meet inclusion criteria, we assessed the first FMO video. After assessment of the FMO videos for each IC, a final sample of 75 index children was identified (8 from the first FMO, 55 from the second FMO, and 12 from the third FMO). The sample included in this analysis (n = 75) did not differ from the sample not included (n = 226) with regard to child sex, child race/ethnicity, birth weight z-score, and maternal age.

5.2.2 Measures

5.2.2.1 Demographic Characteristics

Mothers reported information regarding IC's birthdate, sex, and race/ethnicity (dichotomized for this report as non-Hispanic white vs. not) and mother's birthdate and years of education (dichotomized as more than or equal to a high school education vs. not). Birthdates and dates of visits were used to calculate child and maternal age.

5.2.3 Sibling Characteristics and Birth Order

For each individual living in the household, as well as for each individual on the FMO videotapes, mothers reported age, sex, and relationship to the IC. This information was used to determine the IC's birth order (i.e., younger sibling vs. older sibling) and characteristics of the siblings.

5.2.4 Coding of Interactions between Index Child and Sibling

To evaluate mealtime sibling behaviors that may be most relevant to child obesity risk, we developed a coding scheme based on Bob and Tom's Method of Assessing Nutrition (BATMAN) [10]. The BATMAN is an observational assessment used to evaluate parental behavior around food [10]. Although restrictive feeding behaviors are part of the BATMAN, we did not code these behaviors as they were not observed to occur between siblings with meaningful frequency. Although the BATMAN distinguishes between physical and verbal encouragements to eat, we did not observe frequent physical encouragements to eat between siblings and therefore focused our coding scheme on verbal encouragements to eat. The BATMAN defines verbal encouragements to eat as suggesting, demanding, directing, and making positive statements about food. We adapted some of the operational definitions to be consistent with theoretically important features of sibling interactions (i.e., parent-like interactions or "complementarity" and peer-like interactions or "reciprocity") [12]. For example, food offers (representing complementarity) and statements about eating/ finishing the food (representing reciprocity) were counted as verbal encouragements to eat.

Encouragements to eat delivered by the sibling and directed to the IC were coded in 5-min intervals from the videos. Ten percent of the videos were double coded and inter-rater reliability by intraclass correlation coefficient exceeded 0.80. Number of encouragements was summed across intervals to create the variable "total encouragements delivered to IC by sibling".

5.2.5 Mealtime Maternal Presence

Siblings interact differently when their mother is present [26, 27]. In order to adjust for maternal presence, we coded whether the mother was sitting with the siblings during the meal in each 5-min interval (yes vs. no for each interval). Inter-rater reliability computed as Cohen's kappa was 1.00. We created the variable "proportion of intervals in which mother is present" by dividing the total number of intervals in which the mother was sitting with the siblings by the total number of intervals.

5.2.6 Anthropometry

Staff members measured index children's weight and height during study visits using standardized procedures. BMI was calculated and age and sex specific BMI z-score (BMIz) for the IC was calculated based on the US Centers for Disease Control and Prevention reference growth curves [28]. Mothers reported the IC's birth weight, which was converted to z-scores based on National Centers for Health Statistics Natality Datasets [29]. Birth weight z-scores were missing and were imputed for 26 subjects using multiple imputation.

5.2.7 Statistical Analysis

We conducted statistical analysis using Stata version 13 (StataCorp. 2013. *Stata Statistical Software: Release 13.* College Station, TX: StataCorp LP). First, we calculated descriptive statistics for sample characteristics. Then, to test our hypothesis that encouragements to eat from the sibling is a mediating variable in the association of IC's birth order and the sibling's sex with IC's BMIz, we conducted path analysis, which is an extension of the regression model comprised only of directly observed variables [30]. We ran our path model testing associations between IC's birth order, the sibling's sex, encouragements to eat directed to the IC from the sibling, and IC's BMIz. We included the binary variables IC's birth order (with "older sibling" as the reference category) and sibling's sex (with "male" as the reference category) as predictors in the model. A Poisson distribution was used to model the mediating count variable "total encouragements delivered to IC from sibling", and "number of meal intervals" was set as the offset variable to account for variations in length of the meal. The model was adjusted for maternal presence (i.e., proportion of intervals in which mother is present), sibling's age, and the IC's birth weight z-score. For all statistical analyses, significance level was set at 0.05.

5.3 RESULTS

Mean IC age was 5.3 years (± SD 0.8), and about half (50.70 %) were male (Table 1). Path analysis showed that the IC being the younger sibling in the dyad, as opposed to the older sibling, was associated with receiving more encouragements to eat from the sibling (β: 0.93, 95 % CI: 0.59, 1.26, $p < 0.0001$). The IC having a sister as opposed to a brother was not directly associated with the IC receiving more encouragements to eat from the sibling (β: 0.18, 95 % CI: −0.09, 0.47, $p = 0.20$). The IC receiving more encouragements to eat from the sibling was associated with lower IC BMIz (β: −0.06, 95 % CI: −0.12, 0.00, $p = 0.05$). There was a marginally significant direct positive association between the IC being the younger sibling in the sibling dyad and the IC's BMIz (β: 0.81, 95 % CI: −0.82, 1.70, $p = 0.08$). There was no direct association of the IC having a sister, as opposed to a brother, with the IC's BMIz (β: 0.27, 95 % CI: −0.17, 0.72, $p = 0.23$) (Fig. 1).

TABLE 5.1 Sample characteristics[a]

	Total n = 75
Index child age, M(SD)	5.33 (0.79)
Index child sex, n (%)	
Male	38 (50.70)
Female	37 (49.30)
Index child race/ethnicity, n (%)	
Non-Hispanic white	44 (58.70)
Hispanic or not white	31 (41.30)
Maternal age, M (SD)	30.85 (6.73)
Maternal education, n (%)	
≤ High school education	31 (41.3)
> High school education	44 (58.7)
Sibling age, M (SD)	6.14 (3.49)
Sibling sex, n (%)	
Male	37 (49.3)
Female	38 (50.7)
Index child birth order, n (%)	
Younger sibling	41 (54.7)
Older sibling	34 (45.3)
Total encouragements delivered to index child from sibling, M(SD)	2.81 (3.93)
Proportion of intervals in which mother is present, M(SD)	0.86 (0.30)
Index child BMI z-score, M(SD)	0.81 (1.08)
Index child birth weight z-score, M(SD)	−0.22 (1.03)

[a]Table showing means (M) and standard deviations (SD) or counts (n) and percentages (%)

5.4 DISCUSSION

Findings from this study did not support our hypothesized conceptual model that receiving more encouragements to eat from a sibling is an underlying process for the association between having an older sibling or a sister with higher child BMIz. However, our results do provide support for our hypothesis that siblings play an important role in the family mealtime environment.

Our study suggests that birth order is associated with the number of encouragements a child receives from his/her sibling, with younger siblings receiving more encouragements to eat from their older siblings. We did not detect a statistically significant association between having a sister and receiving more encouragements to eat, though the direction of association was in the expected direction. In summary, in consensus with some of the available literature on sibling interactions in other domains, we found that older siblings may act as potent caregivers and role models during mealtimes [12, 14, 18]. These novel findings regarding how siblings interact around food may contribute to better understanding of how families function during mealtimes.

Contrary to our hypothesis that encouragements to eat directed to the IC from the sibling would be positively associated with the IC's BMIz, we found that encouragements to eat directed to the IC from the sibling was associated with the IC having a lower BMIz. We had based our hypothesis on reports that encouragement to eat from mother to child was positively associated with child overweight [10, 16, 17]. However, others have reported that controlling maternal feeding practices (including encouragement to eat) are inversely associated with child BMI and are a reaction to the child's weight status [15, 31–33]. It is thus not fully understood whether controlling feeding behaviors and encouragements to eat by parents are associated with lower concurrent BMI, or whether they may predict increases in BMI prospectively [6–8, 15, 31, 34]. Since mothers may encourage children who are perceived to be thinner or have a poorer appetite to eat more [15, 32], it is plausible that this kind of feeding behavior might over time reduce the child's ability to self-regulate intake in response to satiety cues and eventually lead to excessive weight gain [6–8]. Whether or not this is the case with regard to the association between encouragements from siblings and child BMI is unknown. However, our data suggest that cross-sectionally, older siblings may be imitating their mothers and encouraging siblings who are thinner to eat more. Prospective studies are needed to better establish the direction of this association.

Strengths of this study include the use of an observational assessment of interactions between siblings during a naturalistic mealtime setting. Limitations of this study include the small sample size, which might have restricted our ability to detect significant associations. Generalizability of our findings may be limited, given that the study cohort only included low-income Head Start families. Furthermore, the study design does not allow us to infer causality or test whether associations may be bidirectional.

5.5 CONCLUSION

Including multiple family members in child obesity programs can be associated with more positive outcomes [2]; including siblings as part of family-based programs represents a novel approach. Future studies are needed to further explore the role of siblings in feeding and the effect of including them in obesity prevention interventions.

REFERENCES

1. Ogden CL, Carroll MD, Kit BK, Flegal KM. Prevalence of childhood and adult obesity in the United States, 2011–2012. JAMA. 2014;311:806–14.
2. Kaplan SG, Arnold EM, Irby MB, Boles KA, Skelton JA. Family systems theory and obesity treatment applications for clinicians. Infant Child Adolesc Nutr. 2014;6:24–9.
3. Rao G. Childhood obesity: Highlights of AMA Expert Committee recommendations. Am Fam Physician. 2008;78:56–63.
4. Stark LJ, Spear S, Boles R, Kuhl E, Ratcliff M, Scharf C, et al. A pilot randomized controlled trial of a clinic and home-based behavioral intervention to decrease obesity in preschoolers. Obesity. 2011;19:134–41.
5. Moens E, Braet C, Soetens B. Observation of family functioning at mealtime: a comparison between families of children with and without overweight. J Pediatr Psychol. 2007;32:52–63.
6. Johnson S, Birch L. Parents' and children's adiposity and eating style. Pediatrics. 1994;94:653–61.
7. Fisher J, Birch L. Restricting access to foods and children's eating. Appetite. 1999;32:405–19.
8. Fisher J, Birch L. Eating in the absence of hunger and overweight in girls from 5–7 y of age. Am J Clin Nutr. 2002;76:226–31.
9. Drucker RR, Hammer LD, Agras SW, Bryson S. Can mothers influence their child's eating behavior? J Dev Behav Pediatr. 1999;20:88–92.
10. Klesges RC, Coates TJ, Brown G, Sturgeon-Tillisch J, Moldenhauer-Klesges LM, Holzer B, et al. Parental influences on children's eating behavior and relative weight. J Appl Behav Anal. 1983;16:371–8.
11. Zeller MH, Reiter-Purtill J, Modi AC, Gutzwiller J, Vannatta K, Davies W. Controlled study of critical parent and family factors in the obesigenic environment. Obesity. 2007;15:126–6.
12. Dunn J. Sibling relationship in early childhood. Child Dev. 1983;54:787–811.
13. Harrist AW, Achacoso JA, John A, Pettit GS, Bates JE, Dodge KA. Reciprocal and complementary sibling interactions: Relations with socialization outcomes in the kindergarten classroom. Early Educ Dev. 2014;25:202–22.
14. Brody GH, Stoneman Z, MacKinnon CE. Role asymmetries in interactions among school-aged children, their younger siblings, and their friends. Child Dev. 1982;53:1364–70.
15. Webber L, Cooke L, Hill C, Wardle J. Child adiposity and maternal feeding practices: a longitudinal analysis. Am J Clin Nutr. 2010;92:1423–8.
16. Hughes SO, Shewchuk RM, Baskin ML, Nicklas TA, Qu H. Indulgent feeding style and children's weight status in preschool. J Dev Behav Pediatr. 2008;29:403.

17. Birch LL, Fisher JO. Development of eating behaviors among children and adolescents. Pediatrics. 1998;101:539–49.
18. Stewart RB, Marvin R. Sibling relations: The role of conceptual perspective-taking in the ontogeny of sibling caregiving. Child Dev. 1984;55:1322–32.
19. Haugaard LK, Ajslev TA, Zimmermann E, Angquist L, Sorensen TI. Being an only or last-born child increases later risk of obesity. PLoS One. 2013;8:e56357.
20. Ochiai H, Shirasawa T, Ohtsu T, Nishimura R, Morimoto A, Obuchi R, et al. Number of siblings, birth order, and childhood overweight: a population-based cross-sectional study in Japan. BMC Public Health. 2012;12:766.
21. Hesketh K, Crawford D, Salmon J, Jackson M, Campbell K. Associations between family circumstance and weight status of Australian children. Int J Pediatr Obes. 2007;2:86–96.
22. Hunsberger M, Formisano A, Reisch LA, Bammann K, Moreno L, De Henauw S, et al. Overweight in singletons compared to children with siblings: the IDEFICS study. Nutr Diabetes. 2012;2:e35.
23. Epstein LH, Paluch RA, Raynor HA. Sex differences in obese children and siblings in family-based obesity treatment. Obes Res. 2001;9:746–53.
24. Mosli RH, Miller AL, Peterson KE, Kaciroti N, Rosenblum K, Baylin A, Lumeng JC. Birth order and sibship composition as predictors of overweight or obesity among low-income 4–8-year-old children. Pediatr Obes 2015. doi: 10.1111/ijpo.12018
25. Goulding AN, Rosenblum KL, Miller AL, Peterson KE, Chen Y-P, Kaciroti N, et al. Associations between maternal depressive symptoms and child feeding practices in a cross-sectional study of low-income mothers and their young children. Int J Behav Nutr Phys Act. 2014;11:75.
26. Lamb ME. Interactions between eighteen-month-olds and their preschool-aged siblings. Child Dev. 1978;49:51–9.
27. Corter C, Abramovitch R, Pepler DJ. The role of the mother in sibling interaction. Child Dev. 1983;6:1599–605.
28. Ogden CL, Flegal KM. Changes in terminology for childhood overweight and obesity. Age. 2010;12:12.
29. Oken E, Kleinman KP, Rich-Edwards J, Gillman MW. A nearly continuous measure of birth weight for gestational age using a United States national reference. BMC Pediatr. 2003;3:6.
30. Acock AC. Discovering structural equation modeling using Stata, revised edition. USA: Stata Press; 2013.
31. Robinson TN, Kiernan M, Matheson DM, Haydel KF. Is parental control over children's eating associated with childhood obesity? results from a population-based sample of third graders. Obes Res. 2001;9:306–12.
32. Powers SW, Chamberlin LA, Schaick KB, Sherman SN, Whitaker RC. Maternal feeding strategies, child eating behaviors, and child BMI in low-income African-American preschoolers. Obesity. 2006;14:2026–33.
33. Galloway AT, Fiorito LM, Francis LA, Birch LL. 'Finish your soup': counterproductive effects of pressuring children to eat on intake and affect. Appetite. 2006;46:318–23.
34. Faith MS, Berkowitz RI, Stallings VA, Kerns J, Storey M, Stunkard AJ. Parental feeding attitudes and styles and child body mass index: prospective analysis of a gene-environment interaction. Pediatrics. 2004;114:e429–36.

CHAPTER 6

Frequency and Socio-Demographic Correlates of Eating Meals Out and Take-Away Meals at Home: Cross-Sectional Analysis of the UK National Diet and Nutrition Survey, Waves 1–4 (2008–12)

Jean Adams, Louis Goffe, Tamara Brown, Amelia A. Lake, Carolyn Summerbell, Martin White, Wendy Wrieden, and Ashley J. Adamson

6.1 BACKGROUND

Out-of-home sources of ready-to-eat food include vending machines, take-aways, cafes, restaurants, supermarkets and convenience stores [1]. Food prepared out-of-home tends to be less healthful than food prepared at home, particularly in terms of energy and fat content [2]. This likely explains the associations found between frequency of eating out-of-home food and both nutritional quality of total diet and body weight [2,3].

Eating food prepared out-of-home is becoming more common across the world and makes a substantial contribution to individual diets and household spending on food [2,4-6]. For example, in 2012, about 10% of total daily energy intake of UK individuals was accounted for by food prepared and consumed out-of-home, with up to an additional 4% accounted for by take-away food eaten at home [7]. Between 2009 and 2012, expenditure on take-away food eaten at home rose by 11%, in real terms, to an average of £1.79 ($US2.86, €2.28) per person per week [7]. Over the same period, spending on eating out (excluding alcoholic drinks) rose by 7% to £8.95 ($US14.29, €11.40) per person per week, accounting for more than one quarter (26%) of total household spending on food and non-alcoholic drinks [7].

In terms of socio-demographic correlates of out-of-home food consumption, the scant, available data from developed countries suggests that men tend to consume more of their total dietary energy away from home [8,9], and obtain more meals from out-of-home sources [5] than women. Consumption of out-of-home food tends to increase with age in children, peak in late adolescence or early adulthood [10], and then drop with increasing age in adulthood [5,8,9,11-13]. An inconsistent relationship between markers of socio-economic position and out-of-home food consumption in developed countries was found in a systematic review [2].

Interventions to improve the nutritional content of food prepared out-of-home have been attempted in the UK and elsewhere [14,15]. Governmental public health and health education agencies are also increasingly urging individuals to cut down on their consumption of food prepared out-of-home, particularly fast food [16]. As reviewed above, some evidence of differences in consumption of out-of-home food according to socio-demographic characteristics [17,18] is emerging. However, little data from the UK exists. Better understanding of socio-demographic patterns of out-of-home eating is needed to more effectively target and tailor interventions.

Two key problems exist within the literature on out-of-home eating. First, variations in the definition of out-of-home eating make comparisons between studies difficult [2,4]. Some authors focus on food consumed out-of-home, irrespective of where it was prepared; (e.g. [8-10,12]) whilst others focus on food prepared out-of-home, irrespective of where it was consumed (e.g. [5,11,13,19]). Second, international differences in dietary intake [20] and out-of-home eating patterns [8] mean data from one country may not be generalisable to others.

To add to the sparse literature on who eats out-of-home food, we explored frequency and socio-demographic correlates of eating meals out and take-away meals at home, using data from a large, UK, population-representative study. We particularly focused on food prepared, rather than consumed, out-of-home as food prepared out-of-home is the subject of current policy focus [16].

6.2 METHODS

We performed a cross-sectional analysis of the first four years of data from the UK National Diet and Nutrition Survey (NDNS).

6.2.1 Data Source and Participants

The NDNS is an annual, cross sectional survey collecting information on the food consumption, nutrient intakes and nutritional status of people aged 1.5 years and older living in private households in the UK. The current programme began in 2008–09 and recruits around 1000 participants per year—500 children aged 1.5-18 years, and 500 adults aged 19 years or older. As far as possible, sampling, recruitment and data collection methods stay constant from year to year allowing data to be combined across survey years.

Households across the UK are selected to take part in the NDNS using a multi-stage probability design. In each wave, a random sample of primary sampling units is selected for inclusion. These primary sampling units are small geographical areas that allow more efficient data collection by enabling it to be geographically focused. Within these primary sampling units, private addresses are randomly selected for inclusion. If, on visiting, it is found that more than one household lives at a particular address, one is randomly selected for inclusion. Within participating households, up to one adult and one child are randomly selected to take part. Data collection involves a researcher interview covering socio-demographics and shopping, cooking and eating habits; participant completion of a four-day food diary; and a nurse visit. Parents, or carers, provide information on children aged 11 years and younger [21].

Overall, 91% of households eligible for inclusion agreed to take part in the first four waves of NDNS. Usable food diaries (three or four completed days) were collected from at least one household member in 58% of eligible households. At an individual level, 56% of those selected to take part completed usable food diaries: 2083 adults and 2073 children [21].

Anonymised data from the first four waves (2008–09 to 2011–12) of the NDNS were obtained from the UK Data Archive—a data sharing service for the UK research community. These data are available to other eligible researchers directly from the Archive.

6.2.2 Variables of Interest

6.2.2.1 Frequency of Eating Meals Out and Take-away Meals at Home

Whilst the NDNS food diary includes information on where food was consumed, it does not collect information on where food was obtained. However, the researcher interview includes two questions on frequency of eating food prepared out-of-home. These are: "On average, how often do you/does child eat meals out in a restaurant or cafe?"; and "On average, how often do you/does child eat take-away meals at home?". In both questions it is specified that "'meals' means more than a beverage or bag of chips" and participants are asked to "include pizza, fish and chips, Indian, Chinese, burgers, kebab etc.". Response options are: "rarely or never", "1-2 times per month", "1-2 times per week", "3-4 times per week", and "5 or more times per week". We believe these questions were designed specifically for the NDNS. Information is not available on the reliability or validity of these questions, but similar frequency-based questions have been used previously [5].

Responses in the two least frequent categories of the above questions (rarely or never, and 1–2 times per month) were collapsed for analysis as previous research indicates that the health risks associated with fast food occur in those with frequent consumption (more than once per week) [22]. As 5% or fewer participants consumed meals out or take-away meals at home more than 1–2 times per week, responses in the three most frequent categories (1–2 times per week, 3–4 times per week, and 5 or more times per week) were also combined for analysis. This led to dichotomous outcome variables with categories of: less than once per week; and once per week or more.

6.2.2.2 Socio-demographic Variables

Three socio-demographic variables were included: age in years, gender, and socio-economic position. Age was collapsed into approximately 5-year categories for children, and 10-year categories for adults.

Socio-economic position (SEP) was measured using household occupational social class and, in adults only, individual age at completion of full time education. Although net household income (another common measure of SEP) [17,18] is collected in NDNS, around 15% of participants refuse the question and this level of attrition was not considered acceptable.

Occupational social class was categorised using the three-level National Statistics Socio-economic Classification [23] of the household as: higher managerial, administrative and professional occupations; intermediate occupations; and routine and manual occupations. This classification assigns all individuals living in the same household according to the occupation of the householder—the individual responsible for owning or renting the accommodation. Where there is more than one householder, the individual with the highest income takes precedence. Where more than one householder has the same income, the oldest individual takes precedence. Unemployed householders are categorised according to their last main occupation. A small number of households are excluded from this classification where the householder has never worked.

Individual age at completion of full time education was categorised as less than 16 years (equivalent to having obtained less than basic school leaving qualifications), 16–17 (equivalent to basic school leaving qualifications), or more than 18 years (equivalent to advanced school leaving qualifications or more). This variable was not calculated for children aged 18 years or younger as many have not completed full time education. Education was used as an individual, rather than household, marker of SEP. As such we did not use parental education as a proxy for children as it would not be clear which parents' educational status to apply.

6.2.3 Data Analysis

Individuals were included in the analysis if they took part in the NDNS in waves 1–4 and information on all of the variables of interest was available.

Logistic regression was used to explore the unadjusted, and mutually adjusted, relationships between likelihood of eating meals out or take-away meals at home once per week or more often across socio-demographic variables. As there was evidence that different patterns in proportion of participants eating these meals once per week or more according to age in adults and children, all analyses were conducted separately for children (18 years or younger) and adults (older than 18 years).

Study weights, prepared by NDNS and provided with the data, were used to account for selective non-response. These weights take account of the fact that whilst sampling for the NDNS is population-representative, response is not. Some population groups are less likely to respond to the invitation to take part in the NDNS than others. Applying study weights corrects for this selective non-response and returns the results to population-representative. The use of study weights mean that percentages (with 95% confidence intervals) are presented rather than raw frequencies.

All analyses were conducted in Stata v13.

6.2.4 Ethics

Ethical approval for collection of NDNS data was provided by Oxfordshire A Research Ethics Committee. Ethical approval for this secondary analyses of anonymised data was not required.

6.3 RESULTS

Of 2083 adults and 2073 children who took part in the NDNS in waves 1–4, 2001 (96.1%) adults and 1963 (94.7%) children were included in the analyses. The distribution of participants across socio-demographic variables is shown in the first data column of Table 1.

The proportion of participants who ate meals out once per week or more, overall and by socio-demographic variables, is shown in Table 1. Just over one-quarter of adults (27.1%) and just less than one-fifth of children (19.0%) ate meals out once per week or more. There were no gender differences in proportions eating meals out once per week or more in adults or children. In adults, eating meals out once per week or more was most common in the youngest age groups (19–29 years), with significantly more participants in this group (41.0%) eating meals out once per week or more than in other groups (20.1%-27.6%) in unadjusted and mutually adjusted analyses. However, there was no evidence of an inverse linear association with age. Significantly fewer children aged 10–14 years ate meals out once per week or more than those in the youngest age group (1.5 – 4 years), but there were no other statistically significant differences by age in children.

Adults living in households in the intermediate and most affluent occupational social class were significantly more likely to eat meals out once per week

TABLE 6.1 Frequency of eating meals out by socio-demographic variables; UK National Diet & Nutrition Survey 2008-12

Variable	Level	Distribution, %[1] (95% CI)	1-2/week or more, % (95% CI)	Unadjusted OR (95% CI)	Mutually adjusted OR (95% CI)
All adults (n = 2001)		100	27.1 (25.0 – 29.4)	–	–
Gender	Male	49.1 (46.7 – 51.6)	28.8 (25.5 – 32.2)	Reference	Reference
	Female	50.9 (48.4 – 53.3)	25.6 (22.8 – 28.6)	0.90 (0.70 – 1.15)	0.89 (0.70 – 1.14)
Age (years)	19-29	18.2 (16.1 – 20.5)	41.0 (34.4 – 47.9)	**Reference**	**Reference**
	30-39	17.4 (15.7 – 19.2)	21.9 (17.7 – 26.7)	**0.39 (0.26 – 0.58)**	**0.35 (0.23 – 0.54)**
	40-49	19.2 (17.4 – 21.1)	24.7 (20.5 – 29.4)	**0.47 (0.32 – 0.70)**	**0.43 (0.29 – 0.65)**
	50-59	15.8 (14.2 – 17.6)	25.7 (21.1 – 31.0)	**0.51 (0.34 – 0.77)**	**0.48 (0.32 – 0.73)**
	60-69	14.0 (12.4 – 15.7)	20.1 (15.3 – 25.8)	**0.36 (0.22 – 0.57)**	**0.34 (0.21 – 0.56)**
	>69	15.4 (13.7 – 17.3)	27.6 (22.3 – 33.7)	**0.58 (0.37 – 0.90)**	**0.57 (0.35 – 0.90)**
NS-SEC	Routine & manual	35.4 (33.1 – 37.8)	20.8 (17.7 – 24.3)	Reference	Reference
	Intermediate	20.5 (18.6 – 22.5)	29.7 (24.8 – 35.0)	**1.76 (1.24 – 2.49)**	**1.89 (1.33 – 2.69)**
	Managerial & professional	44.1 (41.7 – 46.6)	31.1 (27.7 – 34.7)	**1.81 (1.37 – 2.41)**	**1.95 (1.43 – 2.65)**
Age left education (years)	<16	24.1 (21.9 – 26.5)	24.2 (19.8 – 29.3)	Reference	Reference
	16-17	35.5 (33.0 – 38.0)	25.7 (22.0 – 29.7)	1.08 (0.78 – 1.50)	0.97 (0.68 – 1.40)
	>17	40.4 (37.8 – 43.0)	29.5 (25.7 – 33.6)	1.31 (0.95 – 1.80)	1.01 (0.69 – 1.48)
All children (n = 1963)		100	19.0 (17.2 – 21.0)	–	–
Gender	Male	52.0 (49.5 – 54.4)	20.0 (17.4 – 22.8)	Reference	Reference
	Female	48.0 (45.6 – 50.5)	18.0 (15.5 – 20.8)	0.88 (0.67 – 1.14)	0.87 (0.66 – 1.13)

TABLE 6.1 *(Continued)*

Variable	Level	Distribution, %[1] (95% CI)	1-2/week or more, % (95% CI)	Unadjusted OR (95% CI)	Mutually adjusted OR (95% CI)
Age (years)	0-4	19.6 (17.9 – 21.5)	21.0 (17.4 – 25.1)	Comparator	Comparator
	5-9	28.4 (26.2 – 30.6)	17.3 (14.2 – 21.0)	0.82 (0.57 – 1.16)	0.81 (0.57 – 1.16)
	10-14	28.4 (26.2 – 30.8)	13.5 (10.6 – 17.0)	**0.61 (0.42 – 0.89)**	**0.61 (0.42 – 0.89)**
	15-18	23.5 (21.4 – 25.8)	26.1 (21.8 – 31.0)	1.25 (0.87 – 1.81)	1.27 (0.88 – 1.82)
NS-SEC	Routine & manual	37.0 (34.6 – 39.5)	17.9 (15.0 – 21.3)	Reference	Reference
	Intermediate	20.0 (18.1 – 22.1)	21.4 (17.3 – 26.2)	1.34 (0.93 – 1.94)	1.35 (0.93 – 1.96)
	Managerial & professional	43.0 (40.6 – 45.4)	18.8 (16.2 – 21.7)	1.10 (0.81 – 1.48)	1.12 (0.83 – 1.52)

[1]weighted percentages that correct for selective non-response.

OR: odds ratio; CI: confidence intervals; NS-SEC: National Statistics Socio-economic Classification.

Bold indicates statistically significantly different from reference category at $p < 0.05$.

or more than those in the lowest social class in both unadjusted and adjusted analyses. However, there was no difference in the proportion of adults eating meals out once per week or more by individual education in adults, or by household occupational social class in children.

Table 2 shows the proportion of participants who ate take-away meals at home once per week or more. More than one fifth of adults (21.1%) and children (21.0%) ate take-away meals at home this frequently.

There were no gender differences in the proportion of participants who ate take-away meals at home once per week or more in adults, but girls were less likely to eat these meals frequently than boys—in unadjusted and mutually adjusted analyses. In adults, the proportion of participants eating take-away meals at home once per week or more tended to decrease with age. Adults in the oldest group (more than 69 years) were one fifth as likely to eat these meals once per week or more than those aged 19–29 years. In children, the proportion eating take-away meals at home once per week or more increased with age. Children aged older than 9 years were significantly more likely to eat these meals at least once per week than those aged less than 5 years in both unadjusted and mutually adjusted analyses. Children aged 15–18 years were more than twice as likely to eat these meals once per week or more than children aged 1.5 – 4 years.

There was no difference in the proportion of adults eating take-away meals at home once per week or more by household occupation social class or individual education in adults after mutual adjustment. However, children living in households of the highest occupational social class were significantly less likely to eat take-away meals at home once per week or more than those living in the least affluent households.

Table 3 shows cross-tabulations of eating meals out and take-away meals at home in adults and children. There was evidence that both adults and children who ate meals out at least once per week were also more likely to eat take-away meals at home at least once per week.

6.4 DISCUSSION

6.4.1 Statement of Principal Findings

As far as we are aware, this is the first description of frequency and socio-demographic correlates of eating food from out-of-home sources in a UK population-representative cohort. In terms of frequency of consumption, around one

TABLE 6.2 Frequency of eating take away meals at home by socio-demographic variables; UK National Diet & Nutrition Survey 2008-12

Variable	Level	1-2/week or more, % (95% CI)	Unadjusted OR (95% CI)	Mutually adjusted OR (95% CI)
All adults (n = 2001)		21.1 (19.1 – 23.3)	–	–
Gender	Male	23.1 (20.1 – 26.4)	Reference	Reference
	Female	19.2 (16.6 – 22.0)	0.89 (0.68 – 1.17)	0.94 (0.71 – 1.23)
Age (years)	19-29	32.4 (26.3 – 39.1)	Reference	Reference
	30-39	25.8 (21.3 – 30.9)	0.82 (0.54 – 1.26)	0.81 (0.53 – 1.23)
	40-49	26.5 (22.1 – 31.4)	0.96 (0.64 – 1.45)	0.90 (0.59 – 1.36)
	50-59	16.9 (12.9 – 21.8)	**0.50 (0.32 – 0.80)**	**0.49 (0.31 – 0.78)**
	60-69	12.6 (8.6 – 17.9)	**0.38 (0.22 – 0.66)**	**0.36 (0.21 – 0.64)**
	>69	7.9 (4.7 – 12.9)	**0.19 (0.09 – 0.39)**	**0.18 (0.08 – 0.37)**
NS-SEC	Routine & manual	22.1 (18.8 – 25.8)	Reference	Reference
	Intermediate	23.5 (19.0 – 28.8)	1.03 (0.71 – 1.51)	1.09 (0.73 – 1.60)
	Managerial & professional	19.2 (16.4 – 22.3)	0.99 (0.73 – 1.34)	1.03 (0.74 – 1.44)
Age left education (years)	<16	14.5 (10.9 – 19.0)	Comparator	Comparator
	16-17	25.8 (22.0 – 29.9)	**2.04 (1.39 – 3.00)**	1.25 (0.83 – 1.89)
	>17	19.9 (16.8 – 23.5)	1.47 (0.99 – 2.17)	0.83 (0.53 – 1.31)
All children (n = 1963)		21.0 (19.1 – 23.1)	–	–
Gender	Male	23.7 (20.8 – 26.7)	Reference	Reference
	Female	18.2 (15.6 – 21.1)	**0.71 (0.55 – 0.93)**	**0.70 (0.54 – 0.91)**

TABLE 6.2 *(Continued)*

Variable	Level	1-2/week or more, % (95% CI)	Unadjusted OR (95% CI)	Mutually adjusted OR (95% CI)
Age (years)	0-4	14.0 (10.8 – 17.9)	Reference	Reference
	5-9	18.4 (15.1 – 22.1)	1.43 (0.96 – 2.11)	1.44 (0.98 – 2.14)
	10-14	23.1 (19.3 – 27.4)	**1.77 (1.20 – 2.61)**	**1.79 (1.20 – 2.64)**
	15-18	27.7 (23.1 – 32.7)	**2.43 (1.63 – 3.64)**	**2.44 (1.63 – 3.65)**
NS-SEC	Routine & manual	26.0 (22.6 – 29.9)	Reference	Reference
	Intermediate	20.4 (16.1 – 25.4)	0.81 (0.56 – 1.17)	0.82 (0.57 – 1.19)
	Managerial & professional	17.0 (14.4 – 19.9)	**0.59 (0.44 – 0.79)**	**0.60 (0.45 – 0.81)**

[1]weighted percentages that correct for selective non-response.

OR: odds ratio; CI: confidence intervals; NS-SEC: National Statistics Socio-economic Classification.

Bold indicates statistically significantly different from reference category at $p < 0.05$.

TABLE 6.3 Cross-tabulation of frequency of eating meals out and take-away meals at home; UK National Diet & Nutrition Survey 2008-12

Meals out	**Take-away meals at home**			**Chi-squared (df), p-value**
	<1/week	**1-2/week or more**	**Total**	
All adults (n = 2001)	78.9	21.1	100	
<1/week	60.0	12.9	72.9	
1-2/week or more	18.9	8.2	27.1	18.39 (1), <0.001
All children (n = 1963)	79.0	21.0	100	
<1/week	66.9	14.1	81.0	
1-2/week or more	12.1	6.9	19.0	45.66 (1), <0.001

Figures show % of all participants in each cell, weighted for selective non-response.

quarter of adults and one fifth of children ate meals out once per week or more; around one fifth of adults and children ate take-away meals at home once per week or more. In terms of socio-demographic correlates, the only gender differences were that boys were more likely to eat take-away meals at home at least once per week than girls. The proportion of participants who ate both meals out and take-away meals at home at least once per week peaked at age 19–29 years and decreased in older adults. Adults living in households of higher occupational social class were more likely to eat meals out at least once per week, but there was no difference by individual education in adults or household social class in children. Noticeably, there were no socio-economic differences in the proportion of adults eating take-away meals at home at least once per week. But, children living in households of the highest occupation social class were less likely to eat take-away meals at home at least once per week than those in the lowest.

6.4.2 Interpretation and Implications of Findings

In a number of countries, governments provide advice on how to choose more healthful options when eating meals out and choosing take-away meals, but no guidance on the maximum recommended frequency of consumption is provided [24,25]. Studies have found that the health risks associated with fast food occur in those with consumption more than once per week [22]. If 'fast food' and 'take-away' food can be equated, our findings indicate this level of consumption is particularly common in certain population sub-groups. In particular, almost one-third of adults aged 19–29 years ate take-away meals at home this often. Consumers, particularly aged 19–29 years, may benefit from interventions to decrease frequency of consumption.

Differences in methods also make it hard to compare frequency of consumption reported here with previous work. The most comparable previous data reports on frequency of eating meals prepared in restaurants (either sit-in or take-away) amongst adults in the USA—where 41% of US adults ate such meals three times or more per week in 2000 [5]. As 5% or less of participants in the current study consumed meals out or take-away meals at home more than 1–2 times per week, this suggests that consumption is substantially higher in the USA than the UK. Further consideration of why individuals consume meals out and take-away meals at home, and if this differs between the USA and UK, could inform the development of interventions to prevent further increases in, and even reduce, consumption in both settings, and elsewhere.

Changes in consumption of meals out and take-away meals at home over time may also limit comparisons with previous studies. There is evidence that the prevalence of out-of-home eating establishments increased between 1980 and 2000 [26], suggesting that consumption has also increased over recent decades.

Our finding that boys were more likely than girls to eat take-away meals at home, but not meals out, frequently reflects previous findings. Others have reported that men obtain a greater proportion of their total energy from food consumed out-of-home [8,9], and consume commercially prepared foods more often [5]. The distinctions between meals out and take-away meals at home, and gender differences in children, have not been previously studied. Unlike previous work [5,8,9], we did not find the same gender difference in frequency of consumption of either type of meal in adults. It is possible that patterns of out-of-home eating by gender may have changed in recent years.

Our finding that consumption of both meals out and take-away meals at home peak in early adulthood (19–29 years) is similar to previous reports [5,8,9,11-13]. However, few previous studies have explored the relationship with age in children, and only one has included both adults and children [11]. These trends may reflect true changes in consumption over the lifecourse, secular trends in consumption, or a mixture of both. For example, older people may be less likely to eat meals from out-of-home sources because they tend to have less disposable income than others [27]; because they did not develop the habit earlier in their life when such options were less common [5]; or for a combination of these, and other, reasons.

We did not study the nutritional quality of the out-of-home meals consumed by participants. It would be inappropriate to assume that all meals from out-of-home sources are nutritionally equal and there may be systematic differences in what is consumed by socio-demographic characteristics. Interventions seeking to improve dietary intake by reducing consumption of out-of-home food may be more effective if tailored to, and perhaps targeting at, adults aged less than 30 years. It may also be important to develop interventions to help children and adolescents avoid becoming frequent out-of-home food consumers.

Eating meals out at least once per week was particularly high in the youngest children (1.5-4 years) (21.0%). This may reflect that these children spend little or no time in formal educational settings meaning they have more opportunity than others to accompany their parents to lunches out, in particular.

Adults of higher SEP, measured by household occupational class, but not individual education, were most likely to eat meals out at least once per week.

This may reflect the differences in what different measures of SEP capture. Household occupational social class is more often a measure of current status than educational attainment—which may reflect circumstances many years in the past. [17,18] Differences in eating meals out by occupational class may reflect that such meals can be expensive (although comparative data on the cost of meals out, take-away meals, and home cooked meals is not readily available), as well as cultural differences in leisure activities [28].

No differences in consumption of take-away meals at home were seen in adults according to either measure of SEP. However, children living in households of higher occupational class were less likely to eat take-away meals once per week or more than those living in households of the lowest occupational class. This is perhaps contrary to popular beliefs where high take-away consumption in less affluent groups (across the board, and not just in children) is suggested to contribute to socio-economic inequalities in obesity [29,30]. As noted, previous studies have reported inconsistent associations between SEP and out-of-home eating in adults [2]. Our results suggest this may be due to differences in definition of out-of-home eating, with different relationships seen for meals out and take-away meals at home; or differences in operationalization of SEP, with different relationships seen for occupational social class and education (in adults). It is possible that socio-economic trends in take-away consumption in today's children will carry forward to tomorrow's adults.

We studied meals out and take-away meals separately as there is reason to believe these represent different types of eating [28,31]. Whilst the same food can be bought to take-away or eat in-store in some outlets, many outlets will provide only food to take-away or only food to eat in [1]. Furthermore, the prevalence of these different types of outlets varies with socio-economic markers of local areas. In particularly, restaurants for consuming meals out are most common in more affluent areas in the UK [32].

The fact eating take-away meals at home was more common in less affluent children, but not adults, suggests that socio-economic influences on consumption are not consistent across the lifecourse. Take-away outlet density is higher in more deprived UK neighbourhoods [33], and everyday exposure to take-away outlets across home and work neighbourhoods and commuting routes has been associated with consumption in UK adults [34]. It is possible that children are less mobile in their daily lives and so are more exposed to their home neighbourhood environment than adults. Thus, children who live in deprived neighbourhoods may be particularly exposed to the take-away outlets concentrated there, whereas more mobile adults living in the same neighbourhoods may have more variable take-away outlet exposure as they spend time at home, at work, and commuting.

6.4.3 Strengths and Limitations of Methods

The NDNS aims to recruit a population-representative sample at each wave and study weights are provided to take account of selective non-response where this exists. Our results are, therefore, likely to be generalisable across the UK. However, given known international differences in eating patterns [8,20], they may not be generalisable to other contexts. Further work, using consistent methods, is required to provide internationally comparable information. The large sample size of both children and adults means that our analyses are unlikely to be underpowered.

The current data were collected in 2008–12, making this the most up-to-date UK dataset on this topic. Whilst it is possible that more recent data may reveal different trends, there was no evidence of differences in frequency of consumption over the four survey years included (data not shown).

Although NDNS does sometimes include one adult and one child per household and it would be possible, in some cases, to explore household congruence of out-of-home eating patterns, this was out with the scope of the current work. Future work could explore household, and other influences, on eating out-of-home.

The validity and reliability of the questions used to assess frequency of consumption have not been explored. One previous study found that frequency of eating out-of-home food in children aged 5–12 years tended to be under-reported in questionnaire compared to food-diary data [10]. Any systematic differences in interpretations across socio-demographic groups would lead to bias, but the nature of this is difficult to predict. Furthermore, the questions used do not capture the consumption of all food prepared out-of-home. Ideally, the source of all food consumed would be captured alongside food diary data. This could be included in future waves of NDNS.

Out-of-home food outlets are heterogeneous. No information was collected on the specific type of meal out or take-away outlets visited and there may be systematic differences in these across population groups. Similarly, although guidance was given on what a 'meal' is, differences in individual interpretations are likely to introduce error. Future work that disaggregates out-of-home eating using existing tools [32] may reveal further, interesting patterns.

We measured SEP using household occupational social class and, in adults only, age at leaving full time education. These capture two of the three most common measures of individual SEP—occupation, education and income. We were unable to use a marker of individual educational attainment in children as the great majority were still in full time education. Although household income is captured in NDNS, around 15% of the sample refused this particular question—leading to potential non-response bias. We did not include a measure of income for this reason.

It was beyond the scope of the current work to explore the relationships between frequency of eating meals out and take-away meal at home and either dietary quality or adiposity. This has been explored in other (non-UK) cohorts [3,22] and future work could explore these relationships further within NDNS.

CONCLUSIONS

We studied frequency and socio-demographic correlates of eating meals out and take-away meals at home, using data from a large, UK population-representative study. Between a fifth and a quarter of people in the UK eat meals out once per week or more, with one fifth eating take-away meals at home this frequently. Boys were more likely than girls to eat take-away meals at home frequently, but no other gender differences were found. At least weekly consumption of both types of meal peaks in early adulthood. Adults from more affluent households are more likely to eat meals out at least weekly, but children from less affluent households are more likely to eat take-away meals at home at least weekly. Interventions seeking to improve dietary intake by reducing consumption of out-of-home food may be more effective if tailored to, or targeting at, adults aged less than 30 years. It may also be important to develop interventions to help children and adolescents avoid becoming frequent consumers of out-of-home food.

REFERENCES

1. Lake AA, Burgoine T, Greenhalgh F, Stamp E, Tyrrell R. The foodscape: classification and field validation of secondary data sources. Health Place. 2010;16(4):666–73.
2. Lachat C, Nago E, Verstraeten R, Roberfroid D, Van Camp J, Kolsteren P. Eating out of home and its association with dietary intake: a systematic review of the evidence. Obes Rev. 2012;13:329–46.
3. Nguyen BT, Powell LM: The impact of restaurant consumption among US adults: effects on energy and nutrient intakes. Public Health Nutrition 2014, [Epub ahead of print].

4. Bezerra IN, Curioni C, Sichieri R. Association between eating out of home and body weight. Nutr Rev. 2012;70(2):65–79.
5. Kant AK, Graubard BI. Eating out in America, 1987–2000: trends and nutritional correlates. Prev Med. 2004;38(2):243–9.
6. Nielsen SJ, Siega-Riz AM, Popkin BM. Trends in Food Locations and Sources among Adolescents and Young Adults. Prev Med. 2002;35(2):107–13.
7. Department for Environment Food and Rural Affairs: Family Food 2012. In. London: National Statistics; 2013.
8. Orfanos P, Naska A, Trichopoulos D, Slimani N, Ferrari P, van Bakel M, et al. Eating out of home and its correlates in 10 European countries. The European Prospective Investigation into Cancer and Nutrition (EPIC) study. Public Health Nutr. 2007;10(12):1515–25.
9. Vandevijvere S, Lachat C, Kolsteren P, Van Oyen H. Eating out of home in Belgium: current situation and policy implications. Br J Nutr. 2009;102(6):921–8.
10. Burke SJ, McCarthy SN, O'Neill JL, Hannon EM, Kiely M, Flynn A, et al. An examination of the influence of eating location on the diets of Irish children. Public Health Nutr. 2007;10(06):599–607.
11. Guthrie JF, Lin BH, Frazao E. Role of food prepared away from home in the American diet, 1977–78 versus 1994–96: changes and consequences. J Nutr Educ Behav. 2002;34(3):140–50.
12. Kearney JM, Hulshof KF, Gibney MJ. Eating patterns–temporal distribution, converging and diverging foods, meals eaten inside and outside of the home–implications for developing FBDG. Public Health Nutr. 2001;4(2b):693–8.
13. O'Dwyer NA, Gibney MJ, Burke SJ, McCarthy SN. The influence of eating location on nutrient intakes in Irish adults: implications for developing food-based dietary guidelines. Public Health Nutr. 2005;8(3):258–65.
14. Bagwell S. Healthier catering initiatives in London, UK: an effective tool for encouraging healthier consumption behaviour? Critical Public Health. 2013;24(1):35–46.
15. Public Health Responsibility Deal: Food pledges. [https://responsibilitydeal.dh.gov.uk/food-pledges/]
16. Secretary of State for Health. Healthy lives, healthy people: our strategy for public health in England. London: HM Government; 2010.
17. Galobardes B, Shaw M, Lawlor D, Lynch J, Davey Smith G. Indicators of socioeconomic position (part 2). J Epidemiol Community Health. 2006;60:95–101.
18. Galobardes B, Shaw M, Lawlor DA, Lynch JW, Davey Smith G. Indicators of socioeconomic position (part 1). J Epidemiol Community Health. 2006;60:7–12.
19. Adamson A, Rugg-Gunn A, Butler T, Appleton D. The contribution of foods from outside the home to the nutrient intake of young adolescents. J Hum Nutr Diet. 1996;9:55–68.
20. Slimani N, Fahey M, Welch A, Wirfält E, Stripp C, Bergström E, et al. Diversity of dietary patterns observed in the European Prospective Investigation into Cancer and Nutrition (EPIC) project. Public Health Nutr. 2002;5(6b):1311–28.
21. Bates B, Lennox A, Prentice A, Bates C, Page P, Nicholson S, et al. National Diet and Nutrition Survey Results from Years 1, 2, 3 and 4 (combined) of the Rolling Programme (2008/2009 - 2011/2012). London: Public Health England; 2014.
22. Pereira MA, Kartashov AI, Ebbeling CB, Van Horn L, Slattery ML, Jacobs Jr DR, et al. Fast-food habits, weight gain, and insulin resistance (the CARDIA study): 15-year prospective analysis. Lancet. 2005;365(9453):36–42.

23. Rose D, Pevalin D, O'Reilly K. The National Statistics Socio-economic Classification: origins, development and use. Hampshire: Palgrave Macmillan; 2005.
24. Healthier options for eating out and takeaways. [http://www.nhs.uk/change4life/Pages/restaurant-takeaway-healthy-options.aspx]
25. Tips for Eating Healthy When Eating out. [http://www.choosemyplate.gov/healthy-eating-tips/tips-for-eating-out.html]
26. Burgoine T, Lake AA, Stamp E, Alvanides S, Mathers JC, Adamson AJ. Changing foodscapes 1980–2000, using the ASH30 Study. Appetite. 2009;53:157–65.
27. Muriel A, Oldfield Z. Financial circumstances and consumption. In: Banks J, Lessof C, Nazroo J, Rogers N, Stafford M, Steptoe A, editors. Financial circumstances, health and well-being of the older population in England: the 2008 English Longitudinal Study of Ageing (wave 4). London: Institute of Fiscal Studies; 2010.
28. Inglis V, Ball K, Crawford D. Why do women of low socioeconomic status have poorer dietary behaviours than women of higher socioeconomic status? A qualitative exploration. Appetite. 2005;45(3):334–43.
29. Deans J: Jamie Oliver bemoans chips, cheese and giant TVs of modern-day poverty. In: The Guardian. London; 2013.
30. Hardus PM, van Vuuren C, Crawford D, Worsley A. Public perceptions of the causes and prevention of obesity among primary school children. Int J Obes. 2003;27:1465–71.
31. Lupton D. The heart of the meal: food preferences and habits among rural Australian couples. Sociol Health Illn. 2000;22(1):94–109.
32. Lake A, Burgoine T, Stamp E, Grieve R. The foodscape: classification and field validation of secondary data sources across urban/rural and socio-economic classifications in England. Int J Behav Nutr Phys Act. 2012;9(1):37.
33. Macdonald L, Cummins S, Macintyre S. Neighbourhood fast food environment and area deprivation-substitution or concentration? Appetite. 2007;49(1):251–4.
34. Burgoine T, Forouhi NG, Griffin SJ, Wareham NJ, Monsivais P. Associations between exposure to takeaway food outlets, takeaway food consumption, and body weight in Cambridgeshire, UK: population based, cross sectional study. BMJ. 2014;348:g1464.

CHAPTER 7

Feeding Practices of Low-Income Mothers: How Do They Compare to Current Recommendations?

Thomas G. Power, Sheryl O. Hughes,
L. Suzanne Goodell, Susan L. Johnson,
J. Andrea Jaramillo Duran, Kimberly Williams,
Ashley D. Beck, and Leslie A. Frankel

7.1 INTRODUCTION

Overweight and obesity pose significant health problems for children and adolescents [1]. Childhood obesity rates have tripled in the past three decades [2]. These rates are even higher for low-income and minority children [3]. It is well recognized that parents play a fundamental role in shaping the trajectory of eating behaviors in children and thus the development of overweight [4]. Increasingly, parenting styles and practices have been associated with child intake and obesity [5]. Childhood obesity has been linked to both highly controlling and highly indulgent parenting in the eating and non-eating domains [4-6]. Researchers have suggested that these parenting practices can interfere with children's self-regulation of caloric intake, therefore increasing their obesity risk [7].

Currently, researchers and practitioners advocate the use of responsive feeding practices to minimize the likelihood of childhood obesity [8-11]. Responsive feeding, during the preschool years, is characterized by caregiver guidance and recognition of the child's cues of hunger and satiety. Nonresponsive feeding is characterized by a lack of reciprocity between parent and child, with the caregiver taking excessive control of the feeding situation (forcing, pressuring, or restricting food intake), the child controlling the feeding situation (indulgent feeding), or low levels of caregiver involvement (uninvolved feeding) [8-11]. Other feeding practices that researchers and practitioners encourage (mostly to increase child consumption of fruits and vegetables) include: 1) presenting novel foods frequently to encourage liking [12]; 2) encouraging interest in new foods through conversation and granting children opportunities to explore foods [13]; 3) enthusiastic modeling of healthy food consumption [14]; and 4) facilitating the development of independent eating skills and not overemphasizing table manners [15]. Based upon some of this literature, the American Academic of Pediatrics recommended that parents of young children: "provide a healthy array of foods in the correct portion size and allow children to decide what and how much to eat from what they are offered [16]."

Despite these recommendations, few observational studies have examined the degree to which parents adopt responsive feeding behaviors, especially in low-income, minority samples-populations at high risk for childhood obesity [3]. In a systematic review of responsive feeding and child weight published in 2011, most studies relied on parent-report measures [17]. Only four studies employed observational measures, and two were studies of mothers and infants [18,19]. Similarly, Lumeng and colleagues [20], in 2012, noted that "Since 1981, the few studies that have evaluated maternal feeding style by direct observation in association with child weight status have included only ~200 child participants and > 80% of these participants have been white" (p. 640). The reliance on questionnaires is problematic for several reasons—social desirability, under-reporting of negative interactions, parents' limited awareness of their own behavior, and problems in recall [21-25]. Haycraft and Blissett [26], for example, found that mothers' reports of their own feeding practices showed no significant correlations with observed feeding behavior (although some correlations for fathers were significant).

Given than child obesity rates differ as a function of child ethnicity and gender [1,3], a second issue concerns differences in maternal feeding practices as a function of maternal ethnicity, child gender, and child weight status. Previous research on these three variables is limited and inconsistent. Very limited data on ethnic differences are available, for example, because the vast majority of observational studies of feeding practices have examined white, middle class mothers.

In one exception, an observational study of mothers of preschool children feeding their children a snack, Lumeng and colleauges [20] found that non-Hispanic, white mothers used fewer assertive and intrusive feeding prompts than ethnic minority mothers. No other studies of ethnic differences in observed maternal feeding behavior were found. In two self-report studies of maternal feeding practices, Hughes and colleagues [27,28] found that a greater proportion of low-income Latina mothers showed an indulgent feeding style (high responsiveness, low demandingness) compared to mothers from other ethnic groups.

Several observational studies have examined how maternal feeding behavior varies as a function of child gender. In three studies of young children (ages 3-8), mothers of boys encouraged their children to eat more frequently than mothers of girls [29-31]. Similarly, an observational study of 7-13 year olds [32] showed that parents of boys exerted more behavioral control during mealtime than parents of girls. However, one large study that included ethnic minority children [20] found no child gender differences in maternal feeding behaviors.

Research on the effects of child weight status on parental feeding behavior is inconsistent. Two observational studies by Klesges and colleagues found that parents of obese children encouraged their children to eat more frequently than parents of healthy weight children [33,34], whereas other observational studies found no relationship between eating prompts and child weight status [20,35,36]. Interestingly, child and parent self-report studies conclude that parents of obese children report lower levels of pressure to eat [37,38]. Observational studies of the quality of parental control over child eating show that parents of obese children show more assertive, intrusive, authoritarian, or permissive control [20,32]. Finally, Birch and colleagues [35] found that mothers of thinner children (as assessed with skinfold thickness) talked with their children more about nonfood topics during lunch in a laboratory session than mothers of children with higher fat levels.

Without observational data on feeding in low-income families, it is difficult to determine whether or not maternal feeding behaviors might contribute to obesity risk in low-income families, and if so, to determine which practices might best be targeted in education and prevention. The major purpose of this study was to examine the degree to which low-income, ethnic minority parents show feeding practices that are consistent with current recommendations for responsive feeding. The second purpose was to examine differences in maternal feeding behavior as a function of maternal ethnicity, child gender, and child weight status. This was accomplished through direct observations of feeding in a sample of low-income African American and Latina mothers and their preschoolers.

7.2 METHODS

7.2.1 Participants

The videotapes coded for this study came from a larger study of parent-child interaction at dinner [39]. In this larger study of 177 families, observers coded parent-child interactions at three separate meals per family—the results of this live coding are reported in Hughes et al. [39]. These observations had been videotaped for later coding and analysis. To examine differences in maternal behavior as a function of maternal ethnicity, child gender, and child weight status, a subset of the videotapes was coded for the present paper.

Videotapes of eighty mothers and their preschool children were selected. Mothers were chosen from the larger sample to create eight groups (with 10 mothers per group) making up each of the cells of a 2 X 2 X 2 design: maternal ethnicity (African-American vs. Latina) X child gender X child weight status (healthy weight vs. overweight or obese). A cell size of 10 was chosen because the smallest cell was made up of 10 African American mothers of overweight/obese female children. Therefore, 10 mothers were randomly chosen from each of the remaining seven cells. The number of participants in the cells we selected from ranged from 16 to 26 for mothers of healthy weight children and from 10 to 17 for mothers of overweight/obese children. Thirty nine percent of the children in the larger study were classified as overweight or obese. Eighty mother-child pairs was a sufficiently large sample size to detect a medium effect size (f=.25) with a power value of .89 [40].

Sample demographics are presented in Table 1. Children and adults were classified as healthy weight or overweight/obese based upon CDC criteria [41,42]. The second meal was chosen for coding because we expected more reactivity in the first observation and not all families were observed for a third meal.

TABLE 7.1 Characteristics of the Latina and African American mothers of preschoolers in Houston, Texas (n = 80)

	Frequencies
Ethnicity	
Latina	40
African-American	40
Education of Mother	
Less than High School Diploma	21
High School Diploma	19

TABLE 7.1 *(Continued)*

	Frequencies
Some College	32
College Graduate	6
Missing Data	2
Marital Status of Mother	
Married	31
Divorced	1
Separated	13
Never Married	27
Missing	8
Employment of Mother	
Employed Part-time	24
Employed Full-time	20
Not Employed	36
Child Gender	
Female	40
Male	40
Child BMI z score, Mean (SD)	1.02 (1.06)
Child Weight Status	
Healthy Weight (>5th to < 85thBMI percentile)	40
Overweight/Obese (BMI ≥ 85th percentile)	40
Mother BMI, Mean (SD)	31.12 (8.36)
Mother Weight Status	
Healthy Weight (18.5 kg/m^2 < BMI < 25 kg/m^2)	17
Overweight/Obese (BMI ≥ 25 kg/m^2)	63
Age, Mean in Years (SD)	
Parent	32.31 (7.49)
Child	4.51 (0.64)

7.2.2 PROCEDURES

As discussed in Hughes et al. [39], mothers were recruited through Head Start Centers and consented before participating in the study. All mothers were low income because as Head Start participants, families are required to be at or below the federal poverty level. Parents received an incentive (graduated in amount) at the end of each of the three observations. Parents were told to do what they normally do at dinner time and to feed their child as they usually do. Two cameras were placed in the room where the family planned to eat. One camera was directed so that the mother's face could be recorded and the other camera was directed so that mother/child interactions were in view. Cameras were turned on after the family sat down and food was served. Two live coders were also present during the meal while the cameras were recording the parent-child interactions. Although most observations took place at a kitchen or dining room table, five children were observed while eating on a couch or a chair in the living room. In all but eight cases, the mothers sat down and ate the meal with their child. Clearly the families were aware of the cameras; however, after a few minutes the families appeared to no longer pay attention to them. During nine observations, fathers were also present, but only maternal behavior was coded for this study. The study was reviewed and approved by the Institutional Review Board at Baylor College of Medicine.

7.2.3 Videotape Coding

All videotapes were transcribed in the language used by the mother and child (32 of the videotapes were in Spanish). Using the Noldus Observer software (Observer XT, Noldus Information Technology, Wageningen, Netherlands), videotapes were coded by four B.A. level employees (three were bilingual) blind to the purposes of the study. One quarter of the videotapes were coded independently by a second bilingual observer to assess inter-observer agreement. The coders were unaware of which observations had been selected for reliability assessment. Agreement was assessed with Cohen's kappa [43].

Employing event coding, all maternal and child verbalizations, along with a number of nonverbal behaviors, were coded with a system adapted from Baumrind and Black [44] and Cousins, Power, and Olvera [45]. The codes were mutually exclusive and exhaustive. They were developed by expanding on the systems used in these previous studies through examination and discussion of pilot videotapes. Data from only the maternal verbalizations and nonverbal behaviors are presented in the current paper (child verbalizations were not analyzed). As illustrated in Figure 1, all maternal attempts to influence child behavior and child attempts to influence maternal behavior were coded, along with all other verbalizations between mother and child. The maternal behaviors coded included positive strategies representative of responsive feeding practices, as well as controlling feeding strategies.

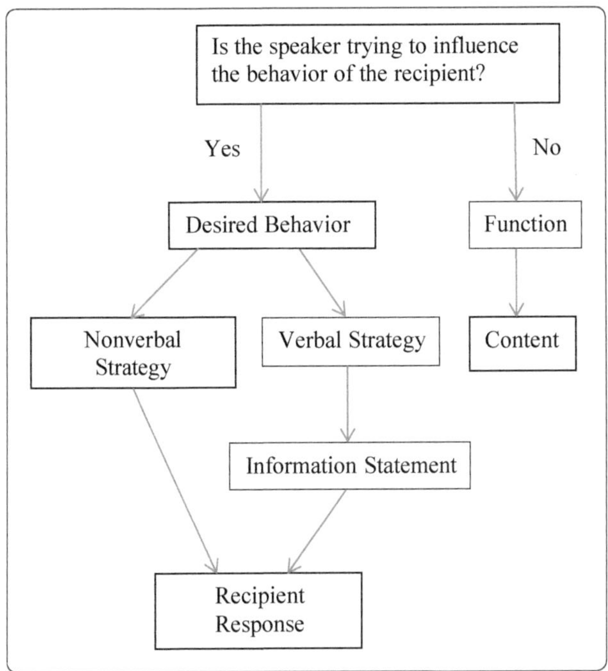

FIGURE 7.1 Flow chart representing videotape coding process.

The maternal behaviors chosen to assess responsive feeding practices in this study were: maternal references to internal hunger and fullness cues; discussion of foods and their characteristics; instruction in independent eating skills; enthusiastic modeling; and the use of non-directive, facilitating strategies to influence child eating (e.g., suggestions, questions, reasoning, helping) rather than more forceful, intrusive strategies (e.g., unelaborated commands, forces eating, spoon feeding). Nonresponsive feeding included frequent prompts to eat, forceful strategies, or a focus on table manners rather than teaching eating skills.

The variables and codes involving influence attempts analyzed for the current paper are listed in the following section. Kappa statistics for the various aspects of the coding system ranged from .72 to .86 with a mean of .77.

7.2.4 Codes Analyzed for Current Paper

I. Total Frequency of Maternal Attempts to Influence Child Behavior During Meal

II. Child Behaviors Mothers were Trying to Influence (i.e., Desired Behaviors)
   A. Encourage Eating
   B. Encourage Child to Eat All the Food on the Plate
   C. Encourage Child to Eat a Different Food
   D. Discourage Eating
   E. Enforce/Teach Table Manners
   F. Teach Eating Skills
   G. Internal Cues Reference to Encourage Eating
   H. Internal Cues Reference to Discourage Eating
   I. Other Food Related Behaviors (e.g., pass food, help sibling serve food)
   J. Non Food-Related Behaviors (e.g., discourage TV watching, be nice to sibling)

III. Maternal Verbal Strategies used to Influence Child Behavior
   A. Hint/Acknowledge
   B. Enthusiastic Modeling
   C. Question/Suggestion
   D. Praise
   E. Reason/Instruct
   F. Unelaborated Command
   G. Verbal Pressure (e.g., "You have to eat it")
   H. Disapprove/Scold
   I. Promise Food Rewards
   J. Threaten Food Punishments
   K. Promise Non-Food Rewards
   L. Threaten Non-Food Punishments

IV. Maternal Non-Verbal Strategies to Influence Child Behavior
   A. Moves Self Closer
   B. Moves Something Closer
   C. Points/Motions
   D. Helps

E. Spoon Feeds
F. Physically Forces

V. Total Frequency of Maternal Non-Influence Attempts

VI. Types of Non-Influence Attempts
A. References to Food Characteristics (e.g., appearance, smell, preparation)
B. References to Other Food-Related Content (e.g., food placement, utensils)
C. References to Target Child
D. References to Mother
E. References to Other People
F. References to Non-Food Related Content (e.g., "It's going to rain tomorrow.")
G. Clarification

7.2.5 Data Analysis

The variables for the analyses were the total frequency of influence and non-influence attempts, along with a number of proportions corresponding to the specific coding categories. Proportions were used for the main analyses because the total number of influence and non-influence attempts varied widely across families. For the influence attempts, separate proportions were calculated for the desired behavior categories, the verbal strategies, and the nonverbal strategies. The numerators for these proportions were the frequencies that a particular code occurred and the dominator for each was the total frequency of influence attempts (verbal plus nonverbal). For example, if a mother encouraged her child to eat 10 times during the observation and the total number of influence attempts was 50, the proportion for that mother was 0.20.

To examine ethnic, child gender, and child weight status differences in maternal behavior, five separate 2 X 2 X 2 MANOVAs (maternal ethnicity X child gender X child weight status) were run. The dependent variables for these five analyses were: 1) the frequencies of influence and non-influence attempts; 2) the proportion measures for eight of the desired behavior codes (the two internal cues references codes were not included due to low frequency of occurrence); 3) the proportion measures for six of the verbal strategy codes (praise, discourage/scold, and the four reward and punishment codes were not included due to low frequency of occurrence); 4) the proportion measures for the six nonverbal strategies; and 5) the proportion measures for the seven non-influence attempts codes. Approximate F statistics were calculated using Wilk's lamda. To help protect against Type I error, univariate effects (ANOVAs) were only examined if the corresponding multivariate effect was significant ($p < .05$).

7.3 RESULTS

Examination of the frequency distributions of the influence and non-influence attempts revealed one extreme outlier—one mother engaged in 200 influence attempts and 117 non-influence attempts during the dinnertime observation. This mother-child pair was dropped because her values were greater than four standard deviations above the mean. After dropping this observation, across families, the mean number of maternal influence attempts per observation was 34.2 and the mean number of non-influence attempts was 13.1 (see Table 2).

TABLE 7.2 Frequency of feeding behaviors of Latina and African American mothers of preschoolers during mealtime observations

Codes	Percent Non-Zero	Mean	SD	Range
Frequency of Influence Attempts	99	34.2	29.6	0-132
Desired Behaviors (proportion of total influence attempts)				
Encourage Eating	99	.42	.19	0-.90
Eat All	44	.03	.05	0-.21
Eat Different Food	45	.06	.11	0-.58
Discourage Eating	78	.09	.11	0-.67
Table Manners	76	.12	.11	0-.35
Eating Skills	60	.09	.12	0-.54
Internal Cues Encourage Eating	13	.01	.02	0-.13
Internal Cues Discourage Eating	18	.01	.02	0-.13
Other Food	70	.10	.11	0-.50
Non-Food	53	.07	.14	0-1.00
Verbal Strategies (proportion of total influence attempts)				
Hint/Acknowledge	62	.05	.06	0-.28
Enthusiastic Modeling	36	.02	.03	0-.15
Question/Suggest	95	.25	.16	0-.71
Praise	27	.01	.04	0-.27
Reason/Instruct	65	.07	.09	0-.50
Unelaborated Commands	99	.54	.18	0-1.00

TABLE 7.2 *(Continued)*

Codes	Percent Non-Zero	Mean	SD	Range
Verbal Pressure	44	.02	.03	0-.14
Discourage/Scold	14	.01	.02	0-.14
Food Rewards	12	.004	.01	0-.09
Food Punishments	9	.003	.01	0-.07
Non-Food Rewards	6	.001	.01	0-.04
Non-Food Punishments	22	.01	.03	0-.18
Non-Verbal Strategies (proportion of total influence attempts)				
Moves Self Closer	44	.04	.07	0-.37
Moves Something Closer	49	.04	.06	0-.33
Points/Motions	76	.11	.12	0-.75
Helps	45	.03	.05	0-.19
Spoon Feeds	22	.02	.05	0-.32
Physically Forces	37	.02	.04	0-.19
Frequency of Non-Influence Attempts	96	13.1	16.1	0-81
Content of Non-Influence Attempts (proportion of total non-influence attempts)				
Food Characteristics	46	.09	.12	0-.50
Other Food Content	64	.34	.31	0-1.00
References to Child	80	.32	.29	0-1.00
References to Mother	28	.03	.07	0-.50
References to Other People	32	.05	.10	0-.50
Non-Food References	32	.06	.13	0-.88
Clarification	54	.11	.18	0-1.00

Meals ranged in duration from seven to forty minutes, with a mean of 18.1 minutes (SD = 7.4). As expected, the frequency of influence attempts, $r(77) = .39$, $p < .001$, and non-influence attempts, $r(77) = .32$, $p < .001$, were positively correlated with the length of the meals.

7.3.1 Descriptive Analyses

7.3.1.1 Influence Attempts: Desired Behavior

Table 2 presents for each code, the percent of mothers who showed that behavior at least once ("percent non-zero"), along with the sample means, standard deviations, and ranges for the measures. The most common desired behavior by far was "encourage eating." This occurred at a mean rate over three times higher than the next desired behavior—"table manners." Other desired behaviors occurring less frequently were "teach the child eating skills," "discourage eating," and "other food-related" desired behaviors. A closer examination of the behaviors making up the discouraging eating category (data not presented in the table) showed that about 60% of these came toward the end of the meal when the parent was trying to get the child to finish the meal and stop eating. Requests for the child to eat all of the food on the plate and references to internal cues were uncommon.

7.3.1.2 Influence Attempts: Verbal Strategies

Table 2 shows that by far, the most common verbal strategy was "unelaborated commands," which occurred about twice as frequently as the next most common strategy, "question/suggestions." The third most common strategy was "reason/instruct" followed by "hint/acknowledge." All of the remaining strategies were very low in occurrence, including bribes and threats, praise and scolding, and enthusiastic modeling.

7.3.1.3 Influence Attempts: Nonverbal Strategies

As shown in Table 2, "points/motions" was by far the most common nonverbal strategy. The next two most common strategies were "moves self closer" and "moves something closer," followed by "helps," "spoon feeds," and "physically forces" which all occurred infrequently. The actual use of rewards and punishments was extremely low—bribes and threats were more common, but as mentioned above, occurred infrequently.

7.3.1.4 Non-influence Attempts: Content

The most common content that mothers referred to in their non-influence attempts was the target child. For example, a mother might say something such as "What did you do in school today?" As shown Table 2, mothers referred to the target child more often than they referred to other people or to themselves. Mothers frequently made references to food, but rarely to "food characteristics."

7.3.2 Differences in Maternal Behavior as a Function of Maternal Ethnicity, Child Gender, and Child Weight Status

The multivariate effect of maternal ethnicity only was significant for the desired behavior codes, $F(8, 63) = 5.26$, $p < .001$, $eta^2 = .40$. As shown in Table 3, examination of the univariate effects showed that Latina mothers scored higher on "encourage eating," "eat a different food," and "teach eating skills," whereas African American mothers scored higher on "eat all food," "discourage eating," "table manners," and "other food" desired behaviors. There was no significant ethnic difference in non-food influence attempts.

TABLE 7.3 Ethnic differences in desired behaviors[a]

Codes	African American M (SD)	Latina M (SD)	F(1, 70)	p ≤	eta²
Encourage Eating	.38 (.19)	.47 (.17)	4.68	.05	.06
Eat All	.04 (.06)	.02 (.04)	2.86	.10	.04
Eat Different Food	.03 (.06)	.09 (.14)	5.52	.05	.07
Discourage Eating	.13 (.13)	.05 (.07)	10.97	.001	.14
Table Manners	.14 (.11)	.09 (.10)	3.88	.05	.05
Eating Skills	.06 (.08)	.12 (.14)	5.18	.03	.07
Other Food	.13 (.11)	.07 (.10)	5.59	.02	.07
Non-Food	.07 (.09)	.08 (.18)	.10	ns	.001

[a]MANOVA significant – see text.

The multivariate effect for child gender only was significant for verbal strategies, $F(6,65) = 2.57$, $p < .05$, $eta^2 = .19$. This was due to two univariate differences: mothers used more unelaborated commands with their boys ($M = .61$, $SD = .18$) than their girls ($M = .47$, $SD = .16$), $F(1, 70) = 14.48$, $p < .001$, $eta^2 = .17$, and more questions/suggestions with their girls ($M = .30$, $SD = .17$) than their boys ($M = .20$, $SD = .14$), $F(1, 70) = 7.04$, $p < .01$, $eta^2 = .09$.

There were three significant multivariate effects involving child weight status: the child weight status main effect was significant for the frequency of influence/non-influence attempts, $F(2,70) = 3.19$, $p < .05$, $eta^2 = .08$, and for the desired behavior codes, $F(8,63) = 2.80$, $p = .01$, $eta^2 = .26$. The child weight status by ethnicity interaction, $F(2,70) = 5.98$, $p < .01$, $eta^2 = .15$, was significant for the frequency of influence and non-influence attempts.

Univariate analyses showed that mothers of healthy weight children engaged in more total influence attempts during the meal ($M = 40.82$, $SD = 32.50$)

than mothers of overweight or obese children ($M=27.72$, $SD=25.30$), $F(1,71)=3.80$, $p=.05$, $eta^2=.05$. Mothers of healthy weight children showed higher levels of encourage eating ($M=.48$, $SD=.19$) than mothers of overweight/obese children ($M=.37$, $SD=.17$), $F(1,70)=8.77$, $p<.01$, $eta^2=.11$. Mothers of overweight/obese children, in contrast, showed higher levels of discourage eating ($M=.12$, $SD=.14$) than mothers healthy weight children ($M=.06$, $SD=.06$), $F(1,70)=8.53$, $p<.01$, $eta^2=.11$.

Finally, the univariate interaction between maternal ethnicity and child weight status was significant for the total number of non-influence attempts, $F(1,71)=4.79$, $p<.05$, $eta^2=.06$. For Latina mothers, mothers of healthy weight children engaged in more total non-influence attempts ($M=16.84$, $SD=19.88$) than mothers of overweight or obese children ($M=8.50$, $SD=9.36$). In contrast, the opposite was true for African American mothers with mothers of healthy weight children engaging in fewer total non-influence attempts ($M=9.70$, $SD=6.97$) compared to mothers of overweight or obese children ($M=17.40$, $SD=21.97$).

There were no significant multivariate effects for the nonverbal strategies or the non-influence attempt content codes.

7.4 DISCUSSION

Together, these observational analyses show that many of the mothers in this sample did not employ feeding practices consistent with current recommendations for the feeding of young children [8-11], including the recommendations by the American Academy of Pediatrics [16]. Rather than providing children with food and then allowing them to decide what and how much to eat, a significant portion of the mothers in this sample spent considerable time encouraging their children to eat—often in spite of their insistence that they were finished (in data not presented here, 84% of the children indicated that they wanted to stop eating at some point during the mealtime observations—often multiple times). Mothers talked little about the food and its characteristics, rarely referred to feelings of hunger and fullness, and focused more on table manners than on teaching children eating skills. In trying to influence child behavior, mothers relied primarily on unelaborated commands and rarely used instruction, helping, reasoning, or praise. Overall, the focus of maternal behavior seemed more on ensuring that the child ate enough food and that the child exhibited proper behavior.

The degree to which mothers encouraged children to eat varied widely across the sample. Combining the frequencies of all of the encouraging eating codes (i.e., encourage eating, eat all, eat different food, and internal cues—encourage eating), the mean number of eating prompts was about 16 occurrences per mealtime observation—about half of all influence attempts observed. Examination of the frequency distributions showed that about one third of the mothers engaged in 16 or more eating prompts (the highest number was 91) (an authoritative or authoritarian feeding style), whereas about one quarter of the mothers engaged in 5 attempts or less (an indulgent or uninvolved style). Discouraging eating was not common—the mean occurrence was about three per dinnertime observation—less than nine percent of all influence attempts.

Several explanations can be offered for why many mothers encouraged eating even after the children indicated that they were done. First, for low income mothers, food security is often an issue [46]. When mothers are in a position to provide their child with a good meal, they may encourage their children to eat, even if the child has indicated that he or she is finished. Second, mothers may believe that it is important that their children consume enough food to meet their daily energy requirements and they may feel that they themselves are in a better position than their child to know when the child has eaten enough. Finally, mothers may encourage child eating at meals to save time, to prevent having to feed a hungry child later, or to ensure that the child does not go to bed hungry.

Examination of the data on non-influence attempts showed that mothers rarely commented on food characteristics—instead they focused primarily on the child's behavior and other food-related topics, such as "Do you want me to put some sauce on it?" By not commenting on food characteristics (getting the child to think and talk about the food's taste, texture, appearance, etc.), these mothers were missing opportunities to encourage children's interest in trying and developing preferences for new foods [13]. The same is true of maternal references to internal hunger or fullness cues. Only about a quarter of the mothers made any references to these internal cues, and among those who did, the vast majority made only one (or sometimes two) per observation (usually at the end of the meal to check to make sure that the child had eaten enough). By frequently encouraging children to eat without making references to these internal cues, mothers may be teaching children to ignore their internal cues of fullness, thereby interfering with the self-regulation of caloric intake [47].

Besides encouraging children to eat, most other maternal influence attempts focused on enforcing table manners. Influence attempts involving manners were common (about 75% of mothers enforced such rules). This is consistent with previous research on the importance of obedience to authority in low-income samples [48-50]. In addition to manners, about 60% of the mothers spent some time teaching eating skills. However, the use of helping and instruction was rare—these mothers relied mostly on unelaborated commands (e.g., "Be careful—don't spill your milk"). Again, the focus on encouraging proper behavior to the exclusion of encouraging independent eating skills is inconsistent with current recommendations.

Examination of how mothers tried to influence children's behavior showed that the only common strategies besides direct commands (about half of all maternal influence attempts) were questions and suggestions (about one quarter of all influence attempts). The high use of direct commands is consistent with other studies of low-income mothers [31,45]. Given that authoritative parenting has been shown to be a protective factor against the development of childhood obesity [4], increasing the use of reasoning, instruction, and praise are teachable skills that could be included in interventions related to parenting and feeding. Moreover, because less power-assertive methods of parental control ultimately elicit better child cooperation by allowing children greater autonomy and giving them the sense that they are involved in a reciprocal relationship [51,52], the use of less directive strategies such as questions and suggestions may be more successful in having a long-term impact on child eating behavior.

Interestingly, several feeding strategies that have received considerable attention in the literature-enthusiastic modeling [14], telling children to clean their plates [53], and using food as a reward [54] were each low frequency, accounting for a very small portion of influence attempts. Only about one third of the mothers made a positive comment about the taste of the food (enthusiastic modeling) or told the child to clean his or her plate, and only 12% of mothers promised food as a reward. So despite the numerous experimental studies that show that these strategies can affect children's self-regulation of intake and the development of food preferences, they may not be the strategies that actually do affect these outcomes in low income populations, given their low frequency of occurrence [55] (most of the experimental studies were conducted with middle class children). This suggests that experimental research on the effectiveness of less directive and more common feeding strategies during mealtimes may be worthwhile.

The only type of modeling examined in this study was "enthusiastic modeling," where mothers paired the eating of a desired food with a positive comment about it. It is likely that other types modeling not studied here (e.g., simply eating a desired food in the child's presence) are effective ways to influence child eating behavior [56]. Moreover, the use of food as a reward might occur more frequently in other situations outside of meals (e.g., motivating child behavior through snacks or treats between meals).

The differences we observed in maternal feeding behavior help replicate and/or extend previous work in this area. The greatest number of differences were for maternal ethnicity. Latina mothers showed higher levels of encouraging eating, getting their child to eat a different food, and encouraging the development of eating skills. African American mothers showed higher levels of discouraging eating, trying to get their children to eat all of the food on their plate, enforcing table manners, and trying to influence "other food-related" behaviors. Despite these ethnic differences in encouraging and discouraging eating, studies on BMI in young children show no significant differences in overweight and obesity rates between African American and Latino preschool children [1,3]. Therefore, the ethnic differences in feeding style identified here may not lead to differences in weight status across the groups (possibly due to ethnic differences in the food served). Similarly, the difference in encouraging eating a different food might be a function of differences in the foods served by mothers of the two ethnicities. This study, to our knowledge, is the first study to examine such ethnic differences in observed feeding behaviors, so it is important to replicate these findings in other samples, as well as examine how feeding behaviors interact with foods served in increasing or decreasing obesity risk.

The findings of this study are inconsistent with three previous studies that found that parents of boys encouraged eating more often in their boys than in their girls [29-31]. However, the finding that mothers of boys used more commands and mothers of girls used more questions/suggestions, is consistent with a study of older children that found that parents exerted more control over their boys than girls during mealtime [32]. A national study [3] showed that for both African American and Latina/o preschoolers, obesity rates were higher for boys than for girls. This difference may be due, in part, to parents' tendency to use more forceful strategies during mealtime with their boys than with their girls—thus overriding children's responsiveness to their internal cues of fullness.

Finally, the differences in child weight status are consistent with several self-report studies that show that parents of healthy weight children pressure their children to eat more frequently than parents of obese children [37,38]. This could be due to mothers of thinner "picky" eaters trying to increase child consumption, to mothers of overweight or obese children not having to pressure eating because their children eat on their own, or to mothers of overweight or obese children not pressuring eating because they are concerned about the child's weight status (or some combination of all three). The results are inconsistent with two smaller-scale studies by Klesges and colleagues who found a positive relationship between child obesity and the frequency of maternal eating prompts [33,34]. The results are also inconsistent with the hypothesis that children are at increased risk for obesity if their parents are highly controlling at mealtime (thereby decreasing children's responsiveness to internal cues of fullness). One possible reason for the studies that find no relationship between child weight status and observed maternal eating prompts [20,35,36] is that in the short run, parents may use high pressure tactics with healthy weight children who are "picky eaters," but in the long run, these high pressure practices—at least for some children—may lead to less child responsiveness to internal cues of fullness and subsequent increased obesity risk. In cross sectional studies such as those reviewed above, the operation of these two conflicting factors might cancel one another out and lead to no correlation between maternal eating prompts and child weight status. Clearly, the relationship between weight status and maternal feeding behavior is complex, and longitudinal research needs to be conducted to further understand these relationships—especially in light of a recent study by Rhee and colleagues who found, in a maternal self-report study, that controlling feeding practices become more common after, not before child weight gain [57].

Although these observational data provide a wealth of information not currently available on the feeding practices of low-income, minority mothers, they should be viewed within the limitations of the study. Only low-income, African-American and Latino mothers whose children were enrolled in Head Start participated. This sampling strategy excluded mothers of other social classes and ethnicities, along with mothers whose children did not participate in center-based childcare (e.g., stay at home mothers, children in family-based care). The fact that so few fathers were present also raises some concerns about representativeness, and future observational studies should investigate more directly the role of fathers e.g., [26].

Observational methods have their limitations as well [58,59]. First, observations of parent-child interactions do not provide insight into the inner thoughts of those observed. Second, parents and children may alter their behaviors just by the nature of being observed, often in a socially desirable direction. Third, observational methods may capture only a small snippet of interactions in time such as family dinners in the home. For example, most observations do not capture interactions in restaurants or fast food outlets and eating while watching TV or in automobiles. Furthermore, low frequency behaviors such as yelling at or punishing children are not usually captured through observations thus limiting the ability to generalize observations to the entire range of behaviors that parents practice. Despite these limitations, observations still comprise an optimal way to measure how parents feed their children (using positive versus negative affect when delivering messages) and what they are doing during eating occasions (e.g. asking questions, giving hints, delivering direct commands). Moreover, observational measures have repeatedly been shown to assess important individual differences in parent-child interaction that are powerful predictors of child development outcomes [21,22].

To address the issue of reactivity, future studies should increase the number of days that videotapes are made, and possibly have parents operate the video camera with no observers present [59]. To explore maternal motivations for adopting these practices, or the barriers that threaten adoption of more responsive feeding practices, future studies should combine observational with self-report methods (e.g., interviews, questionnaires, focus groups) to address these issues. Finally, given the bi-directional nature of mother-child interactions [60-62], future studies and analyses should examine the bi-directional nature of the feeding process.

7.5 CONCLUSIONS

These observational findings provide a detailed picture of mother-child interaction during mealtime in low-income families. They help identify areas that could be addressed in helping mothers engage in feeding practices that might reduce their children's obesity risk. These include: increasing maternal sensitivity and responsiveness to children's satiety cues; addressing over-controlling and indulgent feeding patterns; giving mothers strategies for focusing as much on the teaching of independent eating skills as they do on manners and etiquette; and encouraging greater mother-child conversation about food characteristics. Interventions to do this, however, need to be sensitive to the larger sociocultural context in which these practices occur [59,63].

Future research should examine these feeding practices in other populations that vary in ethnicity (e.g., European American and Asian American parents), education, and social class. Moreover, longitudinal research would help to examine the degree to which the patterns shown here, combined with data on children's diet and activity level, predict the development of childhood obesity. Given that most studies of responsive feeding have been conducted with middle-class, European American mothers, it is possible that different relationships with child health outcomes may emerge in lower income samples. Such information would be useful in helping develop programs that might facilitate healthy eating patterns and promote child health.

REFERENCES

1. Ogden CL, Carroll MD, Kit BK, Flegal KM. Prevalence of obesity and trends in body mass index among US children and adolescents, 1999–2010. J Amer Med Assoc. 2012;307:483–90.
2. Centers for Disease Control and Prevention. Overweight and obesity. Available at: http://www.cdc.gov/obesity/childhood/index.html. (Accessed August 29, 2013).
3. Anderson SE, Whitaker RC. Prevalence of obesity among US preschool children in different racial and ethnic groups. Arch Pediat Adol Med. 2009;163:344–8.
4. Sleddens EFC, Gerards SMPL, Thijs C, DeVries NK, Kremers SPJ. General parenting, child overweight, and obesity-inducing behaviors: a review. Int J Pediatr Obes. 2011;6:e12–27.
5. Hughes S, O'Connor T, Power T. Parenting and children's eating patterns: examining parental control in a broader context. Int J Child and Adolescent Health. 2008;1:323–30.
6. Harrist AW, Topham GL, Hubbs-Tait L, Page MC, Kennedy TS, Shriver LH. What developmental science can contribute to a transdisciplinary understanding of childhood obesity: an interpersonal and intrapersonal risk model. Child Dev Pers. 2012;6:445–55.
7. Frankel LA, Hughes SO, O'Connor TM, Power TG, Fisher JO, Hazen NL. Parental influences on children's self-regulation of energy intake: Insights from developmental literature on emotion regulation. J Obes. 2012;327259:1–12.
8. Black MM, Aboud FE. Responsive feeding is embedded in a theoretical framework of responsive parenting. J Nutr. 2011;141:490–4.
9. DiSantis KI, Hodges EA, Johnson SL, Fisher JO. The role of responsive feeding in overweight during infancy and toddlerhood: a systematic review. Int J Obesity. 2011;35:480–92.
10. Engle PL, Pelto GH. Responsive feeding: implications for policy and program implementation. J Nutr. 2011;141:508–11.
11. Satter E. The feeding relationship. J Am Diet Assoc. 1986;86:352–6.
12. Birch LL, Marlin DW. I don't like it; I never tried it: effects of exposure on two-year-old children's food preferences. Appetite. 1982;3:353–60.
13. View Article
14. Johnson SL, Bellows L, Beckstrom L, Anderson J. Evaluation of a social marketing campaign targeting preschool children. Am J Health Behav. 2007;31:44–55.
15. Hendy HM, Raudenbush B. Effectiveness of teacher modeling to encourage food acceptance in preschool children. Appetite. 2000;34:61–76.
16. Sigman-Grant M, Christiansen E, Branen L, Fletcher J, Johnson SL. About feeding children: mealtimes in child-care in four western states. J Am Diet Assoc. 2008;108:340–6.
17. Kleinman R. Pediatric nutrition handbook. Chapter 7: feeding the child and adolescent. 5th ed. USA: American Academy of Pediatrics; 2004. p. 119–36.
18. Hurley KM, Cross MB, Hughes SO. A systematic review of responsive feeding and child obesity in high-income countries. J Nutr. 2011;141:495–501.
19. Farrow C, Blissett J. Does maternal control during feeding moderate early infant weight gain? Pediatrics. 2006;118:293–8.
20. Worobey J, Lopez MI, Hoffman DJ. Maternal behavior and infant weight gain in the first year. J Nutr Educ Behav. 2009;41:169–75.
21. Lumeng JC, Ozbeki TN, Appugliese DP, Kaciroti N, Corwyn RF, Bradley RH. Observed assertive and intrusive maternal feeding behaviors increase child adiposity. Am J Clin Nutr. 2012;95:640–70.

22. Grotevant H, Carlson C. Family assessment: a guide to methods and measures. New York, NY: Guilford Press; 1989.
23. Kerig P, Lindahl K. Family observational coding systems: resources for systemic research. Mahwah, NJ: Lawrence Erlbaum; 2001.
24. Nisbett RE, Winston TD. Telling more than we can know: verbal reports on mental processes. Psychol Rev. 1977;84:231–59.
25. Straus M. Measuring families. In: Christensen H, editor. Handbook of marriage and the family. Chicago, IL: Rand McNally; 1964.
26. Stansbury K, Haley D, Lee JA, Brophy-Herb HE. Adult caregivers' behavioral responses to child noncompliance in public settings: gender differences and the role of positive and negative touch. Behav Soc Iss. 2012;21:80–114.
27. Haycraft EI, Blissett JM. Maternal and paternal controlling feeding practices: reliability and relationships with BMI. Obesity. 2008;16:1552–8.
28. Hughes SO, Power TG, Fisher JO, Mueller S, Nicklas TA. Revising a neglected construct: parenting styles in a child-feeding context. Appetite. 2005;44:83–92.
29. Tovar A, Hennessy E, Pirie A, Must A, Gute DM, Hyatt RR, et al. Feeding styles and child weight status among recent immigrant mother-child dyads. Int J Behav Nutr Phy. 2012; 9:62.
30. Farrow C, Blissett J, Haycraft E. Does child weight influence how mothers report their feeding practices? Int J Pediatr Obes. 2011;6:306–13.
31. Orrell-Valente JK, Hill LG, Brechwald WA, Dodge KA, Pettit GS, Bates JE. "Just three more bites": an observational analysis of parents' socialization of children's eating at mealtime. Appetite. 2007;48:37–45.
32. Olvera-Ezzell N, Power TG, Cousins JH. Maternal socialization of children's eating habits: strategies used by obese, Mexican-American mothers. Child Dev. 1990;61:395–400.
33. Moens E, Braet C, Soetens B. Observation of family functioning at mealtime: a comparison between families of children with and without overweight. J Pediatr Psychol. 2007;32:52–63.
34. Klesges RC, Coates TJ, Brown G. Parental influences on children's eating behavior and relative weight. J Appl Behav Anal. 1983;16:371–8.
35. Klesges RC, MNarlott J, Boschee P, Weber J. The effects of parental influences on children's food intake, physical activity, and relative weight. Int J Eat Disorder. 1986;5:335–46.
36. Birch LL, Marlin DW, Kramer L, Peyer C. Mother-child interaction patterns and degree of fatness in children. J Nutr Educ. 1981;13:18–21.
37. Khandpur N, Blaine RE, Fisher JO, Davison KK. Fathers' child feeding practices: a review of the evidence. Appetite. 2014;78:110–21.
38. Birch LL, Fisher JO, Grimm-Thomas K, Markey CN, Sawyer R, Johnson SL. Confrimatory factor analysis of the child feeding questionnaire: a measure of parental attitudes, beliefs, and practices about child feeding and obesity proneness. Appetite. 2001;36:201–10.
39. Galloway AT, Fiorita LM, Francis LA, Birch LL. 'Finish your soup': counterproductive effects of pressuring children to eat on intake and affect. Appetite. 2006;46:318–23.
40. Hughes SO, Power TG, Papaioannou M, Cross M, Nicklas T, Hall S, et al. Emotional climate, feeding behaviors, and feeding styles: an observational analysis of the dinner meal in head start families. Int J Behav Nutr Phy. 2011;8:60.
41. Cohen J. Statistical power analysis for the behavioral sciences. Mahwah, NJ: Lawrence Erlbaum; 1988.

42. Centers for Disease Control and Prevention. CDC Growth Charts: United States. Hyattsville, MD: National Center for Health Statistics, U.S. Dept of Health and Human Services; 2000.
43. World Health Organization Expert Committee. Physical status: The Use and interpretation of anthropometry. WHO technical report series: 854. Geneva: World Health Organization; 1995.
44. Cohen J. A coefficient of agreement for nominal scales. Educ Psychol Meas. 1960;20:37–46.
45. Baumrind D, Black AE. Socialization practices associated with dimensions of competence in preschool boys and girls. Child Dev. 1967;38:291–327.
46. Cousins JH, Power TG, Olvera-Ezzell N. Mexican-American mothers' socialization strategies: the effects of education, acculturation, and health locus of control. J Exp Child Psychol. 1993;55:258–76.
47. Alaimo K, Olson CM, Frongillo EA, Briefel RR. Food insufficiency, family income, and health in US preschool and school-aged children. Am J Public Health. 2001;91:781–6.
48. Johnson SL. Improving preschoolers' self-regulation of energy intake. Pediatrics. 2000;106:1429–35.
49. Baumrind D. An exploratory study of socialization effects on black children: some black-white comparisons. Child Dev. 1972;43:261–7.
50. Kelley ML, Power TG, Wimbush DD. Determinants of parenting in low-income, black mothers. Child Dev. 1992;63:573–82.
51. Kohn ML. Class and conformity. Chicago: University of Chicago Press; 1963.
52. Parpal M, Maccoby EE. Maternal responsiveness and subsequent child compliance. Child Dev. 1985;56:1326–34.
53. Power TG, Manire SH. Child rearing and internalization: a developmental perspective. In: Janssens J, Gerris J, editors. Child rearing: influence on prosocial and moral development. Amsterdam: Swets & Zeitlinger B.V; 1992.
54. Birch LL, McPhee L, Shoba BC, Steinberg L, Krehbiel R. "Clean up your plate": effects of child feeding practices on the conditioning of meal size. Learn Motiv. 1987;18:301–17.
55. Birch LL, Birch D, Marlin DW, Kramer L. Effects of instrumental consumption on children's food preference. Appetite. 1982;3:125–34.
56. McCall RB. Challenges to a science of developmental psychology. Child Dev. 1977;48: 333–44.
57. Ventura AK, Birch LL. Does parenting affect children's eating and weight status? Int J Behav Nutr Phy. 2008;5:15.
58. Rhee KE, Coleman SM, Appugliese DP, Kaciroti NA, Corwyn RF, Davidson NS, et al. Maternal feeding practices become more controlling after and not before excessive rates of weight gain. Obesity. 2012;17:1724–9.
59. Gardner F. Methodological issues in the direct observation of parent-child interaction: Do observational findings reflect the natural behavior of participants? Clin Child Fam Psych. 2000;3:185–98.
60. Power TG, Sleddens EFC, Berge J, Connell L, Govig B, Hennessy E, et al. Contemporary research on parenting: conceptual, methodological, and translational issues. Child Obes. 2013;9:S87–94.
61. Bell RQ, Chapman M. Child effects in studies using experimental or brief longitudinal approaches to socialization. Dev Psychol. 1986;22:595–603.

62. Sameroff AJ. Transactional models in early social relations. Hum Dev. 1975;18:65–79.
63. Lollis S, Kuczynski L. Beyond one hand clapping: seeing bidirectionality in parent-child relations. J Soc Pers Relat. 1997;14:441–61.
64. Delormier T, Frohlich KL, Potvin L. Food and eating as social practice: understanding eating patterns as social phenomena and implications for public health. Sociol Health Ill. 2009;31:215–28.

CHAPTER 8

Overweight Among Students Aged 11–15 Years and Its Relationship with Breakfast, Area of Residence and Parents' Education: Results from the Italian HBSC 2010 Cross-Sectional Study

Giacomo Lazzeri, Mariano Vincenzo Giacchi, Angela Spinelli, Andrea Pammolli, Paola Dalmasso, Paola Nardone, Anna Lamberti, and Franco Cavallo

8.1 BACKGROUND

The increase in overweight and obesity among children and adolescents in both developed and developing countries over the past three decades confirm that childhood obesity is a global 'epidemic' [1–4]. The World Health Organization (WHO) considers childhood obesity to be a major public health concern [5]. Childhood obesity is associated with cardiovascular, endocrine, pulmonary, musculoskeletal and gastrointestinal complications, and may have psycho-social consequences (poor self esteem, depression, eating disorders) [6].

One of the most important nutritional factors is breakfast, the first of the three main meals of the day [7]. Skipping breakfast has been associated with increased probability of being overweight both in children and adults [8, 9]. Prospective studies have confirmed this association in adolescents [10].

Obesity is a multi-factorial disorder originating from the interaction between genetics and environment [11–13]. The accumulation of body fat is a very complex phenomenon regulated by a series of physiological mechanisms, some of which are still unknown. Family lifestyles have a big impact on the nutritional and behavioural choices of children, together with social and economic factors, such as place of residence, parental educational level and economic affluence [14]. It is well known that there is an inverse relationship between socio-economic conditions and health status in developed countries [15]. Specifically, studies have also shown an inverse relationship between children's Body Mass Index (BMI) and family educational level [14, 16].

Recent data comparing the Italian national data with the other 13 European countries participating in the WHO Europe Childhood Obesity Surveillance Initiative (COSI) show that Italy had the highest prevalence of overweight and obesity among children aged 8–9 [17]. Moreover, several surveys conducted at local or regional level, in Italy, have found geographic differences in pediatric obesity prevalence [18–20], although its magnitude has been difficult to evaluate because of the differences in methods and definitions, and the limited geographic coverage. The only study that presents estimates of overweight and obesity prevalence in Italian primary school children by regions is "OKkio alla SALUTE", a national surveillance system in which more than 45,000 third-grade (8–9 year old) students are measured every two years [21–23]. These data show a clear geographic trend of overweight and obesity prevalence increasing from North to South and the influence of demographic characteristics. In 2010, for the first time in Italy, the Health Behaviour in School-aged Children (HBSC) study was conducted on regionally representative samples. This paper presents the results on the prevalence of overweight and obesity in 58,928 Italian children (aged 11,13, and 15 years) by geographic area of residence. It also evaluates the association between childhood and adolescent overweight (including obesity) and gender, parental education and breakfast consumption. These results can be compared with those obtained for children aged 8–9 years obtained from "OKkio alla SALUTE" surveillance. It is important to get information at these older ages because most of these adolescents have already had their pubertal development and are more independent in their nutritional and physical activity choices.

8.2 METHODS

Data were collected in accordance with the HBSC international protocol developed and regularly updated by the research group, with the participation of research workers from each member state. HBSC is a WHO collaborative cross-sectional study, involving research teams across Europe and North America, with the aim of gaining insight into adolescents' health and health behaviour. It collects data every four years on 11, 13 and 15-year-old boys' and girls' health and well-being, social environment and health behavior. The protocol describes the methods for performing the survey, the rules to be followed and coding procedures for the data collected [24, 25]. All participating countries must adhere to the detailed version of the protocol. In Italy, in contrast with the two previous rounds of HBSC, all regions decided to have their own representative sample to allow comparisons at regional level.

8.2.1 Sampling

According to the rules agreed internationally, one-stage cluster sampling was used with classes within schools as primary sampling unit. Schools and classes were stratified by region and in each of them by grade (middle and high schools) [26, 27]. The selection of the classes was made using sampling with probability proportional to size and the sample size for each region was about 1,200 children for each age 11, 13 and 15 years, corrected for the general population of students. Over-sampling from 10% to 25% was applied in each age group to compensate for the differences in the children's ages and for those expected to refuse to participate.

8.2.2 Data Collection

Data collection began in late November 2009 and lasted until the end of May 2010. All Italian regions were involved, but Veneto carried out the survey independently and Piedmont, which carried out the survey in 2009, in agreement with the coordination group, did not deem it necessary to repeat it after such a short time. To collect data, a self-reported anonymous questionnaire, prepared by the international HBSC network, was used. Data were collected by trained health workers in collaboration with the school teachers. Further details of the methodology of the Italian HBSC 2010 study are provided elsewhere [27].

8.2.3 Variables

Variables included in the analyses were: children's age, gender, weight, height, region of residence, breakfast consumption and parental educational level.

Children's BMI (kg/m^2) was calculated using self-reported weight and height, and body weight status was assessed according to Cole's classification, as recommended by the International Obesity Task Force [28, 29], in four categories: underweight (U), normal-weight (N), overweight (Ow) and obese (O). In these analyses, we have also considered overweight including obesity (OwO).

Regions of residence were grouped into northern, central and southern areas using the Italian National Statistics Institute classification [30].

On the basis of the strong correlation between educational status and income in Italy [31], the higher educational level of the mother or father was used as a proxy of socio-economic status. Responses to the question on education were grouped: less than high school, high school, university degree or more.

To assess breakfast consumption, adolescents were asked to indicate, in a normal week, how many days in weekdays and in weekends they had breakfast (defined as having more than a glass of milk or fruit juice). Response categories were "never" to "five days" for the weekdays, and "never" to "two days" for the weekend. The number of weekdays and weekend days were summed and dichotomized into "daily breakfast consumption" (seven days in a week) vs. "less than daily" (less than seven days in a week).

8.2.4 Data Analysis

A central automatic data entry system was used. Cases were deleted if gender and/or age were missing. Exclusion criteria in the analyses were age outside the range of ± 6 months compared to the average age of its own stratum, and abnormal values for weight and/or height (5 Kg below 3rd or 30 Kg above the 97th percentile; 5 cm below 3rd or 5 cm above the 97th percentile) [24]. Overweight and obesity prevalence rates and 95% Confidence Intervals (CI) were estimated separately by age and gender [24]. Multiple logistic regressions were performed to assess the relationship between overweight (including obesity) as the dependent variable, and parental education, area of residence and breakfast consumption as independent variables (each model was adjusted simultaneously for parental education, breakfast consumption and children's residence area). All analyses were conducted taking into account the survey design (including stratification, clustering and weighting) using STATA 12.1 SE Surveys routines.

8.2.5 Ethical Aspects

Parents had to consent to the participation of their children in the HBSC survey. The Ethics Committee of the National Institute of Health, which approved the protocol and instruments of the Italian HBSC 2010 study, agreed to the use of an opt-out consent form, in which parents were asked to explicitly refuse permission to participate and the lack of a returned form was taken to imply consent. Since the HBSC survey aims to collect data relating to the population and avoids the identification of individuals, the students answered the questionnaires anonymously. As per protocol, questionnaires, once completed, were collected and immediately placed in a sealed envelope by a health workers. All information collected cannot be traced to the individual student.

8.3 RESULTS

Overall, the Italian HBSC 2010 survey included 2,504 schools and 77,113 students. After data screening and applying the inclusion criteria, over 58,000 students (76.4% of the total) were considered eligible for the analysis. Table 1 shows the main characteristics of the sample. Each age group represented almost one-third of the sample with a 1:1 male:female ratio. Almost half of them were resident in the South (49.6%), a third in the North (33.8%) and 16.6% in Central Italy. Regarding parents' education, 28% of students had at least one parent with a University degree. On average boys were younger, tend to be resident in the north and have more educated parents. Less than 50% of 11-15 yrs schoolchildren had breakfast every day; in particular girls had a lower percentage than boys (44.1% vs. 51.4%). The overall combined prevalence of overweight and obesity was 20.9% according to IOTF criteria, while the prevalence of obesity alone was 3.4%, with higher values among boys (Ow: 21.5% and O: 4.8% vs. Ow: 13.6% and O: 2.0%among girls).

TABLE 8.1 Socio-demographic characteristics of study participants by gender

		Boys		Girls		All	
		N	%	N	%	N	%
Age	**11 y**	10600	37.4	10128	34.1	20728	35.7
	13 y	10244	34.0	10417	35.2	20661	34.6
	15 y	8459	28.6	9080	30.7	17539	29.7
	Total	29303	100	29625	100	58928	100
Geographicarea of residence	**North**	11823	34.2	11954	33.4	23777	33.8
	Centre	6451	17.4	6110	15.8	12561	16.6
	South	11029	48.4	11561	50.8	22590	49.6
	Total	29303	100	29625	100	58928	100
Parental education attainment°	**Less than high school**	7169	33.1	8264	38.0	15433	35.6
	High school diploma	8906	36.4	9038	36.5	17944	36.4
	University degree	7305	30.5	6472	25.5	13777	28.0
	Total	23380	100	23774	100	47154	100
	Missing	5923	20.6	5851	19.0	11774	19.8
	Daily	15487	51.4	13707	44.1	29194	47.8
Breakfast	**Less than daily**	13603	48.6	15717	55.9	29320	52.2
	Total	29090	100.0	29424	100.0	58514	100.0
	Missing	213	0.7	201	0.6	414	0.6
	Underweight	403	1.7	796	3.0	1199	2.4
	Normal-weight	17715	72.1	20200	81.4	37915	76.7
BMI	**Overweight**	4337	21.5	2857	13.6	7194	17.5
	Obese	849	4.8	426	2.0	1275	3.4
	Total	23304	100.0	24279	100.0	47583	100.0
	Missing	5999	20.9	5346	19.2	11345	20.0

°Higher educational level between mother and father.

Table 2 presents weight status prevalence rates by age, gender and geographical area. At every age and in all geographical areas, boys were more likely to be overweight (including obesity). Overall 28.1% of boys and 18.8% of girls aged 11 yrs-old, 24.8% and 16.5% aged 13 yrs, and 25.4% vs. 11.7% aged 15 yrs were overweight or obese. A geographical trend was found in both boys and girls and in all age groups: overweight and obesity rates increase from North to South. Among girls a lower percentage was overweight (including obesity) in the group of 15-year olds (11.7%, 95% CI: 10.6%-13.4%) compared both with the group aged 13 years (16.5%, 95% CI: 15.0%-18.3%) and 11 years (18.8%, 95% CI: 17.1%-20.7%), whereas boys showed the lowest prevalence at thirteen years (24.8%, 95% CI: 22.8%-27.0%), an intermediate prevalence at 15 years (25.4%, 95% CI: 23.1%-27.4%) and then the highest prevalence in youngest, 11 years old (28.1%, 95% CI: 26.0%-30.2%).

The lowest value of overweight including obesity in Italy in 2010 was found in the Northern 15 yrs-old girls (7.1%, 95%CI:5.5%-8.7%) and the highest in the Southern 11 yrs-old boys (36.0%, 95%CI: 33.2%-39.4%). Overall the regions with highest and lowest prevalence were Campania and the Province of Bolzano (Figure 1).

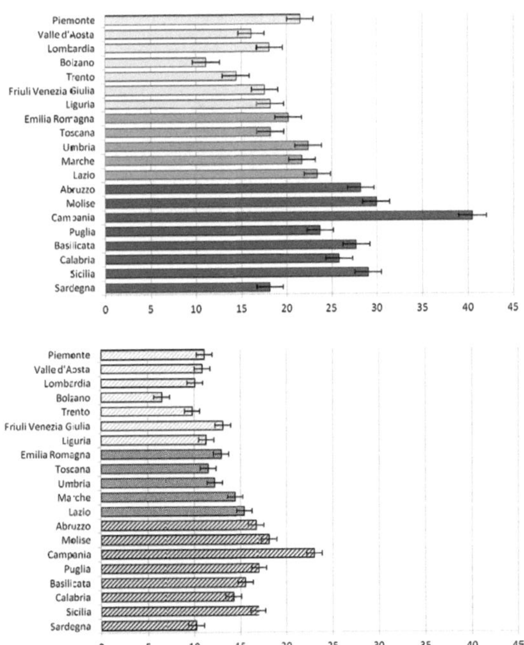

FIGURE 8.1 Prevalence of OwO in the Italian regions by gender.

TABLE 8.2 Prevalence of underweight (U), normal-weight (N), overweight (Ow) and obesity (O) by students' age, gender and residence area, Italy, 2010

Age		Boys				Girls			
		U	N	OW	O	U	N	OW	O
		% (95% CI)	% (95% CI)	% (95% CI)	% (95% CI)	% (95% CI)	% (95% CI)	% (95% CI)	% (95% CI)
11 y									
	North	1.9 (1.17-2.91)	79.3 (76.60-81.77)	14.5 (12.65-16.65)	4.3 (3.17-5.85)	3.3 (2.23-4.72)	83.5 (80.72-85.92)	11.6 (9.39-14.35)	1.6 (1.00-2.62)
	Center	2.3 (1.47-3.72)	72.4 (68.50-75.95)	21.3 (18.41-24.60)	3.9 (2.76-5.59)	3.9 (2.44-6.13)	80.2 (76.65-83.36)	13.5 (10.84-16.72)	2.4 (1.46-3.84)
	South	2.5 (1.78-3.44)	61.5 (58.53-64.43)	28.5 (25.54-31.68)	7.5 (6.01-9.28)	3.4 (2.50-4.65)	72.6 (69.75-75.31)	21.1 (18.66-23.76)	2.9 (2.01-4.07)
	Total	2.2 (1.75-2.82)	69.7 (67.58-71.76)	22.3 (20.41-24.24)	5.8 (4.90-6.85)	3.4 (2.76-4.24)	77.7 (75.85-79.42)	16.5 (14.94-18.28)	2.3 (1.82-3.02)
13 y									
	North	1.5 (0.88-2.60)	80.0 (77.17-82.59)	15.4 (13.24-17.90)	3.0 (2.11-4.35)	2.9 (2.00-4.21)	85.3 (82.90-87.32)	10.1 (8.49-12.01)	1.7 (0.98-3.05)
	Center	1.2 (0.62-2.41)	79.8 (75.84-83.19)	16.2 (13.32-19.51)	2.8 (1.87-4.28)	3.8 (2.52-5.57)	83.0 (79.84-85.66)	12.2 (9.88-15.05)	1.1 (0.53-2.10)
	South	1.7 (1.13-2.67)	67.0 (63.42-70.30)	25.7 (22.70-28.90)	5.6 (3.77-8.32)	2.1 (1.40-3.13)	77.5 (74.80-80.06)	17.2 (14.95-19.72)	3.2 (2.25-4.42)
	Total	1.6 (1.16-2.15)	73.6 (71.39-75.76)	20.5 (18.70-22.48)	4.3 (3.23-5.62)	2.6 (2.05-3.29)	80.9 (79.16-82.49)	14.1 (12.71-15.68)	2.4 (1.81-3.15)
15 y									
	North	1.8 (0.96-3.17)	79.4 (76.58-82.03)	16.3 (13.78-19.25)	2.5 (1.60-3.82)	3.5 (2.44-4.86)	89.5 (87.48-91.22)	6.4 (5.07-7.95)	0.7 (0.36-1.33)
	Center	1.6 (0.85-2.81)	78.4 (75.34-81.25)	18.3 (15.48-21.56)	1.7 (0.94-3.00)	3.6 (2.46-5.32)	82.9 (79.44-85.79)	12.6 (9.83-16.02)	0.9 (0.44-1.90)
	South	1.0 (0.58-1.73)	67.4 (63.60-71.04)	25.9 (22.62-29.56)	5.6 (4.20-7.50)	2.9 (2.14-3.89)	83.2 (80.97-85.18)	12.1 (10.08-14.44)	1.8 (1.21-2.77)
	Total	1.3 (0.95-1.89)	73.3 (71.02-75.40)	21.5 (19.51-23.62)	3.9 (3.08-4.93)	3.2 (2.61-3.88)	85.1 (83.60-86.40)	10.4 (9.14-11.88)	1.3 (0.95-1.86)

The importance of the area of residence is confirmed in the multiple logistic regression models (Table 3). Children living in southern Italy showed a significantly doubled risk of overweight (OwO) compared with those living in North (OR=2.05, CI 1.77-2.38 in boys and OR=2.04, 95% CI 1.70-2.44 in girls). Overweight (OwO) and parent's educational level were inversely associated: students with both parents in the lower educational level are more likely to be overweight than those with at least one parent with the highest educational level (OR=1.63, 95% CI: 1.38-1.91 in boys; OR=2.07, 95%CI: 1.70-2.51 in girls). This relationship is significant and consistent across gender and age groups (Table 3). Among all age groups and both in girls and boys, less than daily breakfast consumption was found to be associated with overweight (OwO) (OR=1.33, 95% CI: 1.16-1.51 in boys; OR=1.58, 95% CI: 1.38-1.82 in girls). Because nearly 20% of replies on educational level were missing, multiple regression analyses were also performed stratified by age and gender including the non-responders recoded as "other" category. The results of these analyses showed the same overall conclusions as main analyses, but with slightly attenuated associations (data not shown).

8.4 DISCUSSION

This study, which used standardized methods and equipment, is the only recent population-based investigation of BMI in 11-15 years old students in Italy where it is possible to make comparisons between regions. In addition to a high prevalence of overweight and obesity in the overall population, which is higher than that of most Western countries [25], there were substantial geographic differences, with the prevalence of obesity twice as high in the South as in the North. Both the overall high prevalence and the geographic disparities have profound implications for the country's healthcare system now and in the future.

Breakfast is not only the first, but also an important meal for both nutritional and familial reason. To take breakfast may be beneficial to the body and mind and to skip it may lead to consumption of snacks and to overeating by lunchtime [32]. Our finding of a negative association between regular breakfast consumption with overweight fits well with the literature. Disparities in breakfast consumption across regions may be explained by differences in cultural practices, socio-economic factors and availability of school-breakfast programs. Daily breakfast consumption (DBC) was related to all socio-demographic factors examined. We found that girls more often skipped breakfast than boys. This is in

TABLE 8.3 Association of parental education, students' residence area and breakfast consumption with overweight (OwO)—(multiple logistic regression), Italy, 2010

	Prevalence of overweight including obesity (OwO)															
	11 y				13 y				15 y				All age group			
	Boys		Girls		Boys		Girls		Boys		Girls		Boys		Girls	
	OwO %	OR (95% CI)	OwO %	OR (95% CI)	OwO %	OR (95% CI)	OwO %	OR (95% CI)	OwO %	OR (95% CI)	OwO %	OR (95% CI)	OwO %	OR (95% CI)	OwO %	OR (95% CI)
Parental educational level																
Less than high school	34.4	1.52* (1.18-1.96)	24.3	2.05* (1.47-2.85)	28.6	1.62* (1.19-2.20)	21.7	2.02* (1.44-2.82)	32.0	1.82* (1.37-2.42)	16.7	2.17* (1.54-3.08)	31.5	1.63* (1.38-1.91)	20.4	2.07* (1.70-2.51)
High school	26.8	1.16 (0.91-1.48)	18.5	1.54* (1.09-2.16)	25.3	1.48* (1.11-1.97)	15.7	1.46* (1.02-2.09)	24.4	1.28 (1.00-1.64)	10.6	1.34 (0.94-1.92)	25.3	1.27* (1.10-1.48)	14.2	1.39* (1.14-1.70)
University	22.9	Referent group	12.5	Referent group	18.3	Referent group	11.3	Referent group	19.8	Referent group	7.9	Referent group	20.5	Referent group	10.4	Referent group
Residence area																
North	18.9	Referent group	13.3	Referent group	18.5	Referent group	11.9	Referent group	18.8	Referent group	7.1	Referent group	18.7	Referent group	10.8	Referent group
Centre	25.8	1.68* (1.20-2.35)	16.3	1.56* (1.09-2.22)	20.3	1.25 (0.91-1.71)	13.7	1.43* (1.01-2.03)	20.3	1.26 (0.97-1.63)	13.8	2.45* (1.73-3.47)	22.1	1.35* (1.14-1.61)	14.5	1.73* (1.40-2.13)
South	36.2	2.49* (1.91-3.24)	24.1	2.07* (1.52-2.82)	31.2	1.77* (1.37-2.27)	20.4	2.03* (1.51-2.73)	31.3	2.02* (1.57-2.58)	14.1	2.08* (1.54-2.80)	33.0	2.05* (1.77-2.38)	19.2	2.04* (1.70-2.44)
Breakfast consumption																
Daily	24.9	Referent group	13.5	Referent group	22.0	Referent group	13.1	Referent group	21.5	Referent group	8.4	Referent group	23.0	Referent group	12.7	Referent group
Less than daily	32.1	1.33* (1.07-1.65)	22.8	1.88* (1.44-2.44)	28.0	1.29* (1.01-1.63)	19.3	1.61* (1.28-2.01)	28.5	1.41* (1.11-1.77)	13.9	1.71* (1.34-2.19)	29.5	1.33* (1.16-1.51)	18.0	1.58* (1.38-1.82)

Odd ratios and 95% CIs were calculated from logistic regression models stratified by age and gender. Each model was adjusted simultaneously for parental education, breakfast consumption and students' residence area.

*$p < 0.05$.

line with previous studies [33] which showed lower prevalence of DBC among girls than boys in most Italian regions [33] and in other countries [14, 15, 34, 35]. The lower DBC in older student compared to 11 year olds is also consistent with previous studies. This age related decline in DBC could be explained by important changes that accompany adolescence including greater autonomy and independence in food choices, decreased frequency of family meals and also increased dieting, especially among girls. These findings emphasize the need for a community-level approach to prevention and health promotion which is not limited to children who are currently overweight or obese.

The geographic gradient in pediatric obesity is also seen for a wide variety of other pediatric health indicators in Italy, with the highest prevalence of most adverse outcomes found in the eight Regions of southern Italy, intermediate levels in the four central regions, and low levels in the seven regions and two autonomous Provinces of the north [22]. Bonati et al., investigating regional inequalities in child health, identified educational level, poverty and access and efficiency of health services as major determinants of this geographic gradient [36].

Our data also show a clear difference in the prevalence of overweight and obesity by age and by gender. As found in all European countries participating in the HBSC international survey, males are more likely to be overweight and obese than females, and this difference increases with increasing age [25]. The total prevalence of overweight including obesity observed in this study in children aged 11, 13 and 15 years are lower than that found in Italian children aged 8–9 years, which was 34.2% [23]. A decrease in prevalence by age is present among girls, reaching about one in ten at age 15. These trends may be due to gender differences in food choices and dietary concerns, as well as overall physical activity levels. Moreover, being thin is highly valued in Western society adolescents, in particular among females for whom it is associated with beauty. This highlights the need for a clearer focus on the environmental influences and gender differences in childhood and adolescent obesity among both researchers and policy makers.

The HBSC Italian study, based on more than 50,000 adolescents, confirms the importance of parents' low educational level as a risk factor for overweight including obesity. The influence of this factor was found in all three age groups and was higher among girls [15]. In addition, we have found a negative association between regular breakfast consumption and overweight, as reported in other studies [7, 8, 37] . Not eating breakfast was especially high in the South and shows a higher prevalence among girls [38, 39].

8.4.1 Strengths and limitations

Our study has some limitations. The cross-sectional design of the study did not allow us to determine clearly the cause/effect of the relationships among the study variables; longitudinal designs might help determine the direction of these relationships. Combining overweight and obesity is another limitation of the study. Behaviors of obese students and their parents may be significantly different from those who are overweight, but not obese, even if the prevalence of obese students is very low. We did not investigate if the parent with higher education attainment was available at home. If he or she were not available at home, the impact of his/her education/knowledge on the child's behavior may be low [40]. In addition, the analyses are not adjusted for other important nutritional factors (for example consumption of high calorific snacks or sugar-sweetened beverages) because data on snacks were not recorded in the survey and many responses to the question on sugar-sweetened beverages were missing. This may lead to the effect of breakfast consumption to be overestimated [37]. The results of our study are based on self reported data that could be subject to socially desirable reporting bias. However, students' responses were anonymous, therefore participants had no reason to deliberately misreport the information, in particular their height or weight. According to some authors, BMI based on self-reported data can produce lower prevalence estimates of overweight and obesity than those based on actual height and weight measurements [41, 42] while others have reported high accuracy for the classification of youth as obese or non-obese based on self-reported data [43, 44]. The problem of the high level of non-responders (nearly 20%) was evaluated using a sensitivity analysis which showed similar results.

The main strength of the study is the use of a large and representative Italian sample which allows regional comparison and also with other countries participating in the HBSC study.

8.5 CONCLUSION

In conclusion, Italy appears to have a major childhood and adolescent obesity problem that is differentially affecting the three areas of the country and is more severe among boys. A comprehensive strategy to prevent obesity in both children and adults has been a central element of the recent initiative "Guadagnare Salute" (Gaining Health) developed by the Ministry of Health [45] which is based on the World Health Organization's initiative of the same name. The strategy calls for the involvement, not only of the health sector, but also schools, transport and agriculture, although the feasibility of the sustained attention and interventions needed through different governments is not clear. Daily breakfast consumption should be encouraged as much as possible within the context of each region and family. Increased attention to DBC is necessary during the transition from childhood to adolescence, especially in girls and young persons from disadvantaged families. Breakfast provision in schools may offer a way to overcome social inequalities in DBC and could serve to yield health benefits associated with breakfast consumption. Although more research is necessary to evaluate intermediate factors and determine which interventions are likely to be most effective to prevent childhood and adolescent obesity, rapid action is needed to avoid both present and future human and financial costs. The HBSC surveys are a useful instrument to monitor the trend of overweight and obesity among 11–15 yrs old children and the effectiveness of the interventions.

REFERENCES

1. Speiser PW, Rudolf M, Anhalt H, Camacho-Hubner C, Chiarelli F, Eliakim A, Freemark M, Gruters A, Hershkovitz E, Iughetti L, Krude H, Latzer Y, Lustig R, Pescovitz O, Pinhas-Hamiel O, Rogol AD, Shalitin S, Sultan C, Stein D, Vardi P, Werther GA, Zadik Z, Zuckerman-Levin ZN, Hochberg Z: Consensus statement: childhood obesity. J Clin Endocrinol Metabol 2005, 90:1871–1887.
2. Branca F, Nikogosian H, Lobstein T: The Challenge of Obesity in the WHO European Region and the Strategies for Response. Copenhagen: World Health Organization Regional Office for Europe; 2007.
3. Flynn M, McNeil DA, Maloff B, Mutasingwa D, Wu M, Ford C, Tough S: Reducing obesity and related chronic disease risk in children and youth: a synthesis of evidence with 'best practice' recommendations. Obes Rev 2006,7(S1):7–66.
4. Lobstein T, Baur L, Uauy R: Obesity in children and young people: a crisis in public health. Obes Rev 2004,5(S1):4–85.
5. WHO: Childhood overweight and obesity. http://www.who.int/dietphysicalactivity/childhood/en/
6. Ebbeling CB, Pawlak DB, Ludwig DS: Childhood obesity: public-health crisis, common sense cure. Lancet 2002, 360:473–482.
7. Rampersaud CG, Pereira AM, Girard LB, Adams J, Metzl DJ: Breakfast habits, nutritional status, body weight, and academic performance in children and adolescents. J Am Diet Assoc 2005, 105:743–760.
8. Keski-Rahkonen A, Kaprio J, Rissanen A, Virkkunen M, Rose RJ: Breakfast skipping and health-compromising behaviors in adolescents and adults. Eur J Clin Nutr 2003, 57:842–853.

9. Utter J, Scragg R, Mhurchu CN, Schaaf D: At-home breakfast consumption among New Zealand children: associations with body mass index and related nutrition behaviors. J Am Diet Assoc 2007, 107:570–575.
10. Niemeier HM, Raynor HA, Lloyd-Richardson EE, Rogers ML, Wing RR: Fast food consumption and breakfast skipping: predictors of weight gain from adolescence to adulthood in a nationally representative sample. J Adolesc Health 2006, 39:842–849.
11. Clement K, Vaisse C, Lahlou N, Cabrol S, Pelloux V, Cassuto D, Gourmelen M, Dina C, Chambaz J, Lacorte JM, Basdevant A, Bougneres P, Lebouc Y, Froguel P, Guy-Grand B: A mutation in the human leptin receptor gene causes obesity and pituitary dysfunction. Nature 1998, 392:398–401.
12. Montague CT, Farooqi IS, Whitehead JP, Soos MA, Rau H, Wareham NJ, Sewter CP, Digby JE, Mohammed SN, Hurst JA, Cheetham CH, Earley AR, Barnett AH, Prins JB, O'Rahilly S: Congenital leptin deficiency is associated with severe early-onset obesity in humans. Nature 1997, 387:903–908.
13. Rankinen T, Perusse L, Weisnagel SJ, Snyder EE, Chagnon YC, Bouchard C: The human obesity gene map: the 2001 update. Obes Res 2002, 10:196–243.
14. Langnase K, Mast M, Muller MJ: Social class differences in overweight of prepubertal children in northwest Germany. Int J Obes Relat Metab Disord 2002, 26:566–572.
15. Keane E, Layte R, Harrington J, Kearney PM, Perry IJ: Measured parental weight status and familial socio-economic status correlates with childhood overweight and obesity at age 9. PLoS One 2012.,7(8): doi:10.1371/journal.pone.0043503
16. Gnavi R, Spagnoli TD, Galotto C, Pugliese E, Carta A, Cesari L: Socioeconomic status, overweight and obesity in prepuberal children: a study in an area of Northern Italy. Eur J Epidemiol 2000, 16:797–803.
17. Wijnhoven TM, van Raaij JM, Spinelli A, Rito AI, Hovengen R, Kunesova M, Starc G, Rutter H, Sjöberg A, Petrauskiene A, O'Dwyer U, Petrova S, Farrugia Sant'angelo V, Wauters M, Yngve A, Rubana IM, Breda J: WHO European childhood obesity surveillance initiative 2008: weight, height and body mass index in 6–9-year-old children. Pediatr Obes 2013, 8:79–97.
18. Cairella G, Casagni L, Lamberti A, Censi L: Prevalenza di sovrappeso ed obesità in Italia nella fascia di età 6–11 anni. Ann Ig 2008, 20:315–327.
19. Albertini A, Tripodi A, Fabbri A, Mattioli M, Cavrini G, Cecchetti R, Dalle Donne E, Cortesi C, De Giorgi S, Contarini V, Andreotti L, Veronesi B, Stefanelli I, Di Martino E: Prevalence of obesity in 6- and 9-year-old children living in central-north Italy. Analysis of determinants and indicators of risk of overweight. Obes Rev 2008, 9:4–10.
20. Lazzeri G, Pammolli A, Pilato V, Giacchi MV: Relationship between 8/9-yr-old school children BMI, parents' BMI and educational level: a cross sectional survey. Nutr J 2011, 10:76. doi:10.1186/1475–2891–10–76.
21. Spinelli A, Baglio G, Cattaneo C, Fontana G, Lamberti A, Gruppo OKkio alla SALUTE; Coorte PROFEA anno 2006: Promotion of healthy life style and growth in primary school children (OKkio alla SALUTE). Ann Ig 2008, 20:337–344.
22. Binkin N, Fontana G, Lamberti A, Cattaneo C, Baglio G, Perra A, Spinelli A: A national survey of the prevalence of childhood overweight and obesity in Italy. Obes Rev 2010, 11:2–10.
23. Spinelli A, Lamberti A, Nardone P, Andreozzi S, Galeone D: Sistema di Sorveglianza OKkio Alla SALUTE: Risultati 2010. Roma: Istituto Superiore di Sanità; 2012. Rapporti ISTISAN 12/14.

24. Roberts C, Freeman J, Samdal O, Schnohr CW, de Looze ME, Nic Gabhainn S, Iannotti R, Rasmussen M, International HBSC Study Group: The health behaviour in school-aged children (HBSC) study: methodological developments and current tensions. Int J Public Health 2009,54(S2):140–150.
25. Currie C, Zanotti C, Morgan A, Currie D, de Looze M, Roberts C, Samdal O, ORF S, Barnekow V: Social Determinants of Health and Well-Being Among Young People. Health Behaviour in School-Aged Children (HBSC) Study: International Report from the 2009/2010 Survey. Copenhagen: WHO Regional Office for Europe, Health Policy for Children and Adolescents, No. 6; 2012.
26. Bennet S, Woods T, Liyanage WM, Smith DL: A simplified general method for cluster-sample surveys of health in developing countries. World Health Stat Q 1991, 44:98–106.
27. Lazzeri G, Giacchi MV, Dalmasso P, Vieno A, Nardone P, Lamberti A, Spinelli A, Cavallo F, and the Italian HBSC 2010 group: The methodology of the Italian HBSC 2010 study (health behaviour in school-aged children). Ann Ig 2013,25(3):225–233.
28. Cole TJ, Bellizzi MC, Flegal KM, Dietz WH: Establishing a standard definition for child overweight and obesity worldwide: international survey. BMJ 2007, 335:194–197.
29. Cole TJ, Flegal KM, Nicholls D, Jackson AA: Body mass index cut offs to define thinness in children and adolescents: international survey. BMJ 2007, 335:194–197.
30. ISTAT. Codici dei comuni, delle province e delle regioni 2008 http://www3.istat.it/dati/catalogo/20090728_00/atlante_geografia_statistica_amministrativa_2009.pdf
31. ISTAT. Disuguaglianze, equità e servizi ai cittadini. In: rapporto annuale 2012: La situazione del paese http://www.istat.it/it/files/2012/05/Capitolo_4.pdf
32. Pereira MA, Erickson E, McKee P, Schrankler K, Raatz SK, Lytle LA, Pellegrini AD: Breakfast frequency and quality may affect glycemia and appetite in adults and children. J Nutr 2011,141(1):163–168.
33. Report nazionale HBSC Italia 2010 http://www.hbsc.unito.it/it/images/pdf/hbsc/report_nazionale_2010.pdf
34. Shaw ME: Adolescent breakfast skipping: an Australian study. Adolescence 1998, 33:851–861.
35. Siega-Riz AM, Popkin BM, Carson T: Trends in breakfast consumption for children in the United States from 1965 to 1991. Am J Clin Nutr 1998, 67:748–756.
36. Bonati M, Campi R: What can we do to improve child health in southern Italy? PLoS Med 2005, 2:e250.
37. Haug E, Rasmussen M, Samdal O, Iannotti R, Kelly C, Borraccino A, Vereecken C, Melkevik O, Lazzeri G, Giacchi M, Ercan O, Due P, Ravens-Sieberer U, Currie C, Morgan A, Ahluwalia N, the HBSC Obesity Writing Group: Overweight in school-aged children and its relationship with demographic and lifestyle factors: results from the WHO-collaborative health behaviour in school-aged children (HBSC) study. Int J Public Health 2009, 54:167–179.
38. Johnson-Taylor W, Everhardt JE: Modifiable environmental and behavioural determinants of overweight among children and adolescents: report of a workshop. Obesity 2006, 14:929–966.
39. Snethen JA, Hewitt JB, Goretze M: Childhood obesity: the infancy connection. J Obstet Gynecol Neonatal Nurs 2007, 6:501–510.
40. Vereecken C, Dupuy M, Rasmussen M, Kelly C, Nansel TR, Al Sabbah H, Baldassari D, Jordan MD, Maes L, Niclasen BV, Ahluwalia N, HBSC Eating & Dieting Focus Group: Breakfast consumption and its socio-demographic and lifestyle correlates in

schoolchildren in 41 countries participating in the HBSC study. Int J Public Health 2009,54(S2):180–190.

41. Himes HJ, Hannan P, Wall M, Neumark-Sztainer D: Factors associated with errors in self-reports of stature, weight, and body mass index in Minnesota adolescents. Ann Epidemiol 2005, 15:272–278.
42. Jayawardene WP, Lohrmann DK, YoussefAgha AH: Discrepant body mass index: behaviors associated with height and weight misreporting among US adolescents from the national youth physical activity and nutrition study. Childhood Obesity 2014,10(3):225–233.
43. Strauss RS: Comparison of measured and self-reported weight and height in a cross-sectional sample of young adolescents. Int J Obes Relat Metab Disord 1999, 23:904–908.
44. Goodman E, Hinden BR, Khandelwal S: Accuracy of teen and parental reports of obesity and body mass index. Pediatrics 2000, 106:52–58.
45. Ministero di Salute. Guadagnare salute: rendere facili le scelte salutarihttp://www.ministerosalute.it/imgs/C_17_pubblicazioni_605_allegato.pdf

CHAPTER 9

Maternal Educational Level and Children's Healthy Eating Behaviour: Role of the Home Food Environment (Cross-Sectional Results from the INPACT Study)

Wilke J. C. Van Ansem, Carola T. M. Schrijvers, Gerda Rodenburg, and Dike Van De Mheen

9.1 BACKGROUND

Dietary behaviour is important for the development and growth of children and also influences health outcomes later in life. Fruit and vegetables and daily breakfast consumption are important components of a healthy diet and their beneficial effects on health are well documented. Diets rich in fruit and vegetables protect against cardiovascular disease (CVD), some types of cancer, and obesity [1],[2]. Regular breakfast consumption is associated with better cognitive performance and a reduced risk of becoming overweight or obese among children and adolescents [3],[4]. Despite the importance of healthy dietary behaviours, the majority of the children in the Netherlands, as in other countries, does not consume the recommended amounts of fruit and vegetables [5]-[8]. In addition, breakfast skipping is highly prevalent in Europe and the United States [9],[10]. Also, because dietary habits track into adulthood, it is important to develop interventions aimed to improve dietary behaviours of children [11],[12].

Children and adolescents with a low socio-economic status (SES) consume less fruit and vegetables than children and adolescents with a high SES [13]-[16]. Furthermore, a Norwegian study found an increase in socio-economic disparities in adolescent's fruit and vegetable consumption between 2001 and 2008 [17]. Studies of socio-economic disparities in breakfast consumption showed inconsistent findings. A literature review found that parental educational level and parental unemployment were unrelated to adolescents and children's breakfast consumption [18]. However, other studies found a positive association between maternal educational level and children's breakfast consumption [9],[19],[20]. Given the inconsistencies in the findings from previous studies and the relative small part of the literature assessing socio-economic disparities in dietary behaviour of children, the first aim of this study is to investigate socio-economic differences in healthy eating behaviours of children (fruit, vegetable and breakfast consumption).

The home food environment is important in the development of children's dietary behaviour [21]. Parents have an important influence on the dietary behaviour of children because they generally determine which food is available at home, they can set rules about what their children are allowed to eat and they act as role models, also with respect to dietary behaviour [22]. Several literature reviews concluded that aspects of the home environment are associated with children's fruit and vegetable intake [16],[23],[24]. Home environmental factors found to be positively related to children's fruit and vegetable intake are home availability, family rules and parental intake. For breakfast consumption, parental breakfast consumption is an important home environmental factor that is positively associated with children's breakfast consumption [18].

As stated before, the first aim of this study is to investigate socio-economic differences (maternal educational level is used as indicator for children's SES) in healthy eating behaviours of children. However, SES does not directly influence dietary behaviour and is not a modifiable correlate of children's dietary behaviour. Thus it is important to identify modifiable determinants that may explain the socio-economic disparities in children's healthy eating behaviour. Therefore, the second aim of this study is to examine whether factors in the home food environment (parental intake of fruit, vegetables and breakfast; rules about fruit and vegetables and home availability of fruit and vegetables) mediate the association between maternal educational level and children's healthy eating behaviours (fruit, vegetable and breakfast consumption). Figure 1 presents the research model.

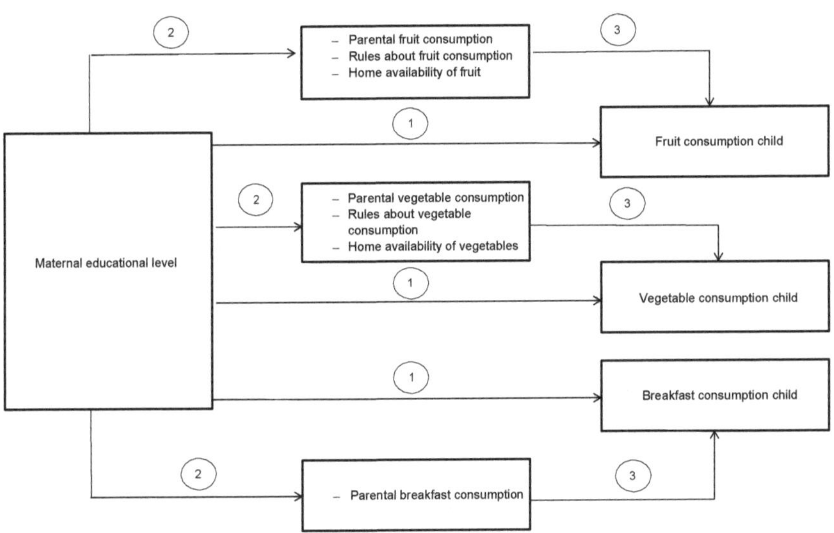

FIGURE 9.1 Research model.

9.2 METHODS

9.2.1 Study Population and Design

The data used in this study are derived from the Dutch INPACT study, INPACT being the acronym for IVO Nutrition Physical Activity Child cohort. This longitudinal study among 8 to 12 year olds and their parents investigated modifiable environmental determinants of children's dietary behaviour. Participants of the INPACT study were recruited through primary schools in the southern part of the Netherlands (Eindhoven and surroundings). The municipal health service invited all general primary schools (n = 265) in this area to participate in this study. Ninety one schools (34.3%) agreed. The response rate of schools in rural and urban areas was similar. A sample of 1844 parent-child dyads (62.5%) gave informed consent. Trained research assistants visited the participating primary schools and measured children's height and weight. Children completed a short questionnaire at school and parents completed a questionnaire at home. The questionnaire topics varied annually. The INPACT study was approved by the Medical Ethical Committee at Erasmus Medical Centre, Rotterdam. The present study was based on cross-sectional data collected in the last wave (2011), in which a questionnaire was completed by 1428 primary caregivers. In most cases (n = 1312, 92.1%) the primary caregiver was the mother.

9.2.2 Measurements

9.2.2.1 Socio-economic Status

The three most commonly used indicators of SES are educational level, income and occupation [25]. Of these three SES indicators, educational level was found to be the strongest and most consistent in predicting health behaviour [25]. In this study, maternal educational level was used as an indicator of children's SES because several studies found maternal educational level to be a reliable determinant of children's dietary behaviour and childhood obesity [9],[19],[20]. In addition, traditionally, in the majority of the households the mother provides the food for the family and, therefore, maternal educational level also impacts the dietary behaviour of the other members of the family and the home availability of foods. Maternal educational level was classified into three groups: 'low educational level' (primary school and lower secondary education), 'intermediate educational level' (intermediate vocational level, higher secondary school and pre-university education) and 'high educational level' (higher vocational education and university). Throughout the remainder of this paper we thus refer to 'low SES' (children of mothers with a low educational level), 'intermediate SES' (children of mothers with an intermediate educational level) and 'high SES' (children of mothers with a high educational level).

Outcome measures (children's fruit, vegetable and breakfast consumption) Children's fruit, vegetable and breakfast consumption were measured with a questionnaire based on a validated Food Frequency Questionnaire [26]-[29]. Parents reported how many days in a normal week their child consumed 1) fruit (fresh or canned fruit), 2) cooked, fried, steamed or otherwise heated vegetables, 3) salad or other raw vegetables and 4) breakfast. Answering categories ranged from 'none or less than one day a week' to '7 days a week'.

Additionally, parents reported the numbers of servings of fruit and vegetables consumed by their child on such a day. For fruit, answer categories ranged from '0 pieces a day' to 'more than 3 pieces a day', by increments of half a piece of fruit. Reported fruit consumption of more than 3 pieces a day (n = 4) was recoded as '4 pieces a day'. For vegetables, answer categories ranged from '0 serving spoons' to 'more than 4 serving spoons a day', by increments of half a serving spoon. Reported vegetable consumption of more than 4 serving spoons (n = 12) was recoded as '5 serving spoons a day'. One serving spoon of vegetables was equivalent to 50 grams of vegetables. Total vegetable consumption was calculated in grams for each child by multiplying consumption frequency (how many days a child consumed vegetables) and serving spoons of vegetables. Subsequently, the vegetable consumption was converted to an amount consumed in a day. Total fruit consumption was calculated in pieces for each child by multiplying consumption frequency (how many days a child consumed fruit) and servings (pieces of fruit). Children's fruit consumption was also converted to an amount consumed in a day.

Breakfast consumption was dichotomized into 'daily' and 'not daily', due to limited variation in the answering categories.

9.2.2.2 Potential Mediating Variables

9.2.2.2.1 Parental Intake of Fruit, Vegetables and Breakfast

Parental fruit, vegetable and breakfast consumption were measured and calculated in the same way as children's fruit, vegetable and breakfast consumption.

9.2.2.2.2 Rules about Fruit and Vegetable Consumption

We assessed whether parents set rules regarding their child's fruit and vegetable consumption with the following questions: 'Do you have the rule that your child should eat 2 pieces of fruit a day?' and 'Do you have the rule that your child should eat 200 grams of vegetables a day?' These specific amounts of fruit and vegetables are consistent with the Dutch guidelines for fruit and vegetables [30]. Response categories were 'yes' and 'no'. These questions were derived from the ENDORSE study [31].

9.2.2.2.3 Home Availability of Fruit and Vegetables

The availability of fruit and vegetables at home was measured using a questionnaire based on the validated Home Environment Survey [32]. Parents were asked about the availability of 1) fruit and 2) vegetables in their home. Response categories were 'yes, always', 'yes, usually', 'sometimes', 'no, usually not' and 'no, never'. Due to limited variability of these variables, we dichotomized both variables into 'always' ('yes, always') and 'not always' ('yes, usually'; 'sometimes'; 'no, usually not'; 'no, never').

9.2.2.2.4 Potential Confounders

The following variables are considered as potential confounders: age, gender, ethnicity and body mass index (BMI) of the child. Age, gender and ethnicity of the child were reported by the parents. A child's age (in years) was calculated on the basis of the date of birth and the date of measurement. For the purpose of analysis we dichotomised child's age into '≤ 11 years' versus '> 11 years. Children's ethnicity was categorised into 'Dutch native' (both parents born in the Netherlands) and 'immigrants' (at least one of the parents was born outside the Netherlands). Children's body mass index (BMI) was calculated on the basis of weight and height, which were measured with clothes but without shoes to the nearest 0.1 kg and 0.1 cm; the measurements were made by trained research assistants. BMI cut-off points for children were used to define overweight and obesity [33]. Subsequently child BMI was dichotomised into 'overweight' ('overweight' and 'obesity') versus no overweight ('underweight and normal weight').

9.2.3 Data Analysis

Respondents who lacked data for maternal educational level were excluded from this study (n = 110, 7.7%). In total, 1318 children and parents were included in this study. Descriptive analyses were performed to describe the characteristics of the study population.

To investigate whether home environmental factors mediated the association between maternal educational level and children's healthy eating behaviour, we used Baron and Kenny's four-step approach [34]. According to Baron and Kenny, there are three criteria for mediation: 1) the predictive variable has to be associated with the outcome variable, 2) the predictive variable has to be associated with the mediator, and 3) the mediator has to be associated with the outcome variable (adjusted for the predictive variable). If all the associations assessed in steps 1-3 are statistically significant, the criteria for mediation have been met. Step four of the approach is to test the mediation model: mediation is supported if the association between the predictive variable and the outcome variable changes after controlling for the mediator.

For each outcome measure (child fruit intake, child vegetable intake and child breakfast consumption) the steps of the mediation approach were conducted separately. Depending on the scale of the outcome measures, logistic regression models or linear regression models were used to test the subsequent steps of the mediation-approach.

Several potential mediators were tested for the outcome measures 'child's fruit consumption' and 'child's vegetable consumption'. If it appeared that more than one potential mediator met the criteria for mediation, the unique contribution of each mediator was determined (single mediator model). Next, a multivariate mediation model was tested. Bootstrapping resampling techniques were used to calculate confidence intervals for the mediated effects.

All regression models were adjusted for the potential confounders. Due to the used sample-strategy (children were recruited trough schools), the data have a nested structure (children within schools). To take into account potential clustering effects, we investigated the associations using multilevel regression analyses. Analyses were performed using R (2013). Cases with missing values were removed per analysis. Due to missing values the computed models for fruit, vegetable and breakfast consumption are based on different numbers of participants.

9.3 RESULTS

Background characteristics of the study population are presented in Table 1. Mean age of the children was 11 years, the majority was native Dutch and not overweight, and about half were boys. Significant differences between the three educational levels were found in the background characteristics: relative to the high and low SES groups there were more girls in the intermediate SES group. More children in the low SES group were overweight, were older than 11 years, and were immigrants compared with children in the intermediate and high SES groups.

TABLE 9.1 Characteristics of the study population: total sample and sample according to socio-economic status (SES)

	Total sample	Low SES	Intermediate SES	High SES	P-value
Mean age N (%)	N = 1317	N = 263	N = 628	N = 426	**0.00**
≤11 years	1119 (85.0)	205 (77.9)	528 (84.1)	386 (90.6)	
> 11 years	198 (15.0)	58 (22.1)	100 (15.9)	40 (9.4)	
Gender %	N = 1318	N = 263	N = 629	N = 426	**0.02**
Boys	50.8	52.5	46.7	55.6	
Girls	49.2	47.5	53.3	44.4	
Child's BMI %	N = 1283	N = 252	N = 616	N = 415	**0.01**
Overweight	11.2	16.7	10.6	8.9	
No overweight	88.8	83.3	89.4	91.9	
Child's ethnicity %	N = 1318	N = 263	N = 629	N = 426	**0.02**
Native Dutch	88.8	84.4	90.9	89.4	
Immigrant	11.2	15.6	9.1	10.6	

9.3.1 Fruit Consumption

Table 2 provides data on children's fruit consumption and determinants of children's fruit consumption stratified by SES. Children with a low SES had the lowest fruit consumption (on average 0.96 pieces per day) while children with a high SES had the highest fruit consumption (on average 1.07 per day). Table 3 presents data on the association between children's SES and their fruit consumption. Children with a high SES consumed more fruit than children with a low SES (B = 0.13, 95% CI: 0.04-0.22). There was no significant difference in fruit consumption between children with an intermediate SES and those with a low SES.

Table 4 presents data on the association between children's SES and possible mediating variables regarding fruit consumption. Parents with a high SES consumed significantly more fruit (B = 0.25, 95% CI: 0.13-0.36), were more likely to have rules about fruit consumption (OR = 1.78, 95% CI: 1.23-2.56) and were more likely to always have fruit available at home (OR = 2.24, 95% CI: 1.25-4.00) than parents with a low SES. Parents with an intermediate SES were also more likely to always have fruit available at home than parents with a low SES (OR = 1.74, 95% CI: 1.05-2.88).

TABLE 9.2 Descriptives of the key study variables

	Socio-economic status (SES)		
	Low	**Intermediate**	**High**
Fruit (N = 1269)	N = 247	N = 607	N = 415
Children's fruit intake, pieces per day (mean, SD)	0.96 (0.65)	0.99 (0.57)	1.07 (0.60)
Parental fruit intake, pieces per day (mean, SD)	0.97 (0.74)	1.04 (0.74)	1.19 (0.73)
Parental rules regarding fruit consumption (%)			
Yes	68.8	72.7	79.5
No	31.2	27.3	20.5
Home availability of fruit %			
Always	88.3	92.8	94.2
Not always	11.7	7.2	5.8
Vegetables (N = 1265)	N = 248	N = 606	N = 411
Children's vegetable intake, grams per day (mean, SD	94.0 (57.7)	100.5 (53.1)	116.9 (60.6)
Parental vegetable intake, grams per day (mean, SD	148.3 (68.1)	158.4 (67.9)	176.7 (68.0)
Parental rules regarding vegetable consumption (%)			
Yes	83.5	85.0	92.0
No	16.5	15.0	8.0
Home availability of vegetables			
Always	83.1	89.4	90.5
Not always	16.4	8.0	9.5
Breakfast (N = 1270)	N = 246	N = 610	N = 414
Children's breakfast consumption (%)			
Daily	91.9	94.3	97.3
Not daily	8.1	5.7	2.7
Parental breakfast consumption (%)			
Daily	83.7	91.3	95.7
Not daily	16.3	8.7	4.3

TABLE 9.3 Associations between socio-economic status (SES) and children's fruit, vegetable and breakfast consumption

Fruit consumption (N = 1269)	**Multivariate regression analyses**†	
SES	**B (95% CI)**	**P-value**
Low (Ref. group)	0.84	
Intermediate	0.04 (−0.05 – 0.13)	0.38
High	0.13 (0.04 – 0.22)	0.01
Vegetable consumption (N = 1265)	**Multivariate regression analyses†**	
SES	**B (95% CI)**	**P-value**
Low (Ref. group)	83.89	
Intermediate	8.33 (0.09 – 16.56)	0.05
High	23.81 (14.93 – 32.69)	0.00
Breakfast consumption (N = 1270)	**Multivariate regression analyses†**	
SES	**OR (95% CI)**	**P-value**
Low (Ref. group)	1.00	
Intermediate	1.39 (0.78 – 2.49)	0.27
High	**2.97** (1.38 -6.39)	0.01

B = unstandardized coefficient, OR = Odds ratio, 95% CI = 95% Confidence Interval. Bold values represent statistically significant association. †Multivariate regression analysis adjusted for: child's age, child's gender, child's ethnicity and child's BMI.

TABLE 9.4 Associations between socio-economic status (SES) and the mediating variables

Fruit consumption (N = 1269)	**Mediators**	**Multivariate regression analyses**†	
SES	**Parental fruit intake**	**B (95% CI)**	**P-value**
Low (Ref. group)		*0.88*	
Intermediate		0.09 (−0.02 – 0.20)	0.10
High		0.25 (0.13 – 0.36)	0.00
SES	**Parental rules regarding fruit intake**	**OR (95% CI)**	**P-value**
Low (Ref. group)		1.00	
Intermediate		1.18 (0.85-1.64)	0.32
High		1.78 (1.23 – 2.56)	0.00
SES	**Home availability of fruit**	**OR (95% CI)**	**P-value**
Low (Ref. group)		1.00	
Intermediate		1.74 (1.05 – 2.88)	0.03
High		2.24 (1.25 – 4.00)	0.01

TABLE 9.4 *(Continued)*

Fruit consumption (N = 1269)	**Mediators**	**Multivariate regression analyses**[†]	
Vegetable consumption (N = 1265)	**Mediators**	**Multivariate regression analyses**†	
SES	**Parental vegetable intake**	**B (95% CI)**	**P-value**
Low (Ref. group)		144.99	
Intermediate		11.29 (1.24 – 21.34)	0.03
High		28.86 (18.05 – 39.67)	0.00
SES	**Parental rules regarding vegetable intake**	**OR (95% CI)**	**P-value**
Low (Ref. group)		1.00	
Intermediate		1.74 (1.13 – 2.69)	0.01
High		2.47 (1.49 – 4.10)	0.00
SES	**Home availability of vegetables**	**OR (95% CI)**	**P-value**
Low (Ref. group)		1.00	
Intermediate		1.18 (0.78 – 1.77)	0.44
High		1.93 (1.19 – 3.11)	0.01
Breakfast consumption (N = 1270)	**Mediator**	**Multivariate regression analyses**[†]	
SES	**Parental breakfast intake**	**OR (95% CI)**	**P-value**
Low (Ref. group)		1.00	
Intermediate		1.94 (1.24 – 3.04)	0.00
High		4.10 (2.28 – 7.37)	0.00

B = unstandardized coefficient, OR = Odds ratio, 95% CI = 95% Confidence Interval. Bold values represent statistically significant association. [†]Multivariate regression analysis adjusted for: child's age, child's gender, child's ethnicity and child's BMI.

Table 5 shows that parental fruit intake, rules about fruit consumption and home availability of fruit were significantly associated with children's fruit consumption. If parents increased their fruit consumption by one piece per day, their children increased their fruit consumption by 0.34 pieces per day. Children of parents who had fruit consumption rules were more likely to consume fruit than children of parents who had no fruit consumption rules. Children of parents who always had fruit available at home were also more likely to consume fruit than children of parents who did not always have fruit available at home.

TABLE 9.5 Associations between possible mediating variables and children's fruit, vegetable and breakfast consumption

Fruit consumption (N = 1269)	**Multivariate regression analyses**†	
	B (95% CI)	**P-value**
Parental fruit consumption	**0.34** (0.30 – 0.39)	**0.00**
Rules about fruit consumption		
No (ref. group)	0.55	
Yes	**0.49** (0.42 – 0.56)	**0.00**
Home availability of fruit		
Not always (ref. group)	0.42	
Always	**0.48** (0.36 – 0.60)	**0.00**
Vegetable consumption (N = 1265)	**Multivariate regression analyses**†	
	B (95% CI)	**P-value**
Parental vegetable consumption	**0.46** (0.42 – 0.47)	**0.00**
Rules about vegetable consumption		
No (ref. group)	63.93	
Yes	**24.94** (15.20 – 34.68)	**0.00**
Home availability of vegetables		
Not always (ref. group)	67.66	
Always	**18.62** (9.72 – 27.51)	**0.00**
Breakfast consumption (N = 1270)	**Multivariate regression analyses**†	
	OR (95% CI)	**P-value**
Parental breakfast consumption		
Not daily (ref. group)	1.00	
Daily	**15.75** (9.04 – 27.44)	**0.00**

B = unstandardized coefficient, OR = Odds ratio, 95% CI = 95% Confidence Interval. Bold values represent statistically significant association. †Multivariate regression analysis adjusted for: child's SES, child's age, child's gender, child's ethnicity and child's BMI.

Table 6 presents the mediation analyses. In the single-mediator models, parental fruit intake explained 66.0% of the difference between children with a low SES and those with a high SES; fruit consumption rules explained 40.9% and home availability of fruit explained 23.2% of the difference in fruit intake. In the multiple-mediator models, parental fruit intake, fruit consumption rules and home availability of fruit together explained 89.5% of the difference in fruit intake between children with a low SES and those with a high SES. Parental fruit intake, fruit consumption rules and home availability of fruit had no significant mediating effect on the difference in fruit intake between children with an intermediate SES and those with a low SES.

TABLE 9.6 Mediation analyses

Fruit consumption (N = 1269)	Direct association between SES and children's fruit consumption B	Mediation models B (95% CI)	P-value	Percentage change	P-value
SES		**Model A**			
Low (ref. group)	0.84	0.54			
Intermediate	0.04	0.01 (−0.07 – 0.09)	0.84	−79.49	0.36
High	0.13	0.04 (−0.09 – 0.17)	0.32	−66.01	**0.02**
SES		**Model B**			
Low (ref. group)	0.84	0.55			
Intermediate	0.04	0.02 (−0.06 – 0.10)	0.58	−42.16	0.42
High	0.13	0.08 (−0.01 – 0.16)	0.09	−40.85	**0.00**
SES		**Model C**			
Low (ref. group)	0.84	0.42			
Intermediate	0.04	0.02 (−0.07 – 0.10)	0.69	−56.10	0.40
High	0.13	**0.10 (0.01 – 0.19)**	**0.03**	−23.15	**0.02**
SES		**Model D**			
Low (ref. group)	0.84	0.23			
Intermediate	0.04	−0.01 (−0.08 – 0.07)	1.12	−114.44	0.40
High	0.13	0.01 (−0.07 – 0.10)	0.75	−89.53	**0.00**

TABLE 9.6 *(Continued)*

Vegetable consumption (N = 1265)	Direct association between SES and children's vegetable consumption B	Mediation models B (95% CI)[†]	P-value	Percentage change	P-value
SES		**Model E**			
Low (ref. group)	83.89	17.91			
Intermediate	8.33	3.19 (−3.66 – 10.05)	0.36	−61.70	0.14
High	23.81	**10.44 (2.97 – 17.93)**	**0.01**	**−56.13**	**0.00**
SES		**Model F**			
Low (ref. group)	83.89	63.93			
Intermediate	8.33	6.75 (−1.42 – 14.92)	0.11	−19.02	0.08
High	23.81	21.47 (12.63 – 30.31)	0.00	−9.85	0.00
SES		**Model G**			
Low (ref. group)	83.89	67.66			
Intermediate	8.33	7.39 (−0.26 – 16.12)	0.06	−4.88	0.56
High	23.81	**22.39 (13.55 – 31.23)**	**0.00**	**−5.98**	**0.00**
SES		**Model H**			
Low (ref. group)	83.89	10.57			
Intermediate	8.33	2.75 (−4.11 – 9.61)	0.43	−66.79	0.06
High	23.81	**9.77 (2.27 – 17.27)**	**0.01**	**−58.89**	**0.00**

TABLE 9.6 *(Continued)*

Breakfast consumption (N = 1270)	Direct association between SES and children's breakfast consumption OR	Mediation model OR (95% CI)[†]	P-value	Percentage change	P-value
SES		**Model I**			
Low (ref. group)	1.00				
Intermediate	1.39	0.99 (0.52 – 1.90)	0.97	- 102.73	0.27
High	2.97	1.63 (0.71 – 3.67)	0.25	**- 67.89**	**0.02**

SES = socioeconomic status; B = unstandardized coefficient, OR = Odds ratio, 95% CI = 95% Confidence Interval. Bold values represent statistically significant association.

Model A: Single mediator model. This model includes the mediator 'parental fruit consumption'.

Model B: Single mediator model. This model includes the mediator 'parental rules regarding fruit consumption'.

Model C: Single mediator model. This model includes the mediator 'home availability of fruit'.

Model D: Multiple mediation model. This model includes the mediators: parental fruit consumption, parental rules regarding fruit consumption and home availability of fruit.

Model E: Single mediator model. This model includes the mediator 'parental vegetable intake'.

Model F: Single mediator model. This model includes the mediator 'parental rules regarding vegetable consumption'.

Model G: Single mediator model. This model includes the mediator 'home availability of vegetables'.

Model H: Multiple mediator model. This model includes the mediators: parental vegetable consumption, parental rules regarding vegetable consumption and home availability of vegetables.

Model I: Single mediator model. This model includes the mediator 'parental breakfast consumption'.

All models are adjusted for: child's age, child's gender, child's ethnicity and child's BMI.

9.3.2 Vegetable Consumption

Table 2 provides data on children's vegetable consumption and determinants of children's vegetable consumption stratified by SES. Children with a low SES had the lowest vegetable consumption (on average 94.0 grams per day) while children with a high SES had the highest vegetable consumption (on average 116.9 grams per day).

Table 3 shows significant socio-economic differences in children's vegetables consumption. Children with an intermediate SES and children with a high SES consumed more vegetables than children with a low SES (resp. B = 8.33, 95% CI: 0.09-16.56; B = B = 23.81, 95% CI: 14.93-32.96).

Table 4 presents data on the association between SES and possible mediating variables regarding vegetable consumption. Parents with a high SES consumed more vegetables (B = 28.86, 95% CI: 18.05-39.67), were more likely to have vegetable consumption rules (OR = 2.47, 95% CI: 1.49-4.10), and were more likely to always have vegetables available at home (OR= 1.93, 95% CI: 1.19-3.11) than parents with a low SES. Parents with an intermediate SES also consumed more vegetables (B = 11.29 95% CI: 1.24-21.34) and were more likely to have rules about vegetable consumption (OR: 1.74, 95% CI: 1.13-2.69) than parents with a low SES.

All potential mediators were significantly associated with children's vegetable consumption (see Table 5). Children consumed more vegetables when their parents consumed more vegetables (B = 0.46, 95% CI: 0.42-0.47), when their parents had rules about vegetable consumption (OR = 24.94, 95% CI: 15.20-34.68), and when vegetables were always available at home (B = 18.62, 95% CI: 9.72-27.51).

Table 6 presents the mediation models. In the single-mediator models, parental vegetable intake explained 56.1% of the difference in vegetable consumption between children with a low SES and those with a high SES; vegetable consumption rules explained 9.9% and home availability of fruit explained 6.0%. In the multiple-mediator model, all the mediators together explained 58.89% of the difference in vegetable intake between children with a low SES and those with a high SES. Parental vegetable intake, vegetable consumption rules and home availability of vegetables had no significant mediating effect on the difference in vegetable intake between children with an intermediate SES and those with a low SES.

9.3.3 Breakfast Consumption

Table 2 presents data on children's and parents breakfast consumption. Children and parents with a high SES more often reported to have breakfast on a daily basis than children and parents with a low and intermediate SES. Table 3 reports on the association between SES and children's breakfast consumption. Children with a high SES were more likely to eat breakfast on a daily basis than children with a low SES (OR = 2.97, 95% CI: 1.38-6.39). There was no significant difference in breakfast consumption between children with an intermediate SES and those with a low SES.

Parents with high and intermediate SES were more likely to consume breakfast on a daily basis than parents with a low SES (see Table 4). Table 5 shows that children were more likely to eat breakfast on a daily basis when their parents ate breakfast on a daily basis (OR = 15.75, 95% CI: 9.04-27.44). Table 6 shows the final mediation model; parental breakfast consumption explained 67.9% of the differences in breakfast consumption between children with a high SES and those with a low SES. Parental breakfast consumption had no significant mediating effect on the difference in breakfast consumption between children with an intermediate and with a high SES.

9.4 DISCUSSION

The first aim of this study was to examine the association between SES and children's fruit, vegetable and breakfast consumption. We found that children with a high SES consumed more fruit and vegetables and consumed more often breakfast on a daily basis, than children with a low SES. These findings are in line with those from the majority of similar studies [9],[13]-[15],[17],[19],[35] and emphasise that children from low socio-economic groups can be considered an important target for interventions to improve dietary behaviour.

However, maternal education level, (and other measures of SES), are not considered to have a direct effect on dietary behaviour and are not easily modifiable. To explain socio-economic disparities in children's dietary behaviour, several studies examined socio-economic differences in the home food environment of children. These studies showed that the home food environment of children of mothers with a low educational level was less supportive than the home food environment of children of mothers with a high educational level [36],[37]. For example, adolescents of mothers with a low educational level were more likely to report that unhealthy foods were always or usually available at home, while adolescents of mothers with a high educational level were more likely to report that fruit was always or usually available at home and that vegetables were always served at dinner time [38]. In addition, a study among 5-6 year old children found comparable results; households of mothers with a low educational level were more likely to watch television while eating dinner and mothers with a low educational level were more likely to have negative perceptions about the quality and variety of fresh fruit and vegetables at their local shops [39]. Furthermore, Hupkens et al. found that mothers with a high educational level more often limited their children's intake of unhealthy foods (e.g. sweets, soft drinks, chips). These differences in the number of restricted foods by educational level were partly explained in health and taste considerations between mothers with a low and high educational level [40]. A more recent study also found socio-economic differences in food parenting practices; frequent consumption of fruit and vegetables, restrictive rules, verbal praise, negotiation and restrain from negative modelling were all more common among mothers with a high educational level [41]. The present study also shows that aspects of the home food environment differed by SES, where low SES had the less supportive home environment.

However, socio-economic differences in determinants of the home food environment do not necessarily account for socio-economic differences in children's dietary behaviour. Therefore, a second aim of this study was to investigate modifiable factors of the home food environment that mediate the association between SES and children's fruit, vegetable and breakfast consumption. We included parental intake, home availability and parental rules about children's fruit and vegetable consumption as possible mediating variables in the association between SES and children's fruit and vegetable intake. Our results indicate that all the studied home environmental factors mediate the association between SES and children's fruit and vegetable intake. Moreover, our results indicate that the difference in fruit and vegetable consumption between children with a low and high SES is explained in particular by parental intake of fruit and vegetables. Very few studies have assessed mediators of the association between socio-economic status and children's fruit and vegetables intake. Vereecken et al. found that differences in children's fruit and vegetable consumption by mother's educational level were completely explained by mother's consumption and parenting practices [41]. Bere et al. concluded that home accessibility was the strongest mediator of the association between maternal educational level and adolescent's fruit and vegetable consumption [13]. Furthermore, Hilsen et al. also found that accessibility of fruit and vegetables mediates part of the association between socio-economic status and adolescent's fruit and vegetable intake [17]. In addition, they found that accessibility of fruit and vegetables explains part of the increase in SES disparities in fruit and vegetable consumption between 2001 and 2008.

To our knowledge, ours is the first study to assess possible explanatory variables of socio-economic disparities in children's breakfast consumption. We found that the difference in breakfast consumption between high SES children and low SES children was mediated by parental breakfast consumption. However, we included only one possible mediator in our analyses (parental breakfast consumption), while other potentially mediating variables were not included. For example, parenting practices are associated with children's breakfast consumption and may also be an explanatory variable of socio-economic differences in children's breakfast consumption.

It is known that aspects of the home environment are associated with children's dietary behaviour. This study indicates that home environmental factors also play a role in the explanation of socio-economic disparities in children's healthy eating behaviour. Given that parental intake was the strongest mediator and that parents shape the home food environment (e.g. they decide which food is available at home and can set food rules), parents play an important role in the development of children's dietary behaviour. Therefore, parents can be important targets for interventions. Moreover, it is necessary to reach parents with a low SES and to increase their own consumption of fruit, vegetables and breakfast, to increase the home availability of healthy products and to set food rules for their children. Campbell et al. found that maternal nutrition knowledge was associated with children's fruit and vegetable consumption and also with the home availability of fruit and vegetables [42]. Therefore, targeting parental nutritional knowledge (especially among those with a low educational level) may be an effective way to improve the home food environment. Besides interventions that aim at the importance of family involvement, also multiple-setting interventions are effective in changing children's dietary behaviour. In the latter case, children receive the messages in more than one setting (e.g. at home, school, and the sports club) thereby increasing the chance that such an intervention will be more effective than a single-setting approach [43]. However, interventions aiming to improve children's dietary behaviour, such as children's fruit and vegetable consumption are also necessary for children from higher socio-economic backgrounds since the majority of all children (including children of higher educational background) does not consume the recommended amount of fruit and vegetables.

The present study has some limitations. First, this study has a cross-sectional design, which does not allow to draw conclusions about causal relationships. However, as educational level is a consistent factor over time, it is highly unlikely that children's food consumption will affect a mother's educational level. Although it is possible that children's fruit and vegetable consumption contributes to the amount of fruit and vegetables available at home, or to parental consumption rules regarding fruit and vegetables, we believe that the impact of the home availability and the consumption rules of fruit and vegetables on children's fruit and vegetable intake are larger. Therefore, we expect the directions of the associations we found to be as presented in Figure 1. Second, assessments of child's fruit, vegetable and breakfast consumption were based on parent's reports instead of child reports. Child reports might be more valid, although this remains unclear. Nevertheless, Tak et al.[44] concluded that parents' reports could be considered as a valid method to measure children's fruit and vegetable consumption, although the use of parent's reports may evoke socially desirable answers. Finally, we measured breakfast frequency and not breakfast quality, which is associated with the nutrient adequacy of diets [45].

9.5 CONCLUSION

This study shows that children of mothers with low educational level have less healthy eating habits than children of mothers with a high educational level. Our study adds to the knowledge on possible mechanisms underlying socio-economic differences in healthy eating behaviour of children. Parent's food intake, home availability of healthy foods and parental rules about children's fruit and vegetable intake mediated the association between maternal educational level and children's healthy eating behaviour. Interventions to improve children's dietary behaviour and to reduce socio-economic disparities in children's eating habits, may benefit by focusing on the role of parents in the development of children's dietary behaviour.

REFERENCES

1. Johnsen SP: Intake of fruit and vegetables and risk of stroke: an overview. Curr Opin Clin Nutr Metab Care. 2004, 7: 665-670. 10.1097/00075197-200411000-00012.
2. Food, Nutrition, Physical Activity and the Prevention of Cancer: A Global Perspective. 2007, AICR, DC

3. Hoyland A, Dye L, Lawton CL: A systematic review of the effect of breakfast on the cognitive performance of children and adolescents. Nutr Res Rev. 2009, 22: 220-243. 10.1017/S0954422409990175.
4. Szajewska H, Ruszczynski M: Systematic review demonstrating that breakfast consumption influences body weight outcomes in children and adolescents in Europe. Crit Rev Food Sci Nutr. 2010, 50: 113-119. 10.1080/10408390903467514.
5. Diethelm K, Jankovic N, Moreno LA, Huybrechts I, De Henauw S, De Vriendt T, González-Gross M, Leclercq C, Gottrand F, Gilbert CC, Dallongeville J, Cuenca-Garcia M, Manios Y, Kafatos A, Plada M, Kersting M: Food intake of European adolescents in the light of different food-based dietary guidelines: results of the HELENA (Healthy Lifestyle in Europe by Nutrition in Adolescence) Study. Public Health Nutr. 2012, 15: 386-398. 10.1017/S1368980011001935.
6. Huybrechts I, Matthys C, Vereecken C, Maes L, Temme EH, Van Oyen H, De Backer G, De Henauw S: Food intakes by preschool children in flanders compared with dietary guidelines. Int J Environ Res Public Health. 2008, 5: 243-257. 10.3390/ijerph5040243.
7. Ocke M, van Rossum C, Fransen H, Buurma E, de Boer E, Brants H, Niekerk E, van der laan J, Drijvers J, Ghameshlou Z: Dutch National Food Consumption Survey Young Children 2005/2006. 2008, RIVM, Bilthoven
8. Van Ansem WJ, Schrijvers CT, Rodenburg G, van de Mheen D: Is there an association between the home food environment, the local food shopping environment and children's fruit and vegetable intake? Results from the Dutch INPACT study. Public Health Nutr. 2013, 16 (7): 1206-1214. 10.1017/S1368980012003461.
9. Vereecken C, Dupuy M, Rasmussen M, Kelly C, Nansel TR, Al Sabbah H, Baldassari D, Jordan MD, Maes L, Niclasen BV-L, Ahluwalia N: Breakfast consumption and its socio-demographic and lifestyle correlates in schoolchildren in 41 countries participating in the HBSC study. Int J Public Health. 2009, 54 (Suppl 2): 180-190. 10.1007/s00038-009-5409-5.
10. Rampersaud GC, Pereira MA, Girard BL, Adams J, Metzl JD: Breakfast habits, nutritional status, body weight, and academic performance in children and adolescents. J Am Diet Assoc. 2005, 105: 743-760. 10.1016/j.jada.2005.02.007. quiz 761-2
11. Kelder SH, Perry CL, Klepp KI, Lytle LL: Longitudinal tracking of adolescent smoking, physical activity, and food choice behaviors. Am J Public Health. 1994, 84: 1121-1126. 10.2105/AJPH.84.7.1121.
12. Craigie AM, Lake A, Kelly S, Adamson AJ, Mathers JC: Tracking of obesity-related behaviours from childhood to adulthood: a systematic review. Maturitas. 2011, 70: 266-284. 10.1016/j.maturitas.2011.08.005.
13. Bere E, van Lenthe F, Klepp K-I, Brug J: Why do parents' education level and income affect the amount of fruits and vegetables adolescents eat?. Eur J Public Health. 2008, 18: 611-615. 10.1093/eurpub/ckn081.
14. Riediger ND, Shooshtari S, Moghadasian MH: The influence of sociodemographic factors on patterns of fruit and vegetable consumption in Canadian adolescents. J Am Diet Assoc. 2007, 107: 1511-1518. 10.1016/j.jada.2007.06.015.
15. Hanson MD, Chen E: Socioeconomic status and health behaviors in adolescence: a review of the literature. J Behav Med. 2007, 30: 263-285. 10.1007/s10865-007-9098-3.
16. Rasmussen M, Krølner R, Klepp K-I, Lytle L, Brug J, Bere E, Due P: Determinants of fruit and vegetable consumption among children and adolescents: a review of the literature. Part I: Quantitative studies. Int J Behav Nutr Phys Act. 2006, 3: 22-10.1186/1479-5868-3-22.

17. Hilsen M, van Stralen MM, Klepp K-I, Bere E: Changes in 10-12 year old's fruit and vegetable intake in Norway from 2001 to 2008 in relation to gender and socioeconomic status - a comparison of two cross-sectional groups. Int J Behav Nutr Phys Act. 2011, 8: 108-10.1186/1479-5868-8-108.
18. Pearson N, Biddle SJH, Gorely T: Family correlates of breakfast consumption among children and adolescents. A systematic review. Appetite. 2009, 52: 1-7. 10.1016/j.appet.2008.08.006.
19. Hallström L, Vereecken C, Ruiz JR, Patterson E, Gilbert CC, Catasta G, Díaz L-E, Gómez-Martínez S, González Gross M, Gottrand F, Hegyi A, Lehoux C, Mouratidou T, Widham K, Aström A, Moreno LA, Sjöström M: Breakfast habits and factors influencing food choices at breakfast in relation to socio-demographic and family factors among European adolescents. The HELENA Study. Appetite. 2011, 56: 649-657. 10.1016/j.appet.2011.02.019.
20. Hallström L, Vereecken CA, Labayen I, Ruiz JR, Le Donne C, García MC, Gilbert CC, Martínez SG, Grammatikaki E, Huybrechts I, Kafatos A, Kersting M, Manios Y, Molnár D, Patterson E, Widhalm K, De Vriendt T, Moreno LA, Sjöström M: Breakfast habits among European adolescents and their association with sociodemographic factors: the HELENA (Healthy Lifestyle in Europe by Nutrition in Adolescence) study. Public Health Nutr. 2012, 15: 1879-1889. 10.1017/S1368980012000341.
21. Tinsley B: How Children Learn to Be Healthy. 2003, Cambridge University Press, Cambridge
22. Lindsay AC, Sussner KM, Kim J, Gortmaker S: The role of parents in preventing childhood obesity. Future Child. 2006, 16: 169-186. 10.1353/foc.2006.0006.
23. Krølner R, Rasmussen M, Brug J, Klepp K-I, Wind M, Due P: Determinants of fruit and vegetable consumption among children and adolescents: a review of the literature. Part II: qualitative studies. Int J Behav Nutr Phys Act. 2011, 8: 112-10.1186/1479-5868-8-112.
24. Pearson N, Biddle SJH, Gorely T: Family correlates of fruit and vegetable consumption in children and adolescents: a systematic review. Public Health Nutr. 2009, 12: 267-283. 10.1017/S1368980008002589.
25. Winkleby MA, Jatulis DE, Frank E, Fortmann SP: Socioeconomic status and health: how education, income, and occupation contribute to risk factors for cardiovascular disease. Am J Public Health. 1992, 82: 816-820. 10.2105/AJPH.82.6.816.
26. Bogers RP, Van Assema P, Kester ADM, Westerterp KR, Dagnelie PC: Reproducibility, validity, and responsiveness to change of a short questionnaire for measuring fruit and vegetable intake. Am J Epidemiol. 2004, 159: 900-909. 10.1093/aje/kwh123.
27. Haraldsdóttir J, Thórsdóttir I, de Almeida MDV, Maes L, Pérez Rodrigo C, Elmadfa I, Frost Andersen L: Validity and reproducibility of a precoded questionnaire to assess fruit and vegetable intake in European 11- to 12-year-old schoolchildren. Ann Nutr Metab. 2005, 49: 221-227. 10.1159/000087276.
28. Dutman AE, Stafleu A, Kruizinga A, Brants HAM, Westerterp KR, Kistemaker C, Meuling WJA, Goldbohm RA: Validation of an FFQ and options for data processing using the doubly labelled water method in children. Public Health Nutr. 2011, 14: 410-417. 10.1017/S1368980010002119.
29. Brants H, Stafleu A, Ter Doest D, Hulshof K: Ontwikkeling van een voedselfrequentievrage nlijst:energie-inneming van kinderen van 2 tot en met 12 jaar. Voeding Nu. 2006, 2: 25-28.
30. The Netherlands Nutrition Centre Foundation: Richtlijnen Voedselkeuze (Dietary Guidelines). The Hague: 2011.

31. Van der Horst K, Oenema A, van de Looij-Jansen P, Brug J: The ENDORSE study: research into environmental determinants of obesity related behaviors in Rotterdam schoolchildren. BMC Public Health. 2008, 8: 142-10.1186/1471-2458-8-142.
32. Gattshall ML, Shoup JA, Marshall JA, Crane LA, Estabrooks PA: Validation of a survey instrument to assess home environments for physical activity and healthy eating in overweight children. Int J Behav Nutr Phys Act. 2008, 5: 3-10.1186/1479-5868-5-3.
33. Cole TJ, Bellizzi MC, Flegal KM, Dietz WH: Establishing a standard definition for child overweight and obesity worldwide: international survey. BMJ. 2000, 320: 1240-1243. 10.1136/bmj.320.7244.1240.
34. Baron RM, Kenny DA: The moderator-mediator variable distinction in social psychological research: conceptual, strategic, and statistical considerations. J Pers Soc Psychol. 1986, 51: 1173-1182. 10.1037/0022-3514.51.6.1173.
35. Johansen A, Rasmussen S, Madsen M: Health behaviour among adolescents in Denmark: influence of school class and individual risk factors. Scand J Public Health. 2006, 34: 32-40. 10.1080/14034940510032158.
36. Sandvik C, Gjestad R, Samdal O, Brug J, Klepp K-I: Does socio-economic status moderate the associations between psychosocial predictors and fruit intake in schoolchildren? The Pro Children study. Health Educ Res. 2010, 25: 121-134. 10.1093/her/cyp055.
37. Neumark-Sztainer D, Wall M, Perry C, Story M: Correlates of fruit and vegetable intake among adolescents. Prev Med (Baltim). 2003, 37: 198-208. 10.1016/S0091-7435(03)00114-2.
38. MacFarlane A, Crawford D, Ball K, Savige G, Worsley A: Adolescent home food environments and socioeconomic position. Asia Pac J Clin Nutr. 2007, 16: 748-756.
39. Campbell K, Crawford D, Jackson M, Cashel K, Worsley A, Gibbons K, Birch LL: Family food environments of 5-6-year-old-children: does socioeconomic status make a difference?. Asia Pac J Clin Nutr. 2002, 11 (Suppl 3): S553-S561. 10.1046/j.0964-7058.2002.00346.x.
40. Hupkens CL, Knibbe RA, Van Otterloo AH, Drop MJ: Class differences in the food rules mothers impose on their children: a cross-national study. Soc Sci Med. 1998, 47: 1331-1339. 10.1016/S0277-9536(98)00211-1.
41. Vereecken C, Keukelier E, Maes L: Influence of mother's educational level on food parenting practices and food habits of young children. Appetite. 2004, 43: 93-103. 10.1016/j.appet.2004.04.002.
42. Campbell KJ, Abbott G, Spence AC, Crawford DA, McNaughton SA, Ball K: Home food availability mediates associations between mothers' nutrition knowledge and child diet. Appetite. 2013, 71: 1-6. 10.1016/j.appet.2013.07.006.
43. Hendrie GA, Brindal E, Corsini N, Gardner C, Baird D, Golley RK: Combined home and school obesity prevention interventions for children: what behavior change strategies and intervention characteristics are associated with effectiveness?. Health Educ Behav. 2012, 39: 159-171. 10.1177/1090198111420286.
44. Tak NI, te Velde SJ, de Vries JHM, Brug J: Parent and child reports of fruit and vegetable intakes and related family environmental factors show low levels of agreement. J Hum Nutr Diet. 2006, 19: 275-285. 10.1111/j.1365-277X.2006.00702.x.
45. Matthys C, De Henauw S, Bellemans M, De Maeyer M, De Backer G: Breakfast habits affect overall nutrient profiles in adolescents. Public Health Nutr. 2007, 10: 413-421. 10.1017/S1368980007248049.

PART III
Education

CHAPTER 10

A Pilot Study of a Pictorial Bilingual Nutrition Education Game to Improve the Consumption of Healthful Foods in a Head Start Population

Veronica Piziak

10.1 INTRODUCTION

The prevalence of overweight and obesity among preschool children has been increasing world wide for over 40 years [1,2,3]. Mexican-American children have a higher prevalence than Caucasian children [4]. Preschool children from low income families are particularly affected with 1 in 7 children noted to be obese in 2009 [5]. The health consequences of obesity such as diabetes, previously limited to adults, are seen in younger age groups [6]. Obesity and ethnicity in Mexican American children markedly increases the risk of early onset Type 2 diabetes and early metabolic syndrome. Recent evidence suggests that obese children also have lower bone mineral density [7].

Many factors lead to increased weight in high risk preschool children but recent evidence suggests that dietary changes particularly increased consumption of sugar sweetened beverages [8], decreased consumption of high fiber foods such as vegetables and increased fat consumption are implicated [9]. Increased screen time as TV watching and computer time leads to decreased exercise. In addition, TV advertising on programming targeted toward children is heavily weighted toward food that is not nutritious and has been shown to influence food choices by children [10]. Targeting nutritional education in preschool children is essential to establish long term eating habits, but the challenges are substantial. The Head Start setting is an important opportunity for nutrition educational activities that are participatory and culturally relevant. This population is also at high risk for obesity because of ethnic and economic composition.

In the border state of Texas the poverty level is high, particularly in the Mexican-American population, and many of the families qualify for Head Start. The prevalence of obesity in the Head Start population surveyed is 20%, far above the national average [11]. In the Head Start Centers of Texas, many children speak Spanish or are bilingual, and reading skills are low at this age. Limited funding can also be a problem. In addition, access to dietary education for families is suboptimal. Studies of dietary habits of the population showed excess calories, fat, concentrated carbohydrates and sodium were taken and insufficient amounts of fiber, potassium, and vitamin A were eaten [12].

The purpose of this study was to test the effectiveness of a bilingual nutrition game to increase the servings of healthful foods particularly vegetables, fruit, and water offered to children and decrease the servings of sugar sweetened beverages in the Head Start population.

10.2 METHODS

10.2.1 Description of Game

The nutrition education game is patterned after Loteria a popular pictorial bingo game in the Mexican-American community. The moderator of the game shows a card with a picture and tells a story or recites a rhyme to describe the picture. The players then put a token on their game boards if they have the picture. This game lends itself to nutrition education. The cards and boards show color images of culturally appropriate food and the reverse side gives the names in English and Spanish which may be used to improve reading skills (Figure 1). Locally popular ethnic foods were included as suggested by the teachers in focus groups. All of the fruits and vegetables in the game are available in the area and popular ethnic foods appear more often on the game boards. The cards contain the name of the food in English and Spanish and a set of rhymes with information in English or Spanish about the foods (Figure 2). There are several ways to use the game in the Head Start setting: the deck may be used as a set of flash cards to acquaint the children with different types of food and their place in a healthy diet; both the game boards and the deck may be used to play a variety of types of nutritional bingo [13]. The teachers were allowed to play the game in either English or Spanish. They could adapt the length of game play for their schedule and attention span of the particular class. The rhymes from the cards could be recited when the children were eating their meals and snacks since many of the foods featured in the game were served by Head Start. Game modifications were made on the basis of suggestions with the teachers at the pilot site in central Texas.

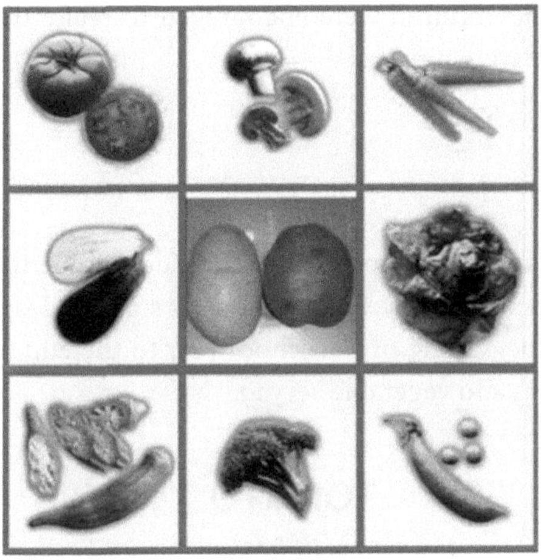

CARROTS *CARROTS*	MUSHROOMS *HONGOS*	TOMATO *TOMATE*
LETTUCE *LECHUGA*	POTATO *PATATA*	EGGPLANT *BERENJENA*
PEAS *GUISANTES*	BROCOLLI *BRO'CULI*	OKRA *BONBOM*

FIGURE 10.1 Game board: Front (pictures), Back (words).

10.2.2 Study Population

The project was approved by the Scott and White IRB. The game was provided to Head Start centers in three Texas border counties and two central Texas counties for use with approximately 10,000 children. Head Start is a government funded locally operated preschool program providing basic education for children of low income families. Most of the children are from 3–5 years of age. The pilot study examines the results in 413 children in one central Texas county where the Head Start population is 57.3% Mexican-American and 56.8%

have a family history of diabetes. The parents were acquainted with the game in a meeting where parents were encouraged to play for prizes and counseled about healthy food choices. At the beginning and end of the school year parents completed a questionnaire about the food offered to the children at home on Monday thru Friday and on the weekends. The parents were asked to document the number of times a day that the children were served milk and soda and water, fruit and vegetables during the week and on weekends. They were not asked to estimate the amount consumed. The parents received instructions about how to complete the questionnaire. The parents were asked to document milk and soda and water, fruit and vegetable served. Head Start provides a healthy diet and structured exercise during the school day on Monday thru Friday. The teachers were instructed about the game and given basic nutrition counseling during a training session before the start of the school year. The game was played by the children at least twice a week and the children were encouraged to recite the rhymes that were on the cards as they were presented.

10.2.3 Data Analysis

To preserve the privacy of the children anonymous aggregate data from the entire county was analyzed. The signed rank test was used to test statistical significance of the difference from the beginning of the school year to the end of the year for the water, milk, soda, fruit, and vegetable served.

LETTUCE
LECHUGA
Lettuce is a vegetable
It grows on the ground
Use it in salads and sandwiches

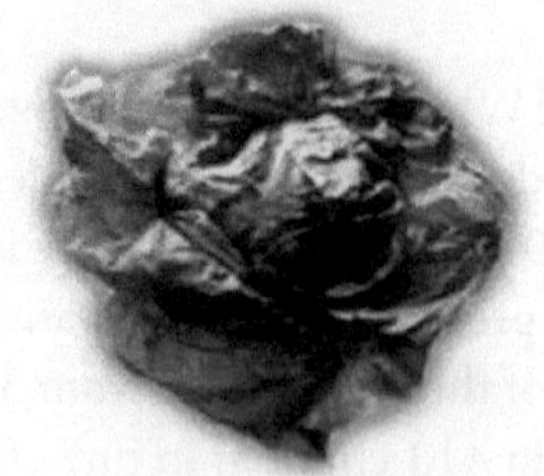

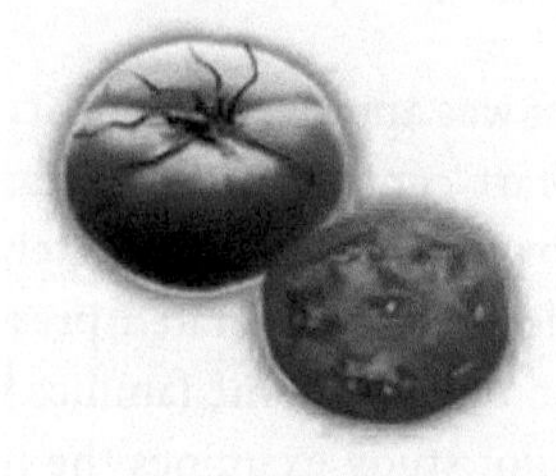

FIGURE 10.2 Game cards: pictures and words.

10.3 RESULTS AND DISCUSSION

Results are shown in Table 1. The mean value for any given parameter was the mean servings of a given food per day for the entire population for the specified time period (Monday–Friday outside of Head Start or on weekends). The difference in the "means" was the difference between the mean value before and after the game was used. Before the intervention 38 parents reported no vegetable served on weekends and 16 reported no vegetable served at all. At the end of the study only 12 families reported no vegetable served on weekends and only 4 reported no vegetable served at any time. There was a statistically significant increase in vegetable served outside of Head Start both after school during the week and on the weekends. There was no change in the amount of exercise in the group over the school year. The study was unable to demonstrate any other statistically significant changes in dietary habits. However, feedback from a focus group of teachers demonstrated that the game was important in promoting recognition of a variety of foods by the children. The repetition of the rhymes could be used to promote the importance of increased water intake and reinforce the desirable decrease in drinking of sugar sweetened beverages and the routine intake of foods with high sugar content which is the policy of Head Start. The teachers felt that they would like to continue to use the game.

TABLE 10.1 Mean Values for Daily Servings of Foods and Water by the Study Population Before and after the Intervention.

Servings per day(Mean for the population)	Before	After	Difference
Water on Saturday and Sunday	3.99	3.97	–0.02
Milk on Saturday and Sunday	3.047	3.046	–0.021
Soda on Saturday and Sunday	1.78	1.62	–0.16
Fruit on Saturday and Sunday	3.03	3.04	0.01
Vegetables on Saturday and Sunday	2.34	2.68	0.34*
Water on Monday through Friday	3.98	4.07	0.09
Milk on Monday through Friday	3.34	3.26	–0.08
Soda on Monday through Friday	1.64	1.57	–0.07
Fruit on Monday through Friday	3.32	3.28	–0.04
Vegetables on Monday through Friday	2.57	2.94	0.37 **

* P value = 0.02; ** P value = 0.009.

Recently, multiple initiatives have been directed toward changing the eating and exercise habits of the preschool population to attempt to decrease obesity and thus prevent the early onset of hypertension, diabetes and metabolic syndrome [14]. A structured education program for preschool children and parents has resulted in an increase in fruit and vegetable consumption [15]. Head Start particularly has made excellent progress in instituting education programs for parents and children [16]. The findings from this pilot study in cooperation with a Texas county Head Start show that vegetable servings may also be improved in the age group by using a simple pictorial nutrition education game that may be played in either English or Spanish and incorporates elements of the Mexican American culture familiar to the majority of the students and their parents. This familiarity simplifies instruction of the teachers and parents. The game is also inexpensive to reproduce helping to control costs. This study only encompasses one of the 5 counties and the data from the total population is still being analyzed. In the future the parents will be asked to play the game with the children and incentives will be provided to families who participate. An exercise initiative using cartoon characters leading the children in age appropriate exercise routines and counseling about healthy foods has been tested and accepted by the teachers and will be studied in the pilot county as well.

REFERENCES

1. Ogden, C.L.; Troiano, R.P.; Briefel, R.R.; Kuczmarski, R.J.; Flegal, K.M.; Johnson, C.L. Prevalence of overweight among preschool children in the United States, 1971 through 1994. Pediatrics 1997, 99.
2. Ogden, C.L.; Flegal, K.M.; Carroll, M.D.; Johnson, C.L. Prevalence and trends in overweight among US children and adolescents, 1999–2000. JAMA 2002, 288, 1728–1732.
3. de Onis, M.; Blössner, M.; Borghi, E. Global prevalence and trends of overweight and obesity among preschool children. Am. J. Clin. Nutr. 2010, 92, 1257–1264.
4. Ogden, C.L.; Carroll, M.D.; Flegal, K.M. High body mass index for age among US children and adolescents, 2003–2006. JAMA 2008, 299, 2401–2405.
5. Pediatric Nutrition Surveilance System. 2009. Available online: www.cdc.gov/obesity/childhood/data.html (accessed on 17 February 2012).
6. Haines, L.; Wan, K.C.; Lynn, R.; Barrett, T.G.; Shield, J.P. Rising incidence of type 2 diabetes in children in the UK. Diabetes Care 2007, 30, 1097–1101.
7. Mughal, M.Z.; Khadilkar, A.V. The accrual of bone mass during childhood and puberty. Curr. Opin. Endocrinol. Diabetes Obes. 2011, 18, 28–32.
8. Nelson, J.A.; Carpenter, K.; Chiasson, M.A. Diet, activity, and overweight among preschool-age children enrolled in the special supplemental nutrition program for Women, Infants, and Children (WIC). Prev. Chronic Dis. 2006, 3, A49:1–A49:12.

9. Barquera, S.; Campirano, F.; Bonvecchio, A.; Hernández-Barrera, L.; Rivera, J.A.; Popkin, B.M. Caloric beverage consumption patterns in Mexican children. Nutr. J. 2010, 9.
10. Dixon, H.G.; Scully, M.L.; Wakefield, M.A.; White, V.M.; Crawford, D.A. The effects of television advertisements for junk food versus nutritious food on children's food attitudes and preferences. Soc. Sci. Med. 2007, 65, 1311–1323.
11. Piziak, V.K.; Morgan-Cox, M.A.; Tubbs, J.; Hasan, M. Elevated body mass index in Texas Head Start children: A result of heredity and economics. South. Med. J. 2010, 103, 1219–1222.
12. Mier, N.; Piziak, V.; Kjar, D.; Castillo-Ruiz, O.; Velazquez, G.; Alfaro, M.E.; Ramirez, J.A. Nutrition provided to Mexican-American preschool children on the Texas-Mexico border. J. Am. Diet. Assoc. 2007, 107, 311–315.
13. Mier, N.; Piziak, V.; Valdez, L. Ultimate nutrition game for Mexican-American preschoolers. J. Nutr. Educ. Behav. 2005, 37, 325–326.
14. Hesketh, K.D.; Campbell, K.J. Interventions to prevent obesity in 0–5 year olds: An updated systematic review of the literature. Obesity (Silver Spring) 2010, 18, s27–s35
15. Witt, K.; Dunn, K. Increasing fruit and vegetable consumption among preschoolers: Evaluation of color me healthy. J. Nutr. Educ. Behav. 2011.
16. Larson, N.; Ward, D.S.; Neelon, S.B.; Story, M. What role can child care settings play in obesity prevention? A review of the evidence and a call for research efforts. J. Am. Diet. Assoc. 2011, 111, 1343–1362.

CHAPTER 11

Blending Better Beverage Options: A Nutrition Education and Experiential Workshop for Youths

Kathy K. Isoldi and Veronika Dolar

11.1 INTRODUCTION

An increase in the consumption of sugar-sweetened beverages (SSBs) and the prevalence of childhood obesity have occurred in tandem. In the United States (US) between 1977 and 2002 the increase in calories consumed from soft drinks and other sweetened beverages increased 230% and 170%, respectively [1]. Concurrently, the prevalence of childhood obesity increased threefold in the US, with those in minority and low-income groups experiencing higher prevalence rates [2, 3]. During this period, many other factors that increase obesity risk changed as well, such as an increase in sedentary activities, purchase of fast food, and sleep debt [4, 5]. However, SSBs are of special concern since the calories contained in this liquid form, for some reason, are not registered by the body, and therefore no dietary compensations are made following intake [6]. Instead paradoxically, researchers have found that when youths drink more SSBs it results in an increase in solid food consumption as well, with choices like pizza, burgers, and savory snacks often chosen [7]. Mathias et al. [7] found through analysis of data collected from the National Health and Nutrition Examination

Surveys (NHANES) conducted between 2003 and 2010 that for every 100 kcalories of SSB consumed by 6–11-year-olds there was an increase in solid food consumed providing an additional 36 ± 14 kcalories. Youths 12–18 years of age revealed an intake of an additional 86 ± 10 kcalories in solid food form for every 100 kcalories of SSB product consumed. Recently, several reviews have illuminated the strong connection between obesity risk and SSB intake [8–10]; however weak potency of effect on interventions has called into question the absolute strength of this association [11].

In addition to an increased risk of obesity from consuming liquid calories, the high sugar content in SSBs has been associated with an increased risk of insulin resistance, dyslipidemia, type 2 diabetes mellitus, and cardiovascular disease [1, 6, 12]. Added sugars consumed from both liquid and solid sources are associated with body weight gain in youths at risk of developing obesity [6]; however Wang et al. [13] found in their group of 564 youths who were followed for two years that consuming sugar from liquid, but not solid, sources predicted a higher risk of developing impaired glucose homeostasis and glucose resistance. Reports spanning the past decade highlight increasing consumption of SSBs among children, adolescents, and teens [1, 4, 14, 15]. Recent estimates of the mean caloric contribution from SSBs range from 117 kcal/day to as much as 356 kcal/day, with calorie contribution variations based upon age category, sex, and ethnicity [14–17]. Those in minority and low-income groups have been identified as drinking greater amounts of SSBs [18]. It has also been found that approximately 5% of children and 16% of adolescents surveyed are heavy consumers of SSBs, with intakes at or exceeding 500 kcal/day [8]. SSBs are available to youths on the school campus as well as on the home front [17, 18]. However, researchers point to data supporting that the majority of SSBs are consumed at home [15, 17].

Public health experts have made a call for action in the form of educational interventions to address the excessive SSB intake in youths and subsequent adverse health issues [1, 9, 10, 14, 16, 17, 19]. The aim of the current study was to gauge impact on knowledge and attitudes regarding SSBs following a hands-on workshop for youths delivered during summer program hours. This experiential workshop addressed the sugar content of commonly consumed SSBs and included preparation and tasting of lower sugar alternatives. The study was given exemption status from Long Island University.

11.2 METHODS

11.2.1 Setting and Participants

A convenience sample of youths who were enrolled in the summer program at a local boys and girls club participated in the nutrition education and blending better beverage options workshop. This program was provided to all attendees of the summer program at one boys and girls club in Long Island in New York State. All 128 summer camp participants were included in the workshop. Participants ranged in age from 5 to 14 years old. The workshop was delivered to approximately 20 participants at a time who were divided into small groups of 6–8 youths of similar age and were seated at one work table together with two undergraduate nutrition student volunteers.

11.2.2 Instrument

The survey instrument was developed by the study investigators and was based upon current literature [8, 16, 18] and designed to explore knowledge and beliefs about SSBs. The survey was modified to be age-appropriate; one version was created for 5–9-year-olds and another was developed for those who were 10–14 years of age. The same questions were asked, but the language was simplified and smile and frown faces were used for improved comprehension on the survey for the younger children. All participants were offered assistance with completion of the program surveys, and the younger participants were given one-on-one assistance when needed from undergraduate nutrition student volunteers. The survey was completed before the workshop began and following the end of the two-hour program for comparison.

11.2.2.1 Usual Intake of SSBs

Each participant was asked to report their usual intake within four commonly consumed beverage categories (soda, sports drinks, sugar-sweetened tea and juice, and energy drinks) before the start of the workshop. For each category the participant was asked to estimate his/her frequency of consumption per week and then to estimate quantity consumed per frequency. Sample cans and bottles and representative glassware were displayed at each table to assist the participants in estimating the quantity of SSBs consumed. Nutrition undergraduate student volunteers assisted the participants in completing the survey.

11.2.2.2 Knowledge of Sugar Content of SSBs

The survey included four questions regarding knowledge of sugar content (in teaspoon counts) of commonly consumed beverage items (16-ounce bottle of one-half sweetened iced tea and one-half lemonade, 12-ounce can of cola beverage, 20-ounce bottle of sweetened fruit punch, and an 8-ounce can of an energy drink). The participants were asked to select the amount (in teaspoons) of sugar from a list of four choices for each SSB item. The choices for each item were 3–5 teaspoons, 7–9 teaspoons, 10–12 teaspoons, or 15 or more teaspoons. The survey created for 5–9-year-olds included assistance in understanding the question by adding qualifying words for each selection with options listed as follows: 3–5 teaspoons, a small amount; 7–9 teaspoons, a medium amount; 10–12 teaspoons, a large amount; and 15 or more teaspoons, a lot.

11.2.2.3 Attitudes Held Regarding SSBs

To record and gauge any change in attitudes held regarding SSB preferences, thoughts about health concerns associated with SSBs, and intention regarding avoidance of SSBs, participants were asked to respond to six statements at baseline and again following the intervention. Following each statement, such as "I should drink less soda and sweetened beverages," participants were directed to choose from a list of responses: strongly agree, agree, disagree, or not sure. The survey instrument completed by 5–9-year-olds included the following choices with accompanying faces to help them better understand and choose their response: yes definitely (broad smile), yes (smile), no (frown), and not sure (neutral).

11.2.2.4 Postprogram Feedback

On the postprogram survey participants were asked to respond to a question asking whether they had enjoyed participation in the program. Attendees were asked to respond to the following statement: "I've enjoyed participating in the beverage workshop." In addition, participants were asked to share their thoughts regarding intention to reduce intake of SSBs in the future by responding to the following statement: "I think I will drink less sugar-sweetened beverages like soda because of what I've learned today." Once again the 10–14-year-old participants were asked to select from the following responses: strongly agree, agree, disagree, and not sure; and 5–9-year-olds chose their answer from yes definitely (broad smile), yes (smile), no (frown), and not sure (neutral), using visual faces to help them better understand and choose their response.

11.2.3 Intervention

Each participant took part in a two-hour workshop held during summer program hours that was composed of two separate, yet related, components.

1. Educational session revealing the sugar content of commonly consumed beverages and demonstration of adding a similar content of table sugar to water. Discussion of the health detriments associated with excessive sugar intake.
2. A hands-on, experiential involvement in blending better beverage options, followed by recipe tastings. A discussion about how to make healthier decisions for beverages.

Undergraduate nutrition student volunteers assisted participants in completing the program surveys and served as facilitators for the workshop. Each volunteer attended a one-hour instructional training session conducted by the Principal Investigator prior to the start of the program.

11.2.3.1 Sugar Content Quiz and Demonstration

After completion of the baseline survey, each table of 6–8 participants took part in a guessing game and discussion about the sugar content of four popular beverage items led by an undergraduate nutrition student. Participants were asked to guess how many teaspoons of sugar were in each of four commonly consumed beverage items. After guessing, the nutrition student revealed the correct answer and asked the participants to count out sugar packets representing the amount of sugar contained in the item. A plate containing all the sugar packages was placed in front of the beverage item to offer a lasting visual image. This process was repeated for each of the four SSBs. When the process was completed for all beverages, the children were asked to view the four items on the table and to consider how much sugar would be consumed if all four SSBs were consumed in one day. The group added the total packages of sugar to achieve a grand total. Then the nutrition undergraduate students at each table led a demonstration showing how much sugar is added to liquid beverages by adding 15 teaspoons of sugar to a 20-ounce glass of water. This item was stirred and passed around for the participants to view the thick, cloudy substance that was created by simulating the amount of sugar often added to SSBs. An interactive discussion regarding the sugar content of SSBs and the health consequences of consuming too much sugar was held. Each nutrition undergraduate student was instructed to pose the following questions to the participants.

1. Is anybody surprised about the amount of sugar in these beverages?
2. Would anyone take a glass of water and add the same amount of sugar to it and then drink it?
3. Do you think drinking so much sugar in these types of beverages is harmful to your health?
   a. Nutrition students were instructed to highlight the association of high sugar intake with weight gain, diabetes, and dental caries.
   b. A review of the concerns associated with the ingredients in energy drinks and why children should not drink these products was conducted.
4. Would you like to make beverages to drink that are lower in sugar?

11.2.3.2 Blending Better Beverage Options: Tasting and Discussion

Participants were led in a hands-on preparation of four recipes: (1) fresh peach and orange infused water, (2) pineapple, mango, peach, and lime slush, (3) cranberry, pineapple, and lime fizzy, and (4) fresh strawberry and banana smoothie. The participants had the opportunity to taste all items they had prepared. The nutrition undergraduate students were instructed to ask for participant feedback about the taste, acceptability, and ease of preparation of lower sugar beverage alternatives. The importance of preparing beverages using diluted versions of 100% fresh fruit juices was stressed.

11.2.4 Analysis

The study, including instruments, protocols, and consent procedures, received exempt approval by the Institutional Review Board at Long Island University. Written parent consent was not required because the student survey portion of this project was classified as exempt. Survey data results were tabulated and compiled into a database and analyzed using STATA (SE 13) to provide descriptive statistics and analysis. In addition to the standard Chi-square tests the analysis includes t-tests for comparing two population proportions. Proportions are among the few measures which can be used for summarizing categorical data and provide an additional dimension to the analysis. Unlike a Chi-square test that tests for the association between qualitative variables using the entire contingency table, the t-test can be applied to test, for example, if the proportion of participants correctly answering the question on the pretest is statistically different from the proportion of participants correctly answering the question on the posttest. The test statistic for comparing two population proportions is $t = ((\widehat{p_1} - \widehat{p_2}) - (p_1 - p_2))/\sqrt{\bar{p}(1-\bar{p})(1/n_1 + 1/n_2)}$, where $\widehat{p_1} - \widehat{p_2}$ are sample proportions estimates, $p_1 - p_2$ are population proportions, and $\bar{p}$ $(x_1 + x_2)/(n_1 + n_2$ is the weighted average of the two sample proportion estimates. All t-tests results are one-tailed tests in order to study if one proportion of respondents is higher than the other, rather than simply being different from each other which would be captured by the two-tailed test. In other words, the tests are to assess if the proportion of participants correctly answering the question on the posttest is higher than the proportion of participants correctly answering the question on the pretest. Level of significance was set at $P < 0.05$.

11.3 RESULTS

11.3.1 Participants

Specific participant sociodemographic data were not obtained due to the study's exemption status. However, study participants were attendees of the local boys and girls club afterschool program. The attendees of the program are predominately Latino and African American and come from single parent (51%) and low-income homes (76% come from families with incomes of less than $33,000/year and 74% receive free or reduced fee lunch). A total of 128 surveys were distributed to participants, 100% were returned, and there were no missing responses or surveys that were deemed incomplete. Of 128 participants, 81 (63.3%) were male and 47 (36.7%) were female, with an average age of 9.3 years. Data were analyzed using the entire sample of 128 participants as well as by two age subgroups: age of 5–9 years and age of 10–14 years. There were 70 participants in the 5–9-year-old age group (41 male and 29 female) with an average age of 7.6 years and 58 participants in the 10–14-year-old age group (40 male and 18 female) with the average age of 11.3 years.

11.3.2 SSB Intake

The average amount of SSBs consumed per week for the entire sample was 125.6 oz. (17.9 oz. per day), with 113.9 oz. (16.3 oz. per day) for the 5–9 year old age group and 139.6 oz. (19.9 oz. per day) for the 10–14-year-old age group. A two-sample mean comparison t-test found no statistically significant difference in total SSB consumption between the two age groups. In addition, the difference in drinking soda and sugar-sweetened teas and juices was not significantly different between the two age groups. However, the older group was found to drink significantly more sports drinks and energy drinks compared to the younger group ($P < 0.05$; Table 1). The drinking habits of males versus females in both the 5–9-year- and 10–14-year-old age groups were not statistically different. However, males in the 10–14-year-old age group reported to drink twice as much soda as females in this age group, 31.1 oz. and 15.6 oz. per week, respectively, and are significantly more likely to drink energy drinks, 45% and 11%, respectively ($P < 0.05$).

11.3.3 Knowledge of Sugar Content in SSBs

To evaluate the level of knowledge obtained by attending the beverage workshop pre- and postintervention survey data were analyzed using the standard Chi-square tests for the association between two qualitative variables. For the entire sample of 128 participants, the Chi-square test for all four knowledge questions rejects the null hypothesis even when the P value is set at $P < 0.01$. Since all the scores have improved, it can be concluded that the intervention was successful in providing information to the participants. The same conclusion is obtained for the 10–14-year-old age subgroup. However, for the 5–9-year-old age group, the Chi-square test failed to reject the null for improvement in knowledge on the question about the sugar content in an 8 oz. can of an energy drink.

TABLE 11.1 Typical consumption of SSBs in youths attending a summer program.

Question	Response	5–9-year-olds number (%)	10–14-year-olds number (%)	Entire group number (%)
I drink soda				
Such as cola, ginger ale, Sprite, and Mountain Dew	Yes	60 (85.7)	51 (87.9)	111 (86.7)
	No	10 (14.3)	7 (12.1)	17 (13.3)
Mean times per week		2.37	2.09	2.25
Mean ounces consumed		9.91	11.1	10.45
Total mean ounces consumed per weeks		26.26	26.28	26.27
I drink sports drinks				
Such as Gatorade and Powerade	Yes	60 (85.7)	49 (84.5)	109 (85.2)
	No	10 (14.3)	9 (15.5)	19 (14.8)
Mean times per week		2.41	2.78	2.58
Mean ounces consumed		15.06	18.28	16.52
Total mean ounces consumed per weeks		42.54	63.03	51.83
I drink sugar-sweetened beverages				
Such as sweetened tea, fruit punch, and Sunny-D	Yes	57 (81.4)	47 (81.0)	104 (81.3)
	No	13 (18.6)	11 (19.0)	24 (18.8)
Mean times per week		2.84	2.81	2.83
Mean ounces consumed		12.16	11.98	12.08
Total mean ounces consumed per weeks		43.59	40.64	42.25
I drink energy drinks				
Such as Red Bull and Rockstar	Yes	11 (15.7)	20 (34.5)	31 (24.2)
	No	59 (84.3)	38 (65.5)	97 (75.8)
Mean times per week		0.3	0.78	0.52
Mean ounces consumed		1.49	3.94	2.6
Total mean ounces consumed per weeks		3.14	9.7	6.11
All beverages mean ounces		113.87	139.64	125.55

Results of the analyses of knowledge data using t-tests revealed that the proportion of participants who correctly answered the questions on the pretest for the entire sample of 128 participants is statistically different from the proportion of participants who correctly answered the questions on the posttest survey for questions 1 and 2 (sugar content in a 16 oz. serving of sweetened one-half iced tea and one-half lemonade; correct answer 10–12 teaspoons and in a 12 oz. can of cola soda; correct answer 10–12 teaspoons, resp.; Figure 1, panels (a) and (b)). However, for questions 3 and 4 (sugar content in a 20 oz. serving of sweetened fruit punch; correct answer 15+ teaspoons and an 8 oz. can of an energy drink; correct answer 7–9 teaspoons, resp., Figure 1, panels (c) and (d)), improvement in knowledge was increased, but not significantly. More precisely, for the age group of 10–14 years the scores on all four questions improved, while for the age group of 5–9 year olds only the scores for questions 1 and 3 (sugar content in a 16 oz. serving of sweetened one-half iced tea and one-half lemonade and the 20 oz. serving of sweetened fruit punch, resp., Figure 1, panels (a) and (c)) improved significantly.

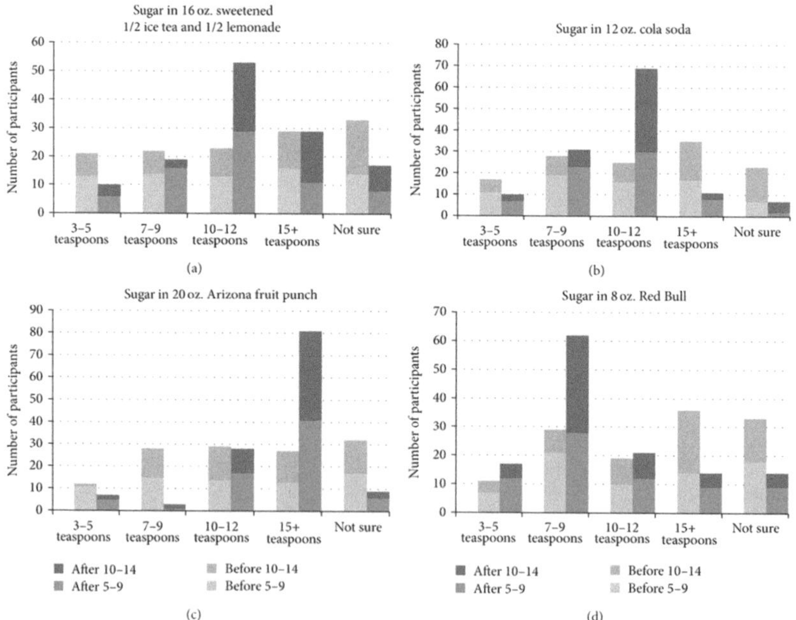

FIGURE 11.1 Baseline and postprogram SSB sugar content knowledge.

11.3.4 Attitudes Regarding SSB Intake

A great majority of participants either strongly agreed or agreed with the statement that they usually choose a glass of water when they are thirsty, that beverages with sugar are not good for them, and that they should drink less soda and sweetened beverages (Figure 2, panels (a), (e), and (f), resp.), both before and after intervention. In addition, most participants disagreed with the statement that soda is their favorite drink, that delicious drinks can be made using fresh fruit and beverages without added sugar, and that energy drinks are healthy (Figure 2, panels (b), (c), and (d), resp.). The differences between the pre- and postintervention responses to comments addressing attitudes, however, are not statistically different when Chi-square tests were applied. In all attitudinal comments posed study participants responded favorably regarding attitudes held on the preprogram survey except when responding to the comment that delicious drinks can be made using fresh fruit without added sugar. The majority of participants disagreed with this comment on the preintervention survey, and although there was an increase in the number of those who strongly agreed or agreed with this comment following the intervention, there was no statistically significant change in response following program completion.

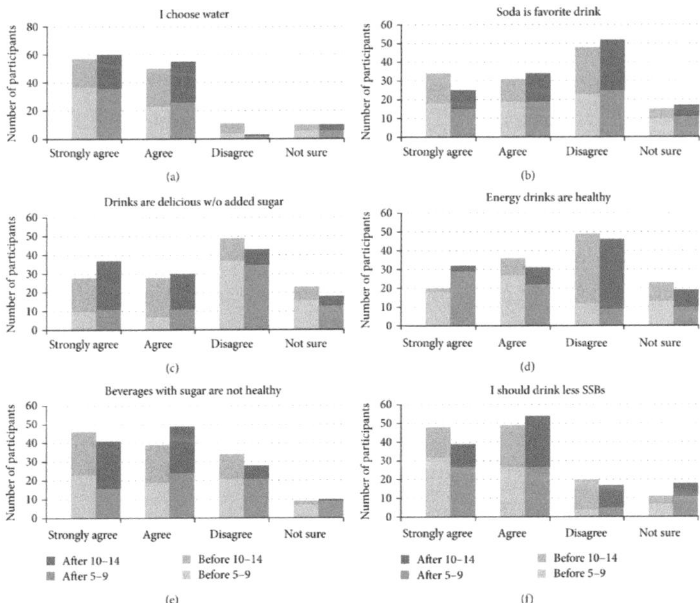

FIGURE 11.2 Baseline and postprogram responses to attitudinal statements.

Responses to one comment went in an unexpected direction for the comment addressing whether an energy drink was a healthy beverage option. The majority of participants disagreed that an energy drink is a healthy beverage option on both the pre- and postintervention surveys; however, unexpectedly less rather than more participants disagreed with the statement after intervention compared with the preprogram surveys. This result was mostly driven by the change observed in the younger participants in the 5–9-year-old age group, where more of them either strongly agreed or agreed that energy drinks are healthy for them after the intervention. One possible explanation for this might be due to their unfamiliarity with this type of SSB.

11.4 DISCUSSION

This interactive workshop conducted during summer program hours held with youths 5–14 years of age queried usual intake of SSBs and focused on transmitting knowledge about the amount of sugar contained in commonly consumed beverage items and the potential health detriments associated with overconsumption. The workshop also included a hands-on preparation and tasting of several lower sugar beverage alternatives. In agreement with current literature [8, 14, 15], the youths attending this workshop reported regular consumption of SSBs. We found that the large majority of the youths who participated in the workshop reported regularly drinking soda (87%), sports drinks (85%), and sweetened teas and juices (81%). Approximately one-quarter of the participants (24%) reported drinking energy drinks, with a significant difference in consumption found in those 5–9 years of age (16%) in comparison with those 10–14 years old (35%). This finding is not surprising given the age of our participants as energy drinks are more commonly consumed by teens and young adults. However, there are many health concerns associated with consuming energy drinks and young children can be influenced by the intense marketing efforts for these products [20, 21]. Therefore, reports of any intake of energy drinks in youths 5–14 years of age are of concern and require further investigation focused on this specific group of SSBs. Of significance is that males were four times more likely than females to consume energy drinks. Based on our results 10–14-year-old males, in comparison with younger children and females, were more likely to consume energy drinks and should be targeted in future interventions aimed at eliminating consumption of this problematic beverage in at-risk youth populations.

Estimated mean intake of soda, sports drinks, sugar-sweetened drinks, and energy drinks per week, rounded to the nearest ounce, was 26, 43, and 44 ounces and 1 ounce, respectively, for 5–9-year-olds and 26, 63, 41, and 4 ounces, respectively, for 10–14-year-olds. We found that the mean intake of fluid ounces of SSBs in our group of participants translated into approximately 17.9 ounces of beverage per day, or a little over two 8-ounce servings. This quantity of SSB translates into approximately 224 kcalories. The mean calorie contribution from SSBs found in this study is similar to what others have reported as usual calorie contribution from SSB in children and adolescents [14–17]. Noted in our data, and in agreement with current trends reported, sports drinks are being consumed with increasing frequency [8]. Researchers have reported that parents in Latino communities may exhibit a misunderstanding regarding sports drinks as some have been found to report that they believe that these drinks are healthy options for their children [18]. This misunderstanding in a community at increased risk of obesity and glucose intolerance is concerning and can promote future health risks. Therefore, outreach to parents, particularly in Latino communities to inform them about the health risks regarding the sugar content of sports drinks, appears advisable [18].

Chi-square tests on the entire sample of participants revealed a significant improvement in knowledge of sugar content for all four commonly consumed beverage items (iced tea/lemonade mix, cola beverage, sweetened fruit punch, and energy drink) between baseline and end of program. Since all the scores improved we conclude that the intervention was successful in providing information to participants.

Results of t-test analysis revealed improvement in knowledge after intervention for all four questions for 10–14-year-olds, but significance for 5–9-year-olds was only established for questions about the sugar content of iced tea/lemonade mix and sweetened fruit punch. These results are expected, since the participants in the age group of 10–14 years are more capable of understanding and retaining learned information. In addition, the older participants are also more likely to either consume and/or be familiar with cola beverages and energy drinks. In other words, the younger participants did improve their knowledge regarding the sugar content in all SSBs; however, for the sugar content in a 12 oz. can of cola and an 8 oz. can of an energy drink; correct answer 7–9 teaspoons, this change was not statistically different from the answers they provided in the pretest. It is not surprising that the younger aged participants did not remember the sugar content in energy drinks reviewed during the workshop as this is not a product that is widely consumed in this age category. It is possible that they did not register the information to memory due to lack of interest and familiarity with the product. Similarly, the younger participants would be more likely to drink sweetened fruit juice than cola beverages and this could explain the lack of significance found in change in knowledge for these beverage items.

Analyses of responses to six questions targeting attitudes about SSBs revealed no significant change in attitudes regarding beverage choice preference, thoughts about health concerns associated with SSBs, and wish to reduce SSBs following program participation. There are several factors that may explain the lack of change in attitude. One reason why there was not a considerable change found in participant attitudes might be that most participants already selected a favorable response prior to the intervention. Baseline surveys revealed that 85.7% of 5–9-year-olds and 81% of 10–14-year-olds reported that they choose water to drink when they are thirsty, and 84.3% of 5–9-year-olds and 65.5% of 10–14-year-olds reported that they knew that they should drink less SSBs. There were 57.1% of 5–9-year-olds and 74.1% of 10–14-year-olds who agreed that they thought beverages with added sugar were not good for them. However, it is possible that this comment may have been misunderstood by some who interpreted "not good for them" as not good in taste rather than not good for health. There were volunteers who read and explained the concept of the comment to the participants, but there may still have been a misunderstanding of the intention. Therefore, response results to this comment need further investigation and when the comment is posed to participants in the future clarity can be enhanced by instead asking for response to "Beverages with added sugar are not healthy for me." Although not statistically significant impact of the program was evident as the results show that, following the intervention, more participants either strongly agreed or agreed with the statement that delicious drinks can be made using fresh fruit and beverages without added sugar (44.5% in the preintervention survey versus 52.3% in the postintervention survey). This trend in change of thought was particularly noticeable for the 10–14-year-old age group.

A significant percentage of children and adolescents seem to know they should reduce their intake of SSBs; however this knowledge does not translate into action. The preference for sweets is innate as well as learned, and so this biological response triggered by environmental availability may help to explain the resistance to behavior change in reducing SSB intake [22]. The strong desire for something sweet to drink and desire for a SSB in spite of known health risks were clearly stated by participants in a qualitative study conducted with college students [23]. College students are in an age category older than our participant sample and so even though they are more mature and should be able to better understand the risks of choosing to drink too many SSBs, the desire to drink what they wanted regardless was evident in the narrative captured by researchers

[23]. Resistance to change in attitude and strong cravings for desired beverages make it difficult to see dramatic behavioral changes in attitudes held following short-term interventions. Despite these obstacles, Ebbeling et al. [24] report success in their study where they provided weekly deliveries of noncaloric beverages for 25 weeks to the homes of 53 children, aged 13–18 years. Compared to the control group the intervention group reduced their intake of SSBs by 84% and experienced a statistically significant reduction in body mass index (BMI) for those participants in the upper tertile for weight at baseline. Similarly, James et al. [25] conducted a year-long, school-based educational program for 644 schoolchildren in England who were 7–11 years old, called *Ditch the Fizz*, and found a small reduction in BMI in the intervention group and a modest reduction in consumption of carbonated drinks. Additionally, Sichieri et al. [26] report a statistically significant reduction in consumption of carbonated beverages in their seven-month-long, school-based intervention (n = 1134) with 9–12-year-olds that focused on increasing water intake. The intervention group received classroom activities and water bottles and had promotional banners hung at the school. A statistically significant reduction in BMI was found only in those who were overweight at baseline and only in females. Evidently, small successes in reducing SSB intake in youth are achievable. However, long-term interventions that address the home, school, and afterschool environments may be needed to realize greater impact.

There were several limitations with this study. A convenience sample was used for the study with all the participants coming from one boys and girls club in one community in the US. The participants were predominately Latino and African American and therefore study results cannot be generalized to other groups. In addition, data collected were self-reported and may be skewed due to participant bias or poor recall. Finally and in hindsight, the comment addressing thoughts about whether sweetened drinks were "not good" for the participant was found to be ambiguously worded and may have been misinterpreted. Study strengths include the use of trained nutrition undergraduate students to assist participants with survey completion and the interactive design of the intervention. We engaged youths in the learning process offering an experiential workshop that allowed the participants to prepare and taste alternatives to SSBs and also provided strong visuals to enhance impact and learning. We did not just tell youth participants to avoid SSBs but instead had them prepare and taste no- and low-sugar alternatives. The results from the program evaluation reveal that participants enjoyed participating in this program, as 87.5% either strongly agreed or agreed with this statement. In addition, almost 80% of the participants either strongly agreed or agreed with the statement I think I will drink less sugar-sweetened beverages like soda because of what I learned today; 81.5% in the 5–9-year-old age group and 77.6% in the 10–14-year-old age group (Table 2).

11.5 CONCLUSION

Childhood obesity and subsequent health detriment remain a formidable public health concern. Weight gain from consuming sugar in liquid form, such as in SSBs, is particularly concerning as liquid calories are not registered by the body and therefore not compensated for with subsequent reduction in food intake. SSBs are ubiquitous and they have made their way into the daily diet of children as they are readily available at home, on the school campus, and at afterschool venues. In this two-hour, hands-on intervention study we found that consumption of SSBs was common in 5–14-year-olds in three major categories: soda, sports drinks, and sugar-sweetened teas and juices. Energy drinks were less commonly consumed; however 24% of the participants reported consumption. Energy drinks should not be consumed by youths and interventions that address avoiding consumption of energy drinks in this age group are needed.

Despite providing a relatively brief intervention we were able to show a significant increase in participants' retention of knowledge regarding the amount of sugar added to commonly consumed SSBs. Postprogram data revealed that the large majority of participants enjoyed the program and intended to reduce intake of SSBs following participation in the program. However, we were unable to significantly influence attitudes held regarding SSBs. Long-term interventions and programs that engage youths and reach out to parents as well as addressing the widespread availability of SSBs are needed in the future to influence resistant attitudes and beverage choosing behaviors in youths.

REFERENCES

1. A. A. Bremer and R. H. Lustig, "Effects of sugar-sweetened beverages on children," Pediatric Annals, vol. 41, no. 1, pp. 26–30, 2012.
2. C. L. Ogden, M. D. Carroll, B. K. Kit, and K. M. Flegal, "Prevalence of obesity and trends in body mass index among US children and adolescents, 1999-2010," Journal of the American Medical Association, vol. 307, no. 5, pp. 483–490, 2012.
3. S. Kumanyika and S. Grier, "Targeting interventions for ethnic minority and low-income populations," The Future of Children, vol. 16, no. 1, pp. 187–207, 2006.

4. P. M. Anderson and K. F. Butcher, "Childhood obesity: trends and potential causes," Future of Children, vol. 16, no. 1, pp. 19–45, 2006.
5. S. R. Patel, "Reduced sleep as an obesity risk factor," Obesity Reviews, vol. 10, no. s2, pp. 61–68, 2009.
6. V. S. Malik, B. M. Popkin, G. A. Bray, J.-P. Despres, and F. B. Hu, "Sugar-sweetened beverages, obesity, type 2 diabetes mellitus, and cardiovascular disease risk," Circulation, vol. 121, no. 11, pp. 1356–1364, 2010.
7. K. C. Mathias, M. M. Slining, and B. M. Popkin, "Foods and beverages associated with higher intake of sugar-sweetened beverages," The American Journal of Preventive Medicine, vol. 44, no. 4, pp. 351–357, 2013.
8. E. Han and L. M. Powell, "Consumption patterns of sugarsweetened beverages in the United States," Journal of the Academy of Nutrition and Dietetics, vol. 113, no. 1, pp. 43–53, 2013.
9. F. B. Hu, "Resolved: There is sufficient scientific evidence that decreasing sugar-sweetened beverage consumption will reduce the prevalence of obesity and obesity-related diseases," Obesity Reviews, vol. 14, no. 8, pp. 606–619, 2013.
10. S. Harrington, "The role of sugar-sweetened beverage consumption in adolescent obesity: a review of the literature,"The Journal of School Nursing, vol. 24, no. 1, pp. 3–12, 2008.
11. K. A. Kaiser, J. M. Shikany, K. D. Keating, and D. B. Allison, "Will reducing sugar-sweetened beverage consumption reduce obesity? Evidence supporting conjecture is strong, but evidence when testing effect is weak," Obesity Reviews, vol. 14, no. 8, pp. 620–633, 2013.
12. L. de Koning, V. S. Malik, M. D. Kellogg, E. B. Rimm, W. C. Willett, and F. B. Hu, "Sweetened beverage consumption, incident coronary heart disease, and biomarkers of risk in men," Circulation, vol. 125, no. 14, pp. 1735–1741, 2012.
13. J. W. Wang, K. Light, M. Henderson et al., "Consumption of added sugars from liquid but not solid sources predicts impaired glucose homeostasis and insulin resistance among youth at risk of obesity," Journal of Nutrition, vol. 144, no. 1, pp. 81–86, 2014.
14. G. Lasater, C. Piernas, and B. M. Popkin, "Beverage patterns and trends among school-aged children in the US, 1989–2008," Nutrition Journal, vol. 10, no. 1, article 103, 2011.
15. Y. C. Wang, S. N. Bleich, and S. L. Gortmaker, "Increasing caloric contribution from sugar-sweetened beverages and 100% fruit juices among US children and adolescents, 1988–2004," Pediatrics, vol. 121, no. 6, pp. e1604–e1614, 2008.
16. R. K. Rader, K. B. Mullen, R. Sterkel, R. C. Strunk, and J. M. Garbutt, "Opportunities to reduce children's excessive consumption of calories from beverages," Clinical Pediatrics, vol. 53, no. 11, pp. 1047–1054, 2014.
17. R. R. Briefel, A. Wilson, C. Cabili, and A. Hedley Dodd, "Reducing calories and added sugars by improving children's beverage choices," Journal of the Academy of Nutrition and Dietetics, vol. 113, no. 2, pp. 269–275, 2013.
18. L. M. Bogart, B. O. Cowgill, A. J. Sharma et al., "Parental and home environmental facilitators of sugar-sweetened beverage consumption among overweight and obese Latino youth," Academic Pediatrics, vol. 13, no. 4, pp. 348–355, 2013.
19. P. B. Crawford, G. Woodward-Lopez, L. Ritchie, and K. Webb, "How discretionary can we be with sweetened beverages for children?" Journal of the American Dietetic Association, vol. 108, no. 9, pp. 1440–1444, 2008.
20. S. M. Seifert, J. L. Schaechter, E. R. Hershorin, and S. E. Lipshultz, "Health effects of energy drinks on children, adolescents, and young adults," Pediatrics, vol. 127, no. 3, pp. 511–528, 2011.

21. K. A. Clauson, K. M. Shields, C. E. McQueen, and N. Persad, "Safety issues associated with commercially available energy drinks," Journal of the American Pharmacists Association, vol. 48, no. 3, pp. e55–e63, 2008.
22. A. K. Ventura and J. A. Mennella, "Innate and learned preferences for sweet taste during childhood," Current Opinion in Clinical Nutrition and Metabolic Care, vol. 14, no. 4, pp. 379–384, 2011.
23. J. P. Block, M. W. Gillman, S. K. Linakis, and R. E. Goldman, "if it tastes good, i'm drinking it: qualitative study of beverage consumption among college students," Journal of Adolescent Health, vol. 52, no. 6, pp. 702–706, 2013.
24. C. B. Ebbeling, H. A. Feldman, S. K. Osganian, V. R. Chomitz, S. J. Ellenbogen, and D. S. Ludwig, "Effects of decreasing sugar-sweetened beverage consumption on body weight in adolescents: a randomized, controlled pilot study," Pediatrics, vol. 117, no. 3, pp. 673–680, 2006.
25. J. James, P. Thomas, D. Cavan, and D. Kerr, "Preventing childhood obesity by reducing consumption of carbonated drinks: cluster randomised controlled trial," British Medical Journal, vol. 328, no. 7450, pp. 1237–1239, 2004.
26. R. Sichieri, A. Paula Trotte, R. A. De Souza, and G. V. Veiga, "School randomised trial on prevention of excessive weight gain by discouraging students from drinking sodas," Public Health Nutrition, vol. 12, no. 2, pp. 197–202, 2009.

PART IV
Future Directions for Self-Regulation

CHAPTER 12

Self-Regulation and the Management of Childhood Obesity

Moria Golan and Rachel Bachner-Melman

12.1 INTRODUCTION

The term *self-regulation* refers to the cognitive processes that govern drives and emotions [1]. *Self-control* refers to the ability to deliberately regulate one's emotions, urges and desires and can be viewed as aspect of self-regulation [2]. Several studies implicate difficulties in selfregulation in the development of overweight and obesity, primarily via deregulated eating behavior [3]. In a prospective longitudinal study, Duckworth et al. [4] found that self-controlled children are protected from weight gain in the transition to adolescence. Francis and Susman [5] found that children with low self-regulation had significantly higher body mass index (BMI) and more rapid weight gain from age 3-12 than other children. These findings suggest that in early childhood, selfregulatory problems are important longitudinal predictors of weight problems in early adolescence.

Children learn to practice self-control skills in the home environment by settling disagreements rationally rather than taking revenge, eating healthy food rather than junk, saving rather than spending, concentrating rather than disrupting the class, being careful rather than thrill-seeking and considerate rather than greedy [6].

With significant burdens of disease attributable worldwide to the obesogenic environment and to weight-related problems, the role of parents has perhaps never been more important in the management of deregulated eating [7,8]. They must find a way to help their children internalize self-regulation, develop coping skills and become physically and emotionally independent.

This paper will explore the relevance of self-control theories to the management of childhood obesity. The relationship of dietary restriction to self-control theories will be examined. The dietary restriction approach [9] will be compared with the trust paradigm, which emphasizes children's internal hunger, satiety cues and a division of responsibilities between parents and children [10].

12.1.1 Self-regulation

"Self-regulation" often refers broadly to the capacity to alter thoughts, feelings, desires, and actions with respect to certain goals. It infers active agency and is vital, since without it we would be helpless spectators. Self-regulation involves self-observation, judgment, and self-reaction [11]. The ability to regulate and control feelings and behaviors is a major accomplishment of the human species, yet the psychological mechanisms involved are incompletely understood. The absence of self-regulation skills is often related to interpersonal difficulties, addictions, emotional eating and weight-related problems [2]. While the capacity to self-regulate may vary across situations, some studies suggest it is more trait-like than state-like [12]. Selfregulation in early childhood has been linked to parental and teacher ratings of self-regulation or impulsivity later in life [13] and recent studies indicate it is both a trait and ability [14]. People with strong self-regulatory abilities can control their impulses much more easily than those without them, and are thus less prone to emotional eating and indulgence when tempted [12].

12.1.2 Self-control

Self-control refers to the capacity to alter one's responses and align them with ideals, values, morals, and social expectations, and the capacity to pursue long-term goals. Whereas 'self-control' and 'self-regulation' are often used interchangeably, those who make a distinction typically consider self-control as a deliberate, conscious, aspect of self-regulation. Self-control facilitates the restraint of overriding of a response, enabling a different response [11].

Self-control comes into play when people are torn between longterm goals to restrain behavior and immediate impulses promising hedonic fulfillment. Like self-regulation in general, it involves selfobservation, monitoring and behavioral control. Monitoring requires awareness of the discrepancy between impulsive reactions and goals or values. Behavioral control includes resisting the urge to respond impulsively to temptation [15].

Self-control deficiencies and *impulsivity* or impulse control problems are related [16], and often imply a failure to consider the consequences of one's actions. Resisting the temptation of immediate pleasure leads to behaviors indistinguishable from those that occur without forethought.

Posner and Rothbart [17] coined the related term "*effortful control*" that is needed to adapt to social demands. Effortful control includes managing attention (*attentional regulation*) and either inhibiting (*inhibitory control*) or activating behavior (*activational control*). It underlies, for example, the ability to focus on health and exert self-control despite a tempting smell of cake, and involves: 1) Alerting (maintaining an alert state); 2) Orienting (focusing on desired information); 3) Executive attention (focusing on goals, planning and decision-making).

Extending this view, Hoffman et al. [18] suggest a *dual system perspective* involving the interplay between: (a) reflection (evaluation of reward value, restraint); (b) impulsive precursors of behavior, such as motor impulsivity; and (c) determination of situational and dispositional boundaries, such as weakness or negative emotionality, which may involve a shift to a different reward value.

In their seminal work [19], Mischel and colleagues define "delay of gratification," as the time individuals wait to obtain a reward of greater value [20]. They explored when children forego a small, immediate reward for a larger future reward. Similar concepts include "delayed reward", "self-discipline" and "self-regulation" [21-23]. Delay of gratification behavior follows different patterns for different people [17]. This interconnection between cognition, behavior and situational/ dispositional boundaries is supported by brain research [24]. There is evidence that positive and negative emotionality activate the prefrontal cortex differently [25], possibly affecting attention and self-control [26].

Moreover, the reward-surfeit model of obesity holds that hyperresponsivity of reward circuitry leads to overeating and substance use [27]. However, findings suggest that obese humans show less activation of reward regions to food receipt, but greater activation in regions that encode the reward value of food cues [28,29]. Stice et al. [30] found that normal-weight adolescents at high-risk versus low-risk for future obesity showed greater activation in the dorsal striatum in response to palatable food receipt. This suggests that the initial vulnerability that gives rise to obesity may be elevated.

12.1.3 Moderators of Self-regulation

Several moderators may be related to difficulties in self-regulation and thus to weight-related problems:

12.1.3.1 Individual Differences and State Variations

Although self-regulation generally develops over the life span, people differ in their degree of impulsivity when faced with temptation [17]. These individual differences no doubt result from genetic, pre-natal and postnatal environmental influences, as well as learning history and current need states [31-34].

12.1.3.2 Hierarchy of Values and Reward Value

A person strongly tempted to accept a piece of chocolate yet wanting to restrain caloric input will experience internal conflict between the value of pleasure and the value of restriction [35]. Immediate value is coded by the *reward system*. The value of sensory stimuli has been called *reward value* [36]. Higgins' regulatory engagement theory [36] related this concept to value estimations and engagement. Overcoming temptation to do something pleasant strengthens engagement and increases the reward value of the *related actions*, as occurs in dieting. Fishbach & Zhang [35] proposed that we represent goal actions either in terms of progress toward a desirable end state, or in terms of commitment to this end state. In a self-control conflict, a high order goal offering delayed but larger benefits conflicts with a low order "temptation goal" offering immediate but smaller benefits [31] For an obese person, for example, food restriction offers delayed long term benefits. Eating large quantities of rich foods, on the other hand, offers immediate, yet smaller benefits. In self-control failures, people diminish the discrepancy between their goals and the temptation ("food restriction won't help slim. I'll never lose weight") and find a "balance" that protects them from a conflict between goals and temptations. These self-control failures result, paradoxically, from a lack of awareness of the intensity of internal conflict [35].

12.1.3.3 Emotional Distress and Ego Depletion vs. Ego Strength

Emotional distress may work against a general pattern of impulse control because it leads to a short-term focus, whereas impulse control requires a long-term focus. Emotional distress probably enhances the tendency to seek immediate sources of good feelings. Many of the common foci of self-regulatory restraints offer immediate pleasure: alcohol, drugs, high-calorie foods, illicit sex, extra sleep, shopping, and entertainment. In weight-related problems, impulse control may fail because distress leads to affect regulation [37], which takes priority over the value of healthy eating.

As a consequence of the short-term need to suppress negative emotions, overeating may deplete long-term self-control resources [37]. According to Baumeister and colleagues' *self-control strength theory* [14], self-control is a limited resource that works like a muscle. Exertion depletes this energy, which replenishes itself periodically [22]. 'Ego depletion' [22] is used to denote low-energy states with impairment of the mental activity necessary for self-control. Baumeister et al. reported that participants who controlled themselves by trying not to laugh while watching a comedian later performed more poorly on a task requiring self-control than participants who did not control their laughter while watching the video [22]. Nevertheless, they continue their muscle analogy by claiming that muscles tire after exercise, but are strengthened by it in the long run. Stice et al. [38] found that a positive mood stimulus helped restore depleted energy.

Actions leading to self-censure are unlikely to be pursued. This idea is of relevance to eating. Vulnerability to overeating in noneating-disordered overweight individuals is associated with increased negative affect [39]. Social-emotional self-regulation and cognitive selfregulation are interconnected; the same neural system is responsible for emotional control and meta-cognitive functions [24]. If the capacity to mentally represent, shield, and update restraint standard is reduced, self-monitoring resources may be depleted [40].

The reflective system is responsible for deliberate judgments, strategic action plans for goal pursuit, and inhibiting or overriding prepotent responses such as impulses or habits [28]. These processes are relatively slow and controlled, based on symbolic representations and operations [41]. Limited control resources may impair the reflective system by undermining its ability to symbolically represent restraint standards and monitor behavior according to those standards. The reflective system may then fail to activate, inhibit or override behavioral schemas. Karpinski & Steinman [42] measured automatic affective reactions to candy under two conditions. Participants drank orange juice with (alcohol condition) or without (control condition) vodka. An intermediate filler task allowed the alcohol to take effect. As expected,only participants in the control condition, but not participants in the alcohol condition, restrained their candy consumption according to their dietary restraint standards. Automatic affective reactions predicted candy consumption for intoxicated but not sober participants. These results indicate that under alcohol intoxication, strong impulses affect the quantities of food we consume.

12.1.3.4 Restrained Eating

Self-regulatory resources also moderate the influence of restraint on eating behavior. Restraint standards normally guide behavior effectively in tempting situations, but not when participants' selfregulatory resources are depleted [43]. Both automatic affective reactions and approach–avoidance tendencies are affected by physical deprivation [33,44]. Dieters, who constantly seek to restrict food intake, therefore eat more when self-regulatory resources are depleted. In contrast, non-dieters, who eat freely according to internal hunger and satiety, do not eat more than usual when their self-regulatory resources are depleted [44]. Nevertheless, choosing not to eat for intrinsic reasons may deplete less strength than feeling compelled by extrinsic reasons to exert self-control when eating [45]. Lowe [46] argues that dieting to reach a weight lower than one's desirable weight for height is potentially harmful. For individuals, overweight or gaining weight, he believes the potential benefits of dietary restriction may outweigh the risks overeating in response to restraint.

12.1.3.5 Exposure to Temptations and Tempters

Exposure to temptation can undermine self-regulatory functioning [22] whereas preschool-age children can self-regulate energy intake in controlled laboratory conditions [23], this ability is easily disrupted by social and situational factors [36].

Contextual factors can suppress the appeal of a temptation. Leander and colleagues [47] found that individuals with chronic self-regulatory problems who were tempted to smoke marihuana were more likely to resist temptation if they had a distant rather than a close relationship with the tempter. So even if no important goal exists, the natural shield of chronic self-regulatory tendencies may sometimes prove sufficient in temptation-laden social contexts. Since obese people tend to control their eating better with company than without, family meals may be a protective factor for obese children.

Fisher & Kral provided evidence that large portion of energydense foods increases energy intake in children as young as two [48]. A reward must be both immediate and self-relevant for people to be tempted by it [49]. Thus, we tend to buy more food when we are hungry. It may be hard for a restrained eater to resist food when it is available and (s)he is hungry. Jansen [50] provided evidence for "cue reactivity": when sensory cues were systematically associated with food intake, they reliably triggered early (cephalic phase) effects of food, such as increased blood sugar and salivary flow. Overweight children fail to regulate their food intake when tempted by the smell and taste of appetizing food. In this case, overeating is related more strongly to induce salivation flow than to psychological factors [50].

12.2 DEVELOPMENT OF SELF-CONTROL

Self-control is a psychological skill involving higher mental processes and attention-focusing abilities that can help prevent weightrelated problems or help manage them. Although biologically based, it can be learned. Research suggests that it develops with the repeated activation of relevant neural systems, just like a muscle [51].

According to Vygotsky's cultural-historical cognitive theory, with the development of self-regulation, we become able to control certain behaviors to acquire "higher mental functions" [52]. Self-regulated behaviors enable children to make the critical transition from "slaves to the environment" to "masters of their own behavior". Vygotsky explains that this process involves the mastery of specific cultural tools like language and other symbolic systems, to gain control of physical, emotional and cognitive functions. Children's self-regulatory abilities originate in social interactions before being internalized [53].

Though influenced by individual temperament, self-regulatory competence involves skills that develop during childhood and adolescence. These are taught formally or informally within the social context and can therefore be enhanced by intervention programs [54]. Values or norms are most effectively transmitted when perceived as a choice rather than a by agents of socialization and are then adhered to in the absence of external surveillance, hope of reward, or fear of punishment.

Vygotsky [53] suggested three conditions for the development of self-regulatory behaviors in children. Firstly, they need the opportunity to engage in "other regulation", to be the subject of others' regulatory behaviors (as in most interaction with adults) as well as agents regulating others' behaviors (as in most interaction with children). Secondly, they learn to master specific cultural tools that allow them to start using selfregulatory behaviors independently. When, for example, they engage in *self-talk* or *"private speech"*, they take words that adults once used to regulate their behavior and use them for self-regulation purposes. Thirdly, well-developed, make-believe play provides opportunities to practice self-regulatory components of mental functions. During play, children fulfill their desires in symbolic form, learn to delay gratification, and adopt different perspectives.

1. Gottman was the first to define "*meta-emotion*" [55] as an organized approach to the understanding of emotions. He said that parental meta-emotion influences children's capacity for physiological and emotional regulation and that talking about emotions develops self-regulation [56]. He claimed that parents can coach their childreBeing aware of their child's emotions
2. Seeing their child's emotion as an opportunity for intimacy or teaching
3. Helping the child to label his/her emotions
4. Empathizing with or validating the child's emotion
5. Trying to understand the feelings underlying misbehavior
6. Helping their child down-regulate emotions
7. Setting clear limits on behaviors, joint problem solving.

Self-regulatory capacities develop optimally when both parents practice meta-emotion coaching and model self-regulation.

According to social cognitive theory, the ability to regulate one's health can be taught via social modeling, support, and feedback. External supports are gradually withdrawn as self-regulation develops. According to Bandura's triadic model [1], we regulate our health by adopting self-care strategies, setting goals, and monitoring feedback on the effectiveness of the strategies used. Perceived self-efficacy in turn enhances motivation to self-regulate health.

The repeated activation of a neural system causes it to expand [51]. Current brain research underscores the importance of the environment (training) in the development of self-regulation. Repeated acts of self-regulation increase our total pool of energy [49]. According to Strayhorn [6], self-control is fostered by: 1. a positive, long-term relationship with a dependable person who communicates the value of this goal; 2. carefully chosen self-control challenges at a suitable level of difficulty; 3. positive self-control models; 4. frequent, graded practice; 5. enjoyment of valued rewards obtained by effort; 6. fantasy rehearsal; 7. compliance skills; 8. relevant verbal concepts (including a term for self-control itself); 8. the art of self-instruction; 9. Removing oneself from temptation; and 10. Self-monitoring skills [6].

Diverse and complex strategies to improve self-control and bolster the value of long-term goals in the face of temptation [20,57- 59] have been suggested. Hoffman et al. [18] suggest that self-control interventions are most effective if they simultaneously (a) change attitudes, beliefs, and control standards via interventions such as cognitive restructuring, education, or persuasion, (b) create situational and dispositional circumstances conducive to effective self-control, and (c) change problematic impulsive precursors of behavior. Recently, they demonstrated that mental self-control strategies such as "cooling" thoughts (imagining chocolate in a non-consummatory manner) and implementation intentions (instructions not to eat the chocolate) reduced the strength of automatically activated affective responses to a tempting stimulus [60]. Baumeister and colleagues [61] posited that self-control skills may be strengthened by exercise and practice just as a muscle is fatigued in the short run but strengthened in the long run by exercise.

12.3 PARENTING, SELF-CONTROL AND WEIGHT-RELATED PROBLEMS

Although self-control is a trait, it can be developed and enhanced [62]. By regularly adopting the above guidelines, parents can help their children develop effortful control and the ability to delay gratification. Gottman [55] suggests placing clear limits on behavior to promote self-control and self-regulation. However, parents who are overweight, who have problems controlling their own food intake, or who are concerned about their children's risk for overweight sometimes adopt controlling child-feeding practices (authoritarian parenting style) in an attempt to prevent overweight in their children [56]. This may be counterproductive in the challenge of developing internalized selfcontrol. According to Baumrind's theory of parenting style, a child is more likely to comply with parental control and internalize it when it is perceived as fair and reasonable [63].

Parenting style is a complex notion denoting specific behaviors that work individually and collectively to influence outcomes in children. It is intended to describe normal variations in parenting, with a focus on issues of control [64]. Two important features of parenting style are [65]: 1. Responsiveness, or "the extent to which parents intentionally foster individuality, self-regulation, and self-assertion by being attuned, supportive, and acquiescent to children's special needs and demands"; and 2. Demandingness, or "the claims parents make on children to become integrated into the family whole, by their maturity demands, supervision, disciplinary efforts and willingness to confront the child who disobeys." Baumrind uses these features to define three parenting prototypes: permissive (indulgent), authoritarian and authoritative styles [64].

12.3.1 Permissive Parents

Permissive parents are more responsive than demanding and essentially allow children to make their own decisions and regulate their own activities. Such parents may avoid setting boundaries recommended by the American Academy of Pediatrics Committee [66]. Parental over-permissiveness, over-protectiveness and a lack of authority can lead to uncertainty, insecurity and self-regulation difficulties in children [67,68]. Since self-regulated eating is difficult in the obesogenic environment, it is hardly surprising that the permissive parenting style has been shown to be counterproductive in the management of weight-related problems [67].

12.3.2 Authoritarian Parents

Authoritarian parents are high in demandingness and low in responsiveness [69]. This style correlates negatively with children's psychosocial well-being [70] and positively with obesity [71,72] and eating disorders [73]. Authoritarian parents lack the sensitivity to assess their child's self-regulating ability before making behavioral demands and may expect behaviors beyond the child's developmental ability. Authoritarian parenting style, negatively associated with healthy child development [74,15], involves overt psychological control via parenting practices such as the induction of guilt or shame and the withdrawal of love, which hinders children's psychological and emotional development and control over food intake [74]. Faith et al. [75] found that parental restriction of their child's food intake predicted increase in BMI two years later. Parental style was not measured in this study, so we do not know whether psychological control was an element of the parental restriction.

Authoritarian and authoritative parenting styles seem to impact children's eating behaviors and responses differently. The association between authoritarian parenting and poor internalization of selfcontrol [76], and between authoritative parenting and successful internalization [77] appear to be strongest in middle-class Anglo-Europeans. In other cultural contexts, authoritarian parenting is more likely to be the norm and less likely to be associated with negative outcomes. Since individualism is a supreme value in North American and Western European societies, authoritarian parenting style is perceived psychologically controlling. Yet in collectivist cultures, which value socialization, parents promote interdependence, cooperation, and unconditional compliance. They aim not to facilitate autonomy, and tend to inhibit a child's personal wishes [78].

In Western cultures, overt authoritarian parenting may also enhance children's greediness for food. According to Winnicott [79] the word 'greed' brings together the psychical and the physical, love and hate. He suggested greed appears in disguised form, even in infants, and that greediness is a symptom secondary to anxiety. Anxiety and greediness may be one outcome of authoritarian parenting, which lacks warmth [63], a factor important in motivating children to follow parental wishes [80]. Authoritarian parents also tend to make dispositional attributions for children's misdeeds [81]. They tend to be angry, use reasoning to teach appropriate behaviors, and humiliate their children, which may lower the children's capacity for selfregulation [82]. Many people in Western consumer society are highly anxious. Hypervigilance, attention bias and lack of self-regulation have been found to be key features of anxiety [83,84]. Greediness, emotional eating, disordered eating and lack of self-control may form a part of a coping mechanism with the anxiety associated with our society.

12.3.3 The Authoritative Parenting

The authoritative parenting style, characterized by high levels of warmth and low levels of coercive control, has been associated with positive outcomes in child development across gender, ethnic and socioeconomic backgrounds [9]. Expectations from children are balanced by responsiveness to their needs. Authoritative parents are neither intrusive nor restrictive and tend to maintain an authoritative stance and to view the parental role as more collaborative and supportive than the authoritarian parents. Authoritative parenting has consistently been linked with social competence and with a lack of behavioral problems in children of all ages [69]. Findings suggest that children raised in authoritative homes ate more healthily, were more physically active and had lower BMI levels, compared to children who were raised with other styles (authoritarian, permissive/indulgent, uninvolved/neglectful). General parenting has a differential impact on children's weight-related outcomes, depending on child and parental characteristics [85,86].

To prevent the counterproductive impact of authoritarian parenting style and its negative influence on children's ability to focus on their internal needs and develop self-control, Satter [87] suggests health care providers and parents rely on a "trust" paradigm instead of the currently widespread "control" paradigm. She proposes a division of responsibilities [87] between parents and children. Parents provide structure (e.g. regular mealtimes, sitting during meals), support, and new foods that children can reject or accept, and children choose how much to eat. According to this "authoritative feeding style", parents communicate age-appropriate demands to their children and model self-control while maintaining a non-intrusive stance. The risk for overweight in first graders is five times greater for those with authoritarian versus authoritative mothers [88]. Children of permissive or neglectful parents are twice as likely as children of authoritative parents to be overweight. Caregivers generally know what foods are healthy for their children but do not apply this knowledge during meal times [89].

Satter's trust paradigm appears to provide support for permissive parenting since parents trust their children to consume appropriate amounts of food. This may, however, be counterproductive in a childcentered environment, when career-oriented parents feel guilty for being insufficiently available. Despite good intentions, obese children may experience subjective failure when offered too many choices [9]. When permissive parents trust their children's ability to choose from many food options, they may be overlooking a tendency to feel overwhelmed and experience a lapse in self-control [90]. Parental trust in their children's eating behavior is warranted when the child has healthy eating habits and effective self-regulation [91]. However, when children are not offered a varied enough diet, they may make a habit of always eating the same foods. The tendency of morbidly obese children to overeat also presents parents with challenging decisions about when and how to intervene. With experience, we can learn to override innate self-control in order to obtain various short-term rewards, and develop creative control strategies.

The ability of three- to five-year-olds to determine appropriate portion sizes was examined in a study by Leahy et al. [92]. Breakfasts, lunches, and afternoon snacks were served two days per week for two weeks. During the first week, energy density of the foods served was low. During the second week, energy density was increased by adding fat and sugar and decreasing fruit and vegetable intake during the day. Dinner and an evening snack of constant energy density were sent home with children. Children consumed a consistent weight of foods and beverages over two days in both conditions, and their energy consumption was therefore 72 kcal (14%) less in the lower energy density condition, a significant result ($P = 0.0001$). Reducing the energy density of children's diets may therefore be an effective strategy for reducing energy intake.

Kirschenbaum and Kelly [9] argue that dietary restriction is often an ineffective weight control strategy. Nevertheless, there is evidence that excessive restrictiveness leads to poor self-regulation and may contribute to child obesity [93]. Arguably, there is insufficient evidence to determine the effectiveness of dietary interventions in treating excessive weight gain in children and adolescents [93]. However, a meta-analysis supports the effectiveness of some interventions including dietary modification, though effectiveness may decline over time. Luttikhuis et al. concluded in their review that childhood obesity interventions works, but only if combined with behavior modification [94]. The most effective interventions may be those that encourage parents to decide what is served (reducing energy density rather than food quantities) and children to decide how much they eat [91].

12.4 CONCLUSION

Self-control and self-regulation can be developed and serve as buffers against emotional dysregulation and problematic eating behavior. There are no empirically-based guidelines for effective parenting practices or for external interventions promoting weight control. Not all children need to moderate their energy intake, so the need for reductions in energy density should be "weighed" carefully. Neither inappropriate levels of trust nor extensive restriction of food intake are effective in fostering self-control and self-regulation in eating.

Since restrictive feeding practices increase children's preferences for restricted and palatable foods [95] and promote overeating when restricted foods are freely available [4], parents should aim to control the environment rather than children's behavior. Moderate restrictions should be imposed on less nutritional foods. Social contexts promoting alertness (rather than vigilance) to long- versus short-term rewards should be provided to enhance self-regulation and self-control. This can be achieved without overt psychological control in most cultures via an authoritative parenting style and effective communication.

Self-regulation is built via effective communication at home, at school and in the health system. Three interrelated processes, in which language skills are paramount, contribute to it: information exchange, behavior influence, and problem solving [96]. As language is internalized, competent children and adolescents make increasing use of self-talk to describe and evaluate their thoughts, feelings and actions, and monitor their own behavior [97]. This enables children to acquire the foundations of self-regulation, on which affective, social and cognitive competence depend. A growing sense of competence enhances the development of self-regulation that paves the way to complex abilities that surpass mere compliance. These abilities include delay of gratification, impulse and affect control, modulation of motor and linguistic activities, and the ability to act in accordance with social norms in the absence of external monitors [98].

12.5 RECOMMENDATIONS FOR FUTURE RESEARCH

Additional research is needed to further study the association between self control mediating and moderating factors and child's weight status.

The next generation of programs should engage new models such as behavioral economics to foster self control among children with hyper or hypo sensitivity of reward circuitry. Future research needs to identify the components or types of treatments that achieve the most comprehensive and persistent effects on child's self control. How parenting programs address the need to train parents to enforce self regulation and self control in their children.

Given the lack of current intervention studies addressing general parenting and their impact on child's self control and weight status, further development and testing of theory and practice based interventions is strongly recommended, preferably employing a longitudinal design with more extended follow-up periods to establish causation.

REFERENCES

1. Bandura A (1986) Social foundations of thought and action: A social cognitive. Englewood Cliffs, NJ, Prentice Hall (1986).

2. Baumeister RF (1998) The self; in Gilbert D, Fiske ST & Lindzey G (eds): Handbook of social psychology. Boston, McGraw-Hill: 680-740.
3. Fisher JO, Birch LL (2002) Eating in the absence of hunger and overweight in girls from 5 to 7 y of age. Am J Clin Nutr 76: 226-231.
4. Duckworth Al, Tsukayama E, Geier AB (2010) Self-controlled children stay leaner in the transition to adolescence. Appetite 54: 304-308.
5. Francis LA, Susman EJ (2009) Self-regulation and rapid weight gain in children from age 3 to 12 Years. Arch Pediatr Adolesc Med 163: 297-302.
6. Strayhorn JM (2002) Self-control: toward systematic training programs. J Am Acad Child Adolesc Psychiatr 41: 17–27.
7. Murphy NF, MacIntyre K, Stewart S, Hart CL, Hole D, et al. (2006) Longterm cardiovascular consequences of obesity: 20-year follow-up of more than 15,000 middle-aged men and women (the Renfrew-Paisley study). Eur Heart J 27: 96–106.
8. Golan M, Crow S (2004) Parents are key players in the prevention and treatment of weight-related problems. Nutrition Reviews 62: 39–50.
9. Kirschenbaum DS, Kelly KP (2009) Five reasons to distrust the trust model. Obesity 17: 1107–1111.
10. Eneli IU, Crum PA, Tylka TL (2008) The trust model a different feeding paradigm for managing childhood obesity. Obesity 16: 2197–2204.
11. Baumeister RF, Vohs KD, Tice DM (2007) The strength model of self-control. Curr Dir Psycholo Sci 16: 351–355.
12. Mischel W, Shoda Y, Rodriguez ML (1989) Delay of gratification in children. Science 244: 933–938.
13. Tremblay RE, Masse B, Perron D, Leblanc M, Schwartzman AE, et al. (1992) Early disruptive behavior, poor school achievement, delinquent behavior, and delinquent personality: longitudinal analyses. J Consult Clin Psychol 60: 64–72.
14. Baumeister RF, Heatherton TF (1996) Self-Regulation Failure: An Overview. Psychol Inq 7:1–15.
15. Barber LK, Munz DC, Bagsby PG, Grawitch M (2009) When does time perspective matter? Self-control as a moderator between time perspective and academic achievement. Pers Indiv Differ 46: 250–253.
16. Strayhorn JM (2002) Self-Control: theory and research. J Am Acad Child Adolesc Psychiatry 41: 7–16.
17. Posner MI, Rothbart MK (1998) Attention, self-regulation and consciousness. Philosophical transactions of the Royal Society of London Series B-Biological Sciences 353: 1915–1927.
18. Hoffman W, Friese M, Strack F (2009) Impulse and self-control from a dualsystems perspective. Perspect Psychol Sci 4: 162–176.
19. Mischel W, Shoda Y, Rodriguez S (1989) Delay of gratification in children. Science 244: 933–938.
20. Mischel W, Cantor N, Feldman S (1996) Principles of self-regulation: The nature of willpower and self-control; in Higgins ET, Kruglanski WK(eds): Social psychology: Handbook of basic principles. New York, Guilford Press: 329–360.
21. Kochanska G (1993) Toward a synthesis of parental socialization and child temperament in early development of conscience. Child Dev 64: 325–347.
22. Baumeister RF, Bratslavsky E, Muraven M, Tice DM (1998) Ego depletion: Is the active self a limited resource? J Pers Social Psychol 74: 1252–1265.

23. Birch LL, Deysher M (1986) Caloric compensation and sensory specific satiety: evidence for self-regulation of food intake by young children. Appetite 7: 323– 331.
24. Blair C (2002) School readiness: Integrating cognition and emotion in a neurobiological conceptualization of children's functioning at school entry. Am Psychol 57: 111–127.
25. Davidson RJ, Jackson DC, Kalin NH (2000) Emotion, plasticity, context, and regulation: Perspectives from affective neuroscience. Psychol Bull 126: 890– 909.
26. Davidson RJ (1999) Perspectives on affective styles and their cognitive consequences; in Dalgleish T & Power M (eds): Handbook of Cognition and Emotion. Chichester, England: Wiley: 103–123.
27. Dawe S, Loxton NJ (2004) The role of impulsivity in the development of substance use and eating disorders. Neurosci Biobehav Rev 28: 343–351.
28. Stice E, Yokum S, Bohon C, Marti N, Smolen A (2010) Reward circuitry responsivity to food predicts future increases in body mass: moderating effects of DRD2 and DRD4. Neuroimage 50: 1618 –1625.
29. Stice E, Yokum S, Burger KS, Epstein LH, Small DM (2011) Youth at risk for obesity show greater activation of striatal and somatosensory regions to food. J Neurosci 31: 4360–4366.
30. Burger KS, Stice E (2011) Variability in Reward Responsivity and Obesity: Evidence from Brain Imaging Studies. Curr Drug Abuse Rev 4: 182-189.
31. Gross J, Thompson RA (2007) Emotion regulation: Conceptual Foundations; in Gross JJ (ed): Handbook of emotion regulation. NY, Guilford Press: 3–24.
32. Strack F, Deutsch R (2004) Reflective and Impulsive Determinants of Social Behavior. Pers Soc Psychol Rev 8: 220–247.
33. Seibt B, Hafner M, Deutsch R (2007) Prepared to eat: How immediate affective and motivational responses to food cues are influenced by food deprivation. Eur J Soc Psychol 37: 359–379.
34. Wiers RW, Dictus M, Houben K, Van den Wildenberg E, Rinck M (2009) Strong automatic appetitive action tendencies in heavy drinkers with a g-allele in a functional polymorphism of the Mu-opioid receptor gene (OPRM1). Genes Brain Behav 81: 101–106.
35. Fishbach A, Zhang Y (2009) The Dynamics of Self-Regulation: When goals commit versus liberate; in Wvnke M (ed): The Social Psychology of Consumer Behavior (in the series Frontiers of Social Psychology), NY, Psychology Press: 365–386.
36. Higgins ET (2006) Value from hedonic experience and engagement. Psychol Rev 113: 439-460.
37. Stice DM, Bratslavsky E, Baumeister RF (2001) Emotional distress regulation takes precedence over impulse control. J Pers Soc Psychol 80: 53–67.
38. Stice DM, Baumeister RF, Shmueli D, Muraven M (2007) Restoring the self: Positive affect helps improve self-regulation following ego depletion. J Experiment Soc Psychol 43: 379–384.
39. Jansen A, Vanreyten A,Van Balveren T, Roefs A, Nederkoorn C, et al. (2008) Negative affect and cue-induced overeating in non-eating disordered obesity. Appetite 51: 556–562.
40. Carver CS, Scheier MF (1998) On the self-regulation of behavior. New York, Cambridge University Press.
41. Smith ER, De Coster J (2000) Dual process models in social and cognitive psychology: Conceptual integration and links to underlying memory systems. Pers Soc Psychol Rev 4: 108–131.

42. Karpinski A, Steinman RB (2006) The single category implicit association test as a measure of implicit social cognition. J Pers Social Psychol 91: 16–32.
43. Vohs KD, Heatherton TF (2000) Self-regulatory failure: A resource-depletion approach. Psychol Sci 11: 249–254.
44. Baumeister R F, Gailliot M, DeWall CN, Oaten M (2006) Self-regulation and personality: How interventions increase regulatory success, and how depletion moderates the effects of traits on behavior. J Pers 74: 1773–1801.
45. Muraven M (2008) Autonomous self-control is less depleting. J Res Pers 42: 763–770.
46. Lowe MR (2003) Self-regulation of energy intake in the prevention and treatment of obesity. Is it feasible? Obes Res 11: 44S–59S.
47. Leander NP, Shah JY, Chartrand TL (2009) Moments of Weakness: The Implicit Context Dependencies of Temptations. Pers Soc Psychol Bull 35: 853- 866
48. Fisher OJ, Kral TVE (2008) Super-size me: children's eating. Physiol Behavior 94: 39-47.
49. Muraven M, Baumeister RF (2000) Self-regulation and depletion of limited resources: Does self-control resemble a muscle? Psychol Bull 126: 247–259.
50. Jansen A, Merckelbach H, Oosterlaan Cognitions and self-talk during food eaters. Behav Res Ther 26: 393–398.
51. Bialystok E, Craik FIM, Grady C, et al. (2005) Effect of bilingualism on cognitive control in the Simon task: Evidence from MEG. NeuroImage 24: 40–49.
52. Bialystok E, Craik FIM, Grady C, et al. (2005) Effect of bilingualism on cognitive control in the Simon task: Evidence from MEG. NeuroImage 24: 40–49.
53. Zimmerman BJ, Schunk DH (1996) Vygotskian view; in Zimmerman BJ, & Schunk DH (eds): Self-regulated learning and academic achievement, 2nd ed. Hillsdale, NJ, Lawrence Erlbaum: 227–252.
54. Vygotsky L (1978) Mind in society: The development of higher psychological processes. Cambridge, MA: Harvard University Press (M Cole, V John-Steiner, S Scribner, E Souberman, eds. & trans.).
55. Schunk DM, Zimmerman BJ (1997) Social origins of self-regulatory competence. Educ Psychol 32: 195-208.
56. Gottman JM, Katz LF, Hooven C (1996) Parental meta-emotion philosophy and the emotional life of families: Theoretical models and preliminary data. J Fam Psychol 10: 243–268.
57. Gottman J, Katz L, Hooven C (1997) Meta-emotion: How families communicate emotionally. Mahwah, NJ, Lawrence Erlbaum.
58. Fishbach A, Friedman RS, Kruglanski AW (2003) Leading us not unto temptation: Momentary allurements elicit overriding goal activation. J Personal Soc Psychol 84: 296–309.
59. Mischel W, Ayduk O (2004) Willpower in a cognitive-affective processing system: The dynamics of delay of gratification; in Baumeister RF & Vohs KD (eds): Handbook of Self-regulation. research, theory, and applications. New York, Guilford : 99–129.
60. Gailliot MT, Baumeister RF, DeWall CN, Maner JK, Plant EA, et al. (2007) Selfcontrol relies on glucose as a limited energy source: willpower is more than a metaphor. J Personal Soc Psychol 92: 325–336.
61. Hofmann W, Deutsch, Lancaster K, Banaji MR (2010) Cooling the heat of temptation:mental self-control and authomatic evaluation of tempting stimuli. Eur J Soc Psychol 40: 17–25.
62. Baumeister RF, Heatherton TF, Tice DM (1994) Losing control: How and why people fail at self-regulation. San Diego, Academic Press.

63. Strayhorn J (2002) Self-Control: Theory and research. J Am Acad Child Adolesc Psychiatry 41: 7–16.
64. Baumrind D (1967) Child care practices anteceding three patterns of preschool behavior. Genet Psychol Monogr 75: 43–88.
65. Baumrind D (1991) The influence of parenting style on adolescent competence and substance use. J adolesc 11: 56–95.
66. Maccoby EE, Martin JA (1983) Socialization in the context of the family: Parentchild interaction; in Mussen PH (Series Ed) & Hetherington EM (eds.): Handbook of child psychology: Socialization, personality, and social development (4th ed). New York, NY: Wiley.
67. American Academy of Pediatrics (1995) Committee on Communications. Children, adolescents and television. Pediatrics 96: 786–787.
68. Chen JL, Kennedy C (2004) Family functioning, parenting style, and Chinese children's weight status. J Fam Nurs 10: 262–279.
69. Damon W (1995) Greater expectations: Overcoming the culture of indulgence in our homes and schools. New York, The Free Press.
70. Darling N, Steinberg L (1993) Parenting style as context: An integrative model. Psychol bull 113: 487–496.
71. Olvera-Ezzell N, Power TG, Cousins JH (1990) Maternal socialization of children's eating habits: Strategies used by obese Mexican-American mothers. Child Dev 61: 395–400.
72. Wardle J, Sanderson S, Guthrie CA, Rapoport L, Plomin R (2002) Parental feeding style and the inter-generational transmission of obesity risk. Obes Res 10: 453–462.
73. Enten RS, Golan Rev 66: 65–75.
74. Enten RS, Golan M (2009) Parenting styles and the eating disorder pathology. Appetite 52: 784–787.
75. Barber LK (1996) Parental psychological control: revisiting a neglected construct. Child Develop 67: 3296–3319.
76. Faith MS, Berkowitz R, Stallings VA, Kerns J, Storey M, et al. (2004) Parental feeding attitudes and styles and child body mass index: Prospective analysis of a gene environment interaction. Pediatrics114: 429–436.
77. Dekoviç M, Janssens JMAM (1992) Parents' child-rearing style and child's sociometric status. Dev Psychol 28: 925–932.
78. Grolnick WS, Ryan RM (1989) Parent styles associated with children's selfregulation and competence in school. J Educ Psychol 81: 143–154.
79. Markus HR, Kitayama S (1991) Culture and the self: Implications for cognition, emotion, and motivation. Psychol Rev 98: 224–253.
80. Winnicott DW (1978) Appetite and emotional disorder. (Originally published in 1936). Republished in Through Paediatrics to Psycho-Analysis. The International Psychoanalytical Library. The Hogarth Press and the Institute of Psychoanalysis.
81. Grusec JE, Goodnow JJ (1994) Impact of parental discipline methods on the child's internalization of values: A reconceptualization of current points of view. Dev Psychol 30: 4–19.
82. Dix T, Ruble DN, Zambarano RJ (1989) Mothers' implicit theories of discipline: Child effects, parent effects, and the attribution process. Child Dev 60: 1373– 1391
83. Dix TH, Grusec JE (1985) Parental attribution processes in child socialization; in: Sigel IE (ed): Parental belief systems: Their psychological consequences for children. Hillsdale, NJ, Lawrence Erlbaum: 201–233.

84. Mogg K, Bradley BP (1998) A cognitive motivational analysis of anxiety. Behav Res Ther 36: 809–848.
85. Harvey AH, Watkins E, Mansell W, Shafran R (2004) Cognitive behavioural processes across psychological disorders: A transdiagnostic perspective to research and treatment. Oxford, OUP.
86. Sleddens EF, Gerards SM, Thijs C, de Vries NK, Kremers SP (2011) General parenting, childhood overweight and obesity-inducing behaviors: a review. Int J Pediatr Obes 6: e12-27.
87. Gerards SM, Sleddens EF, Dagnelie PC, de Vries NK, Kremers SP (2011) Interventions addressing general parenting to prevent or treat childhood obesity. Int J Pediatr Obes 6: e28-45.
88. Satter E (2005) Your child's weight, helping without harming. Madison, WI, Kelcy Press: 16.
89. Rhee K, Lumeng JC, Appugliese DP, Kaciroti N, Bradley RH (2006) Parenting styles and overweight status in first grade. Pediatrics 117: 2047–2054.
90. Hoerr S, Utech AE, Ruth E (2005) Child control of food choices in head start families. J Nutr Educ Beh 37: 185–190.
91. Vohs KD, Baumeister RF, Twenge JM, et al. (2008) Making choices impairs subsequent self-control: A limited resource account of decision making, selfregulation, and active initiative. J Pers Soc Psychol 94: 883–898.
92. Golan M (2008) The PATCH program – parental agency towards child's health, leaders guide. Maxanna Press, Israel.
93. Leahy KE, Birch LL, Rolls BJ (2008) Reducing the energy density of multiple meals decreases the energy intake of preschool-age children Am J Clin Nutr 88: 1459–1468.
94. Collins CE, Warren J, Stokes BJ (2006) Measuring effectiveness of dietetic interventions in Child Obesity. A Systematic Review of Randomized Trials. Arch Pediatr Adolesc Med 160: 906–922.
95. Oude LH, Baur L, Jansen H, Shrewsbury VA, O 'Malley C, et al. (2009) Interventions for treating obesity in children. Cochrane Database Syst Rev 1:CD001872.
96. Dumas JE, Prinz RJ, Smith EP, Laughlin J (1999) The Early Alliance Prevention Trial: An integrated set of interventions to promote competence and reduce risk for conduct disorder, substance abuse, and school failure. Clin Child Psychol Rev 2: 37–54.
97. Weiss LH, Schwartz JC (1996) The relationship between parenting types and older adolescents personality, academic achievement, adjustment and substance abuse. Child Dev 67: 2101–2114.
98. Greenberg MT, Kusche CA, Speltz ML (1991) Emotional regulation, self-control, and psychopathology: The role of relationships in early childhood; in Cicchetti D & Toth SL (eds): Rochester Symposium on Developmental Psychopathology. New York, Cambridge University Press: 21–66.
99. Kopp CB (1991) Young children's progression to self-regulation; in Bullock M (ed). The development of intentional action: Cognitive, motivational, and interactive processes. Basel, Switzerland, Krager: 38–54.

CHAPTER 13

Weight Self-Regulation Process in Adolescence: The Relationship Between Control Weight Attitudes, Behaviors, and Body Weight Status

Jordi Pich, Maria del Mar Bibiloni, Antoni Pons, and Josep A. Tur

13.1 INTRODUCTION

Results from US National Health and Nutrition Examination Surveys (NHANES) pointed out that the obesity prevalence remained stable over past 10 years (1). However, several cross-surveys in Western countries showed that around 30% of adolescents boys and 25% of girls are still overweighed (2, 3), mainly due to high-calorie food intake and sedentary lifestyle.

The increased prevalence in adolescent overweight contrasts paradoxically with the prevailing social appreciation of thinness (4–6), which is more pronounced among females (7, 8). The flip side of that appreciation is society's rejection of obesity, whether expressed openly or through implicit attitudes (9).

Longitudinal surveys and psychiatric studies have long warned that adolescents' weight self-regulation practices promoted by thinness goals sometimes fuel unhealthy habits such as smoking, alcohol and drug use, purges, or vomits, or even result in anorexia and bulimia disorders (10).

Comprehensible alarm resulting from these potential hazards has tended to obscure the positive role that body weight self-regulation processes, motivated by concern with body image, may represent by promoting a more balanced food intake and regular physical activity during adolescence. In our view, the relationship between ideal body image and weight self-regulation process can be connected through Higgins' (11, 12) regulatory focus theory (RFT). Essentially, RFT describes the processes by which individuals try to self-regulate or adjust their attitudes and behaviors to achieve a positive goal by means of two differentiated strategies: promotion focus goals ("making good things happen") or prevention focus goals ("avoiding bad things happen"). Some studies on adults have explored the relationship between individuals' dominant focus and several dimensions of eating behavior, such as fruit consumption (13), restrained eating (14), emotional, external and restrained eating (15), or food choice motives (16).

In this theoretical framework, we consider that adolescents' weight self-regulation efforts either by losing excessive weight, or by maintaining it in reasonable magnitudes, would involve a motivational "promotion focus" (i.e., the desire to show an attractive personal body image in alignment with present beauty standards) as well as a "prevention focus" (i.e., to avoid social rejection linked to deviance of body standards).

However, as any human motivated behavior, weight-control may turn into a serious mental illness (17). Anorexia would represent the most dramatic case of healthy weight self-regulation failure. On the other side, adolescents' hypothetical involvement in a promotion focus, a prevention one, or both can contribute to initiating positive attempts to eat a more balanced diet and/or practice regular physical activity. In this direction, after remarking that during adolescence, body attractiveness tends to be a stronger motive than health when adopting healthy habits; Nowak (18) observed that boys and girls who attempted weight loss reduced consumption of sweet foods and snacks, while concurrently increasing consumption of healthy foods, such as fruit and yogurt. More recently, another study has also recorded that most obese and overweight boys and girls who manifested their desire to slim reported a congruently healthy lower consumption of several high-calorie food groups (19).

Until now, many cross-sectional surveys have assessed the relationship between losing weight behaviors and body image attitudes. These studies have pointed out the common inclination of the obese and overweight population to underestimate their weight (20–23). On the same lines, some longitudinal studies also have pointed out a propensity to judge their body image as not being excessively overweight, which seems to be consistent with a general decline in students' dissatisfaction with their body-image (24). In particular, Anglo-American countries have registered a significant increase in the percentage of overweight subjects, in both adults (25, 26) and adolescents (27, 28), who defined their weight as "normal." In previous studies, roughly half of the overweight boys and a quarter of obese ones also claimed to be normal weight, a belief that was not shared and dropped sharply among girls (20, 21).

With reference to measured body fat, half of the girls with above-average values also considered themselves to be normal weight (29), and 4% even defined themselves as underweight. Contrarily, 33% of normal-weight girls overestimated their weight (30).

In agreement with these unexpected findings within a context of obesity rejection, one longitudinal study found a dip in interest among teenagers in controlling their weight (31). Moreover, in a multi-ethnic sample of British adolescents, 65% of overweight boys and 36% of obese boys stated that they have never tried to lose weight, and these proportions fell to 41 and 23%, respectively, among girls (21). By contrast, the ideal of being slim has been shown to spur girls with normal weight to perceive themselves as "fat" (20, 23), and most of them admit to have dieted on some occasions (21).

Incongruences between self-regulatory theoretical predictions and empirical findings demand a better understanding of self-weight goals among adolescents. The aim of this study was to assess the relationship between body mass status, body image perception, self-weight concern, and the personal motivation to actually engage in healthy weight control behaviors through cutting down food intake and/or regular exercise in a representative sample of adolescents living in a Mediterranean area. Body image satisfaction according to weight status, age, and gender was also assessed.

13.2 MATERIALS AND METHODS

13.2.1 Study Design and Population

The study is part of a broader population-based cross-sectional survey carried out on Balearic Islands' 12- to 17-year-old adolescents between 2007 and 2008. The sample was selected by means of a multiple-step, simple random sampling, taking into account, first, the location, with towns from all over the Balearic Islands being represented (Palma de Mallorca, Calvià, Inca, Manacor, Maó, Eivissa, Llucmajor, Santa Margalida, S'Arenal, Sant Jordi de Ses Salines), and then by random selection of schools within each town. Sample size was stratified by age and gender.

To calculate a representative number of adolescents, a variable BMI was selected with the greatest variance for this age group, based on data from the literature at the time of the study (32). Sampling was determined for the distribution of this variable, with a confidence interval (CI) established at 95% with a ±0.25 error. The total number of subjects (2400) were uniformly distributed within the towns and proportionally distributed by gender and age. Exclusion criteria were: type 2 diabetes, pregnancy, alcohol or drug abuse, and non-directly related nutritional medical conditions.

The sample was oversized to prevent loss of information and was needed to do the fieldwork in complete classrooms. In each school, classrooms were randomly selected from among those of the same grade, or level, and all the adolescents in one classroom were asked to participate in the survey. A letter informing the nature and purpose of the study was sent to parents or legal guardians. After receiving their written consent, the adolescents were then considered for inclusion in the study. All responses to questionnaires were filled in by the adolescents. Once the field study had been completed, the adolescents who did not fulfill the inclusion criteria were excluded. Finally, the sample was adjusted by a weighting factor in order to balance the sample according to the distribution of the Balearic Islands' population and to guarantee that each of the groups, already defined by the previously mentioned factors (age and gender), were representative. The final number of subjects included in the study, 1961 adolescents (82% participation; 47.9% male), were a representative sample of the Balearic Islands' adolescent population. Reasons for not taking part were: (a) the subject declined to be interviewed, and (b) the parents did not authorize the interview.

The study was conducted according to the guidelines laid down in the Declaration of Helsinki, and all procedures involving human subjects were approved by the Balearic Islands' Ethics Committee (Palma de Mallorca, Spain) under number IB-530/05-PI. Written informed consent was obtained from all subjects and also from the next of kin, careers, or guardians on the behalf of the minors involved in the study.

13.2.2 Body Composition

Height was calculated to the nearest millimeter using a mobile anthropometer (Kawe 44444, Kirchner & Wilhelm GmBH Co., KG, Asperg, Germany), with the subject's head placed in the Frankfurt plane. Body weight was determined to the nearest 100 g using a digital scale (Tefal, sc9210, Groupe SEB, Rumilly, France). The subjects were weighed barefoot, wearing light underwear, as previously described (33). BMI was computed as weight (kg) divided by height (m2), and study participants were specifically categorized by age and gender using the BMI cut-offs developed and proposed by the International Obesity Task Force (IOTF) (34) and Cole et al. (35, 36): normal weight: $18.5 \geq$ BMI < 24.9; overweight: $25.0 \geq$ BMI < 29.9; obesity: BMI ≥ 30.

13.2.3 Self-Reported Body Weight

The subjects were asked to estimate their current height and weight prior to measurement. Estimates within ±2 kg of real weight were classified as correct, <2 kg under real weight were considered as an underestimate, and >2 kg than real weight were considered as an overestimate.

13.2.4 Body Image Perception

Subjects had to choose the most similar silhouette to their image ("real silhouette"), and the silhouette they would like to have from other similar series ("ideal silhouette") using Stunkard's Figure Rating Scale (Figure 1), which includes nine different body silhouettes (37). The difference between the two values was classified as acceptance of body image (ideal = real), dissatisfaction with being overweight (ideal thinner than real), and dissatisfaction with being underweight (ideal weightier than real).

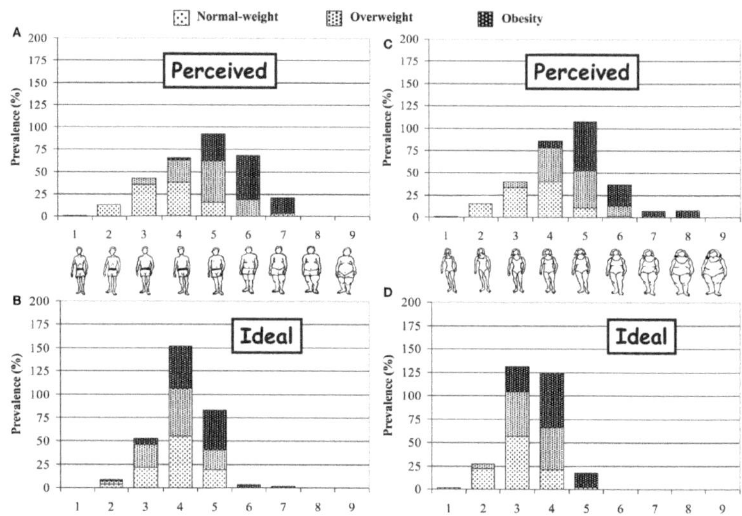

FIGURE 13.1 Perceived and ideal silhouettes chosen by boys (A,B) and girls (C,D).

13.2.5 Attitudes toward Self-Body Weight

The subjects were given multiple choice answers to the question, "Would you say that to gain weight is something that worries you? Not at all—Somewhat—A lot," followed by the question and multiple choice answers, "I consider myself obese: Yes—No."

13.2.6 Behaviors toward Body Weight Self-Control

The subjects responded to the question, "Have you ever tried to control your weight? (Yes—Never)" followed by the question, "If you answered yes, have you done so by: dieting (Yes—No); regular sport practice (Yes—No)."

13.2.7 Statistics

Analyses were performed with the Statistical Package for the Social Sciences, version 21.0 (SPSS, Inc., Chicago, IL, USA). Significant differences in prevalence were calculated by means of χ^2. The level of significance for acceptance was $P < 0.05$.

13.3 RESULTS

As shown in Table 1, a quarter of the sample showed higher weight than recommended. Around 20% of adolescents were overweight and around 6% were obese, and the incidence in both categories did not differ between genders and ages. Underweight adolescents just represented 0.8% of total sample. Therefore, they were analyzed together with normal weight adolescents.

TABLE 13.1 BMI distribution in the sample of adolescents according to the different variables in the study.

Variables	n	BMI(kg/m2)			p
		Normal weight (18.5 ≥ BMI < 24.9)	Overweight (25.0 ≥ BMI< 29.9)	Obese (BMI ≥ 30)	
Total	1961	74.5	19.6	5.9	
Gender					
Male	939	72.4	20.9	6.7	0.103
Female	1022	76. 5	18. 4	5.1	
Age (years)					
12-13	495	72 .3	21.2	6.5	0.096
14-15	948	73.1	20.5	6.4	
16-17	518	79.1	16.5	4.4	

Values are %. Significant trends evaluated by $\chi 2$.

Figure 1 shows body image self-perceptions. Adolescents tended to attribute silhouettes to themselves with lower signs of body fat than was inferred from the BMI measured. Around 35% of overweight girls ranked themselves as a 4—normal weight appearance—while almost half of the boys ranked themselves as a 5, a more robust size, but still with no clear signs of being overweight. The same parameters increased by one size among obese adolescents. Moreover, the choice of ideal silhouettes tended to be a larger size in boys, and rose consistently in line with BMI.

Table 2 shows that one-tenth of the subjects did not specify their weight. "Don't know" answers increased with age and BMI, reaching the 27.8% in the obese group. Weight underestimations increased as BMI increased but decreased with age, and the opposite occurred with overestimation. Girls estimated their weight better than boys, a knowledge that increased with age.

TABLE 13.2 Weight estimation, weight gain concern, and body image satisfaction by gender, age, and BMI group.

Variables[a]	N	Weight estimation					Weight gain concern				Body image satisfaction			
		Under-estimate	Correct	Over-estimate	Don't know/ don't answer	p[b]	Not at all	A little	A lot	p[b]	Thinner	Satisfied	Bigger	p[b]
Total	1961	27.8	51.9	9.2	11.1		50.4	36.5	13.1		46.8	37.0	16.2	
Gender						<0.001				<0.001	35.4	38.9	25.7	<0.001
Male	939	29.6	48.0	11.7	10.7		65.9	28.0	6.1		57.4	35.2	7.4	
Female	1022	26.1	55.4	6.9	11.5		36.1	44.3	19.6					
Age (years)						0.011				0.071				0.095
12–13	495	32.7	49.6	8.8	8.8		53.6	36.2	10.3		44.4	41.7	14.0	
14–15	948	26.8	52.6	8.6	12.0		47.5	37.9	14.6		48.4	35.4	16.2	
16–17	518	25.1	52.9	10.5	11.5		52.5	34.2	13.2		46.2	35.6	18.3	
BMI (kg/m^2)						<0.001				<0.001				<0.001
Normal weight	1462	22.1	58.7	10.9	8.3		58.1	31.5	10.4		33.7	44.9	21.4	
Malec	680	23.6^{NS}	53.7**	14.3***	8.4^{NS}		76.5***	19.5***	4.0***		18.1***	46.6^{NS}	35.3***	
Female	782	20.8	62.9	8.1	8.2		42.4	41.7	15.9		47.1	43.3	9.6	
Overweight	384	43.6	39.7	5.6	11.1		28.7	50.1	21.1		82.9	16.6	0.6	
Male[c]	196	42.9^{NS}	42.3^{NS}	7.1^{NS}	7.7*		42.2***	48.3^{NS}	9.4***		75.7***	23.2**	1.1^{NS}	
Female	188	44.4	37.1	3.9	14.6		14.9	52.0	33.1		90.3	9.7	0.0	
Obese	115	51.9	19.4	0.9	27.8		19.8	55.7	24.5		98.1	0.9	0.9	
Male[c]	63	54.2^{NS}	16.9^{NS}	0.0^{NS}	28.8^{NS}		23.2^{NS}	58.9^{NS}	17.9^{NS}		96.5^{NS}	1.8^{NS}	1.8^{NS}	
Female	52	49.0	22.4	2.0	26.5		16.0	52.0	32.0		100.0	0.0	0.0	

[a] Values are expressed as percentages.

[b] Significant trends between weight estimation, weight gain concern, and body image satisfaction groups have been evaluated by $\chi 2$.

[c] Significant trends between males and females have been evaluated by $\chi 2$.

*P < 0.05; **P < 0.01; ***P < 0.001; NS: not significant.

The difference between the real and ideal silhouette selected by each subject is shown in the body image satisfaction columns, which reveal that nearly half of the teenagers would like to be thinner. However, 25.7% of boys would like to have a larger silhouette.

The percentages of satisfied boys and girls were similar among subjects of normal weight, but girls still wished to be thinner and boys to be larger. Acceptance of being overweight was significantly higher amongst boys.

The Weight gain concern columns in Table 2 clearly reflect girls' greater concern about gaining weight, which was not affected by age but increased with BMI. Specifically, 47 and 21% of overweight and obese boys, respectively, stated that they were "Not at all" worried about weight concern. These percentages were significantly lower in girls. This unexpected lack of concern about their weight helps to explain the matching lack of any behavior attempt to lose weight in the corresponding column. In effect, 41% of overweight boys and 25% of obese boys stated that they had "Never" attempted to lose weight, and these percentages decreased significantly among females.

Table 3 shows that half of adolescents declared that they had tried to lose weight at least once. This general pattern to lose weight fits for the combination of diet and exercise, but the evolution is quite different when focus is just addressed to exercise, them most of the youngest age group (12-13), and normal weight boys tried more to lose weight with physical activity only.

13.4 DISCUSSION

Among the Balearic Islands' adolescents, the prevalence of overweight is higher and the prevalence of obesity is lower than in the Spanish adolescent population (38). Our study points to important gender differences in weight self-regulation attitudes and behaviors arose in the adolescent period. These findings agree with previous research (39, 40), and are in line with the superior worth given to thinness among girls, a phenomenon usually attributed to different beauty standards in boys and girls (8).

Our data confirm that girls have a more accurate knowledge of their weight than boys (probably by checking it frequently at home); they desire a thinner ideal body image; are much more concerned about weight gain and; as in adults (41), they make more efforts to keep their weight under control. At the studied ages, it was more likely to underestimate than overestimate, similarly to previous findings (42). The obtained results showed that underestimation decreased and overestimation increased with adolescent age. It could be inferred that as much

TABLE 13.3 Influence of gender, age, and gender within each BMI group on the intention to lose weight and the start of diet and/or exercise.

Variables[a]	N	Intention	p[b]	Do nothing	Diet	Exercise	Diet + Exercise	p[b]
Total	1961	48.4		0.6	24.2	38.2	36.9	
Gender			<0.001					<0.001
Male	939	32.9		1.3	11.2	56.8	30.7	
Female	1022	62.7		0.3	30.4	29.3	39.9	
Age			0.004					<0.001
12–13	495	41.8		1.5	18.0	52.5	28.0	
14–15	948	50.3		0.4	26.8	33.3	39.5	
16–17	518	51.2		0.4	24.3	36.1	39.2	
BMI (kg/m^2)			<0.001					0.001
Normal weight	1462	38.7		0.8	23.9	41.7	33.6	
Male[c]	680	19.2***		1.7	6.7	69.2	22.5***	
Female	782	55.3		0.5	29.0	33.7	36.9	
Overweight	384	74.6		0.0	25.3	37.0	37.7	
Male[c]	196	62.8***		0.0	12.4	48.7	38.9***	
Female	188	86.9		0.0	34.9	28.3	36.8	
Obese	115	88.7		0.0	23.4	20.2	56.4	
Male[c]	63	82.1*		0.0	19.6	37.0	43.5***	
Female	52	96.0		0.0	27.1	4.2	68.8	

[a] Values are expressed as percentages.
[b] Significant trends between intention to lose weight and the start of diet and/or exercise groups have been evaluated by $\chi 2$.
[c] Significant trends between males and females have been evaluated by χ^2.
*$P < 0.05$; ***$P < 0.001$.

older the adolescent is, as much worried on body weight may be. However, obtained answers on weight gain concern and body image satisfaction did not show it.

According to RFT, the personal motivation to weight self-control may be triggered by the wish to be attractive and/or to avoid to be rejected, being last case more influential, as an individual perceives himself/herself more deviant from social body standard.

However, it is a well-known psychological principle that losing weight is an objective hard to attain, as our adolescents' figures actually reveal. Clearly, changing comforting habits requires difficult psychological skills, which include an ability to tolerate uncomfortable internal reactions due to hunger or fatigue and a reduction of pleasure, as well as and a behavioral commitment to clearly defined values (43). Therefore, cognitive and emotional expectations about the sacrifices demanded by weight self-regulatory behaviors may dissuade many male and female candidates, while unpleasant experiences from diet and exercise probably lead others to surrender in their first attempts.

This failure may result in frustration and anger (44), a decrease in self-efficacy (45), or even to eat more (46, 47). These psychological outcomes usually arise when people feel unable to control themselves as they wish, or as societal rules dictated (17). In fact, changes in self-regulatory cognitive processes have been demonstrated in the context of adult overeating problems (48, 49).

However, in a social context where the stigma of obesity is a long way of being relaxed (50), the high percentages particularly of overweight males seemingly unconscious of their weight status, unconcerned about weight gain, and consequently unwilling to lose weight, were not. Accordingly, in agreement with similar studies, it can be concluded that most overweight and many obese boys seem to be satisfied with their physical appearance. Therefore, according to the Transtheorical Model (TTM) stages of change (51, 52), this adolescent population should be located in the "pre-contemplation step," i. e., healthy weight loss practices are not to be expected if subjects do not recognize excess weight, do not consider overweight to be a problem, or that is not a problem serious enough to engage in demanding weight self-regulatory behaviors.

Looking for alternative explanations, one may conjecture that the obese stigmatization actually threatens the self-esteem, particularly of the most weighted individuals, thus setting up subconscious ego self-defense denial mechanisms to protect self-esteem (53–55). High percentage of obese who declared that they did not know their weight would fit this interpretation.

Moreover, social stigma may also pose a cognitive dissonance conflict to overweighed population. Thus, biased body image perception and weight underestimations might be a reflection of a compromise between the social "ought" to body self-image and the perceived body self-image. In other words, self-indulgent weight judgments would be attempts to restore cognitive consonance by claiming "I'm not so fat!" This would explain why half of overweight and obese boys underestimated their weight.

However, our data reveal that most overweight and obese girls do not seem to be affected by the same emotional and cognitive processes. Therefore, beyond the superior worth given to thinness among girls, other psychological parameters are needed to explain the high percentage of boys not concerned about weight gain, or even willing to gain it (65.9 and 25% respectively). Because in male population, masculinity is frequently correlated with a big body, many boys may have considered that to look "manly," one should better be "well built" than "slim." This aim at looking "strong" parallels the girls' concern at looking "pretty." Thus, in the case of males, being overweight is not always associated to a negative social value, but rather to a positive one if associated to strength. Accordingly, to be a very thin boy may trigger more negative social consequences that to be moderately overweight (luckily, the percentage of underweight boys in our sample was irrelevant). Indeed, a silhouette that represents a slightly overweight boy could be interpreted as a silhouette representing a muscular boy (i.e., a "well-built" boy). This could also explain the discrepancy between the ideal silhouettes chosen by boys and girls.

In conclusion, "the lesser of two evils principle" is somewhat pertinent in this context: when confronted to the choice "being a bit overweight" vs. being a "bit too thin," perhaps, most boys would choose the first option.

Complementarily, our results could indicate the emergence of a process of social habituation to people exhibiting signs of overweight, a phenomenon comparable to the familiarity with shaved heads, which made it acceptable to be bald. In this direction, Rand and Resnick (56) not only asked teenagers to choose a real and ideal silhouette from a series, but also to check those that were socially acceptable. This study reported that 85% of overweight teenagers and 54% of obese ones considered that their current shape was within the socially acceptable margins of body size, regardless of whether or not they would like to have a slimmer figure. These results are compatible with the social habituation process hypothesis, which deserves further research including estimations of the "regular" or "average" silhouette. Moreover, new researches on body image attitudes demand a better methodology, thus substituting the classical but rather imprecise drawings we employed (e.g., silhouette that represents a slightly overweight boy could be interpreted as a silhouette representing a muscular boy). Instead, the employ of distorted pictures of the subjects (57) asking them to adjust on a computer screen should be encouraged.

Beyond the influence of body image attitudes on weight self-control, it has recently been suggested that personality factors, such as impulsivity and reward/punishment sensitivity, may also play a role in the observed gender motivational and behavioral differences in weight self-monitoring and control (58). The perfectionism personality trait has also previously been related to weight self-regulation, with adult women, who are highly perfectionistic, being more likely to see themselves as overweight and to be more dissatisfied with their bodies (59).

Nowadays, when public efforts to prevent overweight are multiplying (60–62), and many specific school-based interventions have been addressed to cope with the problem (63, 64), a deeper comprehension of factors involved in adolescent weight self-control may contribute to increase their efficiency. Accordingly, our results suggest that to stimulate the use of tailored messages regarding different boys and girls, body image attitudes could be beneficial to obesity epidemics.

Moreover, messages must face the fact that many overweight and obese boys do not actually feel the necessity to lose weight, rather to attribute their physical status to laziness, lack of will-power, or other common negative social stereotypes of overweight people (50).So, in the field of obesity prevention, researches should bear in mind Obelix's [a character from a well-known French comic book, (65)] famous denial, "I'm not fat. My chest just slipped a bit!," and adapt their messages suitably.

Another practical finding of our study is the important gender difference we observe in behaviors to achieve a healthy weight. In fact, girls typically used diet and exercise to lose weight, and boys used only exercise. The different competing body image motivations between boys and girls (e.g., to "look like strong" vs. to "look like pretty") probably boosts the males' link between sport and muscles and the females' one between diet and slenderness, thus explaining the girls' increased confidence in diet and the boys in exercise. Moreover, boys are perhaps more reluctant to go hungry, and girls have a greater fear of having their figures criticized. Therefore, interventions to prevent obesity should suitably accommodate and highlight the benefits of diet among boys, and physical activity among girls.

Afterward, interventions should focus on the advantages of maintaining a reasonable weight by healthy eating and exercise habits by means of presenting well described, attractive strategies to achieve that goal.

REFERENCES

1. Yanovski SZ, Yanovski JA. Obesity prevalence in the United States – up, down or sideways? N Engl J Med (2011) 11:987–91. doi: 10.1056/NEJMp1009229
2. Ogden CL, Carroll MD, Curtin LR, McDowell MA, Tabak CJ, Flegal KM. Prevalence of overweight and obesity in the United States, 1999-2004. J Am Med Assoc (2006) 295:1549–55. doi:10.1001/jama.295.13.1549
3. Bibiloni MM, Martínez E, Llull R, Juárez D, Pons A, Tur JA. Prevalence and risk factors for obesity in Balearic Islands adolescents. Br J Nutr (2010) 103:99–106. doi:10.1017/S000711450999136X
4. Grogan S. Body Image: Understanding Body Dissatisfaction in Men, Women and Children. London: Routledge (1999).
5. Gómez-Peresmitre G, Acosta MV. Valoraci6n de la delgadez. Un estudio transcultural (México/España). Psicothema (2002) 14:221–6.
6. Smolak L. Body image in children and adolescents: where do we go from here? Body Image (2004) 1:15–28. doi:10.1016/S1740-1445(03)00008-1
7. Silverstein B, Peterson B, Purdue L. Some correlates of the then standard of physical attractiveness of women. Int J Eat Disord (1986) 5:898–905. doi:10.1002/1098-108X (198607) 5:5$<$895:AID-EAT2260050510$>$3.0.CO;2-W
8. Poppe HG, Olivardia R, Borowiecki JJ, Cohane GH. The growing commercial value of the male body: a longitudinal survey of advertising in women's magazine. Psychother Psychosom (2001) 7:189–92. doi:10.1159/000056252
9. Vartanian LR, Herman CP, Polivy J. Implicit and explicit attitudes toward fatness and thinness: the role of the internalization of societal standards. Body Image (2005) 2:373–81. doi:10.1016/j.bodyim.2005.08.002
10. Neumark-Sztainer RD, Wall M, Guo J, Story M, Haines J, Eisenberg M. Obesity, disordered eating, and eating disorders in a longitudinal study of adolescents: how do dieters fare 5 years later? J Am Diet Assoc (2006) 106(4):559–68. doi:10.1016/j.jada.2006.01.003
11. Higgins ET. Beyond pleasure and pain. Am Psychol (1997) 52:1280–300. doi:10.1037/0003-066X. 52.12.1280
12. Higgins ET. Promotion and prevention: regulatory focus as a motivational principle. In: Zanna MP, editor. Advances in Experimental Social Psychology. San Diego, CA: Academic Press (1998). p. 1–46.
13. Spiegel S, Grant-Pillow H, Higgins ET. How regulatory fit enhances motivational strength during goal pursuit. Eur J Soc Psychol (2004) 34:39–54. doi:10.1002/ejsp.180
14. Vartanian LR, Herman CP, Polivy J. Does regulatory focus play a role in dietary restraint? Eat Behav (2006) 7:333–41. doi:10.1016/j.eatbeh.2005.11.007
15. Pfattheicher S, Sassenrath C. A regulatory focus perspective on eating behavior: how prevention and promotion focus relates to emotional, external, and restrained eating. Front Psychol (2014) 5:1314. doi:10.3389/fpsyg.2014.01314
16. Pula K, Parks CD, Ross CF. Regulatory focus and food choice motives. prevention orientation associated with mood, convenience, and familiarity. Appetite (2014) 78:15–22. doi:10.1016/j.appet.2014.02.015
17. Strauman TJ, Goetz EL. Self-regulation failure and health: pathways to mental and physical illness. In: Leary MR, Tangney JP, editors. Handbook of Self and Identity. New York, NY: The Guildford Press (2012). p. 247–67.

18. Nowak M. The weight-conscious adolescent: body image, food intake, and weight-related behavior. J Adolesc Health (1998) 23(6):389–98. doi:10.1016/S1054-139X(97)00263-2
19. Bibiloni MM, Pich J, Pons A, Tur JA. Body image and eating patterns among adolescents. BMC Public Health (2013) 13:1104. doi:10.1186/1471-2458-13-1104
20. Strauss RS. Self-reported weight status and dieting in a cross-sectional sample of young adolescents. National Health and Nutrition Examination Survey III. Arch Pediatr Adolesc Med (1999) 153:741–7. doi:10.1001/archpedi.153.7.741
21. Viner RM, Haines MM, Taylor SJC, Head J, Booy R, Stansfeld S. Body mass, weight control behaviours, weight perception and emotional well-being in a multiethnic sample of early adolescents. Int J Obes (2006) 30:1514–21. doi:10.1038/sj.ijo.0803352
22. Sherry B, Jefferds ME, Grummer-Strawn LM. Accuracy of adolescent self-report of height and weight in assessing overweight status: a literature review. Arch Pediatr Adolesc Med (2007) 161:1154–61. doi:10.1001/archpedi.161.12.1154
23. Standley R, Sullivan V, Wardle J. Self-perceived weight in adolescents: over-estimation or under-estimation? Body Image (2009) 6:56–9. doi:10.1016/j.bodyim.2008.08.004
24. Cash TF, Morrow JA, Hrabosky JI, Perry AA. How has body image changed? A cross-sectional investigation of college women and men from 1983 to 2001. J Consult Clin Psychol (2004) 72(6):1081–9. doi:10.1037/0022-006X.72.6.1081
25. Johnson-Taylor WL, Fisher RA, Hubbard VS, Staerke-Reed P, Eggers OS. The change in weight perception of weight status among the overweight: comparison of NHANES III (1988-1994) and 1999–2004 NHANES. Int J Behav Nutr Phys Act (2008) 2008(5):9. doi:10.1186/1479-5868-5-9
26. Johnson F, Cooke L, Croker H, Wardle J. Changing perceptions of weight in Great Britain: comparison of two population surveys. Br Med J (2008) 337:a494. doi:10.1136/bmj.a494
27. Brener ND, Eaton DK, Lowry R, McManus T. The association between weight perception and BMI among high school students. Obes Res (2004) 12(11):1866–74. doi:10.1038/oby.2004.232
28. Elgar FJ, Roberts C, Tudor-Smith C, Moore L. Validity of self-reported height and weight and predictors of bias in adolescents. J Adolesc Health (2005) 37(5):371–5. doi:10.1016/j.jadohealth.2004.07.014
29. Scott DJ, Duncan EK, Scholfiels G. Associations between weight perception, weight control and body fatness in a multiethnic sample of adolescents girls. Public Health Nutr (2011) 14:93–100. doi:10.1017/S1368980010000236
30. Deschamps V, Salanave B, Chan-Chee C, Vernay M, Castetbon K. Body-weight perception and related preoccupations in a large national sample of adoelscents. Pediatr Obes (2015) 10:15–22. doi:10.1111/j.2047-6310.2013.00211.x
31. Jones DC. Body image among adolescent boys and girls: a longitudinal study. Dev Psychol (2004) 40:823–35. doi:10.1037/0012-1649.40.5.823
32. Moreno LA, Fleta J, Mur L, Feja C, Sarriá A, Bueno M. Indices of body fat distribution in Spanish children aged 4.0 to 14.9 years. J Pediatr Gastroenterol Nutr (1997) 25:175–81. doi:10.1097/00005176-199708000-00008
33. WHO. Physical status: the use and interpretation of anthropometry. Technical Report Series. Geneva: World Health Organization (1995).
34. International Association for the Study of Obesity (IASO). (2013). Available from: http://www.iaso.org/resources/aboutobesity/child-obesity/newchildcutoffs/ (accessed July 15, 2013)

35. Cole TJ, Bellizzi MC, Flegal KM, Dietz WH. Establishing a standard definition for child overweight and obesity worldwide: international survey. Br Med J (2000) 320:1240–3. doi:10.1136/bmj.320.7244.1240
36. Cole TJ, Flegal KM, Nicholls D, Jackson AA. Body mass index cut-offs to define thinness in children and adolescents: international survey. BMJ (2007) 335:194–202. doi:10.1136/bmj.39238.399444.55
37. Stunkard AJ, Sorensen T, Schulsinger F. Use of the Danish adoption register for the study of obesity and thinness. In: Kety SS, Rowland LP, Sidman RL, Matthysse SW, editors. Genetics of Neurological and Psychiatric Disorders. New York, NY: Raven Press (1983). p. 115–20.
38. Serra-Majem L, Ribas-Barba L, Aranceta-Bartrina J, Pérez-Rodrigo C, Saavedra-Santana P, Peña-Quintana L. Childhood and adolescent obesity in Spain. Results of the enKid Study (1998-2000). Med Clin (Barc) (2003) 121:725–32.
39. Boutelle K, Neumark-Sztainer D, Story M, Resnick M. Weight control behaviors among obese, overweight, and non-overweight adolescents. J Pediatr Psychol (2002) 27(6):531–40. doi:10.1093/jpepsy/27.6.531
40. Halvarsson K, Lunner K, Westerberg J, Anteson F, Sjödén P. A longitudinal study of the development of dieting among 7-17-year-old Swedish girls. Int J Eat Disord (2002) 31:32–42. doi:10.1002/eat.10004
41. Lemon SC, Rosal MC, Zapka J, Borg A, Andersen V. Contributions of weight perceptions to weight loss attempts: differences by body mass index and gender. Body Image (2009) 6:90–6. doi:10.1016/j.bodyim.2008.11.004
42. Park E. Overestimation and underestimation: adolescents' weight perception in comparison to BMI-based weight status and how it varies across socio-demographic factors. J Sch Health (2011) 81:57–64. doi:10.1111/j.1746-1561.2010.00561.x
43. Forman EM, Butryn ML. A new look at the science of weight control: how acceptance and commitment strategies can address the challenge of self-regulation. Appetite (2015) 84:171–80. doi:10.1016/j.appet.2014.10.004
44. Hofmann W, Vohs KD, Baumeister RF. What people desire, feel conflicted about, and try to resist in everyday life. Psychol Sci (2012) 23(6):582–8. doi:10.1177/0956797612437426
45. Bandura A. Self-Efficacy: The Exercise of Control. New York, NY: Freeman (1997).
46. Herman CP, Polivy J. Restrined eating. In: Stunkard A, editor. Obesity. Philadelphia, PA: Saunders (1980). p. 208–25.
47. Lowe MR, Doshi SD, Katterman SN, Feig EH. Dieting and restrained eating as prospective predictors of weight gain. Front Psychol (2013) 4:557. doi:10.3398/fpsyg.2013.00577
48. Polivy J, Herman CP, McFarlane T. Effects of anxiety on eating: does palatability moderate distress-induced overeating in dieters? J Abnorm Psychol (1994) 103:505–10. doi:10.1037/0021-843X.103.3.505
49. Scholz U, Nagy G, Gohner W, Lusczynska A, Kliegel M. Changes in self-regulatory cognitions as predictors of changes in smoking and nutrition behavior. Psychol Health (2009) 24:545–61. doi:10.1080/08870440801902519
50. Puhl RM, Heuer CA. The stigma of obesity: a review and update. Obesity (2009) 17:941–64. doi:10.1038/oby.2008.636
51. Prochaska JO, DiClemente CC. Trans-theoretical therapy – toward a more integrative model of change. Psychother Theor Res Pract (1982) 19:276–88. doi:10.1037/h0088437

52. Prochaska JO, DiClemente CC. The transtheoretical approach. 2nd ed. In: Norcross JC, Goldfried MR, editors. Handbook of Psychotherapy Integration. New York, NY: Oxford University Press (2005). p. 147–71.
53. Freud A. The Ego and the Mechanisms of Defense. London: Hogarth Press and Institute of Psycho-Analysis (1937).
54. Baumeister RF, Dale K, Sommer KL. Freudian defense mechanisms and empirical findings in modern social psychology: reaction formation, projection, displacement, undoing, isolation, sublimation, and denial. J Pers (1998) 66(6):1081–124. doi:10.1111/1467-6494.00043
55. Zoccalia R, Brunoa A, Muscatelloa MR, Micòa U, Coricab F, Meduria M. Defense mechanisms in a sample of non-psychiatric obese subjects. Eat Behav (2008) 9:120–3. doi:10.1016/j.eatbeh.2007.06.005
56. Rand CSW, Resnick JL. The "good enough" body size as judged by people varying age and weight. Obes Res (2008) 8:309–16. doi:10.1038/oby.2000.37
57. Docteur A, Urdapilleta I, Defrance C, Raison J. Body perception and satisfactions in obese, severely obese, and normal weight female patients. Obesity (2010) 18(7):1464–5. doi:10.1038/oby.2009.418
58. Dietrich A, Federbusch M, Grellmann C, Villringer A, Hortsmann A. Body weight status, eating behavior, sensitivity to reward/punishment, and gender: relationships and interdependencies. Front Psychol (2014) 5:1073. doi:10.3398/fpsyg.2014.01073
59. Vohs KD, Bardone AM, Joiner TE Jr, Abramson LY, Heatherton TF. Perfectionism, perceived weight status, and self-esteem interact to predict bulimic symptoms: a model of bulimic symptom development. J Abnorm Psychol (1999) 108:695–700. doi:10.1037/0021-843X.108.4.695
60. Brug J, Oenema A, Ferreira I. Theory, evidence and Intervention Mapping to improve behavior nutrition and physical activity interventions. Int J Behav Nutr Phys Act (2005) 2:2. doi:10.1186/1479-5868-2-2
61. US Department of Health and Human Services. The Surgeon General's call to action to prevent and decrease overweight and obesity. Rockville, MD: US Department of Health and Human Services, Office of the Surgeon General (2001). Available from: http://www.surgeongeneral.gov/topics/obesity/
62. Sassi F. Obesity and the Economics of Prevention. Fit not Fat (2013). Available from: http://www.oecd.org/els/health-systems/obesity-and-the-economics-of-prevention-9789264084865-en.htm (accessed September 13, 2013)
63. Campbell K, Waters E, O'Meara S, Summerbell C. Interventions for preventing obesity in children. A systematic review. Obes Rev (2001) 2(3):149–57. doi:10.1046/j.1467-789x.2001.00035.x
64. Traill WB, Shankar B, Brambilla-Macias J, Bech-Larsen T, Aschemann-Witzel J, Strand M, et al. Interventions to promote healthy eating habits: evaluation and recommendations. Obes Rev (2010) 11(12):895–8. doi:10.1111/j.1467-798X.2010.0017.x
65. Goscinny A, Uderzo R. Astérix the Gaul. Paris: Dargaud (1961).

CHAPTER 14

The Role of Self-Regulating Abilities in Long-Term Weight Loss in Severely Obese Children and Adolescents Undergoing Intensive Combined Lifestyle Interventions (HELIOS); Rationale, Design and Methods

Jutka Halberstadt, Sabine Makkes, Emely de Vet, Anita Jansen, Chantal Nederkoorn, Olga H. van der Baan-Slootweg, and Jacob C. Seidell

14.1 BACKGROUND

14.1.1 Prevalence and Consequences of Obesity

The prevalence of obesity in the Netherlands increased 6-fold in the period 1980–2009 in boys (0.3% to 1.8%) and 4.5-fold in girls (0.5% to 2.2%) [1].

Generally, when there is an increase in prevalence of obesity, there is a greater relative increase in severe obesity [2].

Childhood and adolescent obesity are associated with serious comorbidities including type 2 diabetes mellitus, hyperlipidemia, hypertension, respiratory and musculoskeletal conditions and liver abnormalities [3–5]. The increase in obesity-associated diseases leads to a significant increase in direct and indirect medical costs [6]. In addition to physical health problems, obese children and adolescents also are more likely to suffer from a variety of psychosocial problems [7–9]. They are more likely than non-obese children to be a target of societal stigmatization, including teasing and bullying [10, 11], to be socially isolated [5, 12], to have relatively high rates of disordered eating, anxiety, and depression [5], and to suffer from suicidal thoughts and making suicide attempts [9]. When they reach adulthood, they are less likely than their thinner counterparts to complete college and more likely to live in poverty [5]. They are also less likely to get married [13]. A further illustration that obesity has a large impact on young people's lives is reflected in the finding that severely obese children and adolescents reported to have similar quality of life as those diagnosed with cancer [14, 15]. Therefore adequate management of severe childhood obesity may contribute to reduce their current and future social, psychological and physical impairment.

14.1.2 Intensive Combined Lifestyle Interventions

It is generally recognized that the more severe forms of obesity may well warrant more intensive therapeutic interventions [16] than less severe obesity [17]. Because regular outpatient treatment appears to be insufficiently effective for the specific patient group of severely obese children and adolescents [18–20], it has been proposed that there is a need for experienced, specialized pediatric obesity centers that can provide intensive treatment by a multidisciplinary team with expertise in childhood obesity and its comorbidities [18–20]. According to several guidelines, the treatment team should include a physician, dietician, exercise specialist and psychologist or other mental health care provider that is able to offer behavioral counseling [17–22].

A promising alternative to regular outpatient treatment is so called "immersion treatment" that places patients in a therapeutic and educational environment for extended periods of time, for example a residential summer camp or inpatient setting [21, 23]. Immersion programs described in a recent review included the components controlled diet, physical exercise/activity, nutrition education and therapy and/or education regarding behavior change. The participants in the reviewed treatments that included a follow up lost an average of 23.9% of their overweight during treatment and 20.6% pre-immersion to follow up (ranging from 4 months to 3.6 years later) [23]. Inclusion of cognitive behavioral therapy (CBT), defined as including "regular group and/or individual meetings with a therapist utilizing CBT techniques for managing behavior change, such as self-monitoring, motivational interviewing/decisional counseling and problem-solving", seems especially promising, resulting in an average of 29.9% loss of overweight in total at follow-up, compared to 9.4% for programs without cognitive behavioral therapy [23].

Heideheuvel (part of Merem Treatment Centers) is a specialized clinic in the Netherlands offering a form of immersion treatment, by means of an intensive inpatient combined lifestyle intervention, focusing on nutrition, physical activity and behavior change of the severely obese participants and their parents. Improving self-regulation of eating behavior is one of the main goals of the treatment at Heideheuvel. The clinic uses cognitive behavioral techniques to improve self-regulation.

Although the need for combined lifestyle interventions targeting nutrition, physical activity and behavior change is widely acknowledged, long-term follow-up studies of obesity interventions are lacking, especially for severely obese youth [17, 24, 25].

According to Yanovski and Yanovski the known long-term results for children and adolescents are generally disappointing, because the weight reduction is often not maintained [18]. However, there appear to be remarkable individual differences in treatment success [26]. For some patients treatment is highly successful, while others continue to gain weight despite treatment. This raises the question what determines inter-individual variability in intervention success.

Currently there is little insight in the psychosocial factors that may be crucial in determining the long-term outcome. The ability to self-regulate dietary intake has been proposed as an important factor in weight loss and weight loss maintenance [8, 27–32].

14.1.3 The Role of Self-regulation

Severe obesity results from a sustained chronic positive energy balance. This implies that there is an underlying inability to regulate food intake in such a way that it matches energy expenditure. Volkow and others have postulated that this inability to regulate food intake can be seen as a brain-related dysfunction whereby reward-driven urges for food override the cognitive ability to limit food intake [33]. Especially children and adolescents are vulnerable to problems arising due to self-regulatory failure, because the neurocognitive structures that link reward systems to the executive control system are still in development [34]. The inability to self-regulate is particularly problematic for children who are overwhelmed with an abundance of food and food cues due to their socioeconomic and cultural environments or who grow up in families where the parents have insufficient parenting skills to teach their children self-regulation in response to food cues [35].

Self-regulation encompasses any, conscious and non-conscious, efforts by people to alter their thoughts, emotions, attention, impulses and behavior [36] in the service of attaining and maintaining personal goals [37]. Self-regulation reflects the ability to resist immediate rewards (e.g. a chocolate cake) in the face of long-term goal pursuit (e.g. losing weight and maintaining the weight loss) [38]. It is known that people differ greatly in their ability to self regulate [39].

Not many studies examined self-regulation of food intake in obese individuals, but the few studies that did consistently showed that obese people generally are less able to self-regulate than lean people [27, 28, 40, 41].

Two distinct aspects of self-regulation that are particularly relevant to controlling food intake, are sensitivity to reward and inhibitory control [40, 42, 43]. Sensitivity to reward is associated with the mesolimbic dopamine system [44]. It reflects the sensory pleasure associated with the reward and the motivation to obtain the reward. Inhibitory control is regulated by the prefrontal cortex, and refers to the executive function by which impulses or responses are controlled [43, 44].

Research has indeed indicated that food is more rewarding for overweight children than for lean children, making it therefore harder for them to resist food temptations and possibly increasing the chance of excessive food intake and resulting further weight gain [45, 46]. Obese children are found to have a higher sensitivity to reward and less response inhibition than lean children [29, 41, 47–52]. For example, Nederkoorn and colleagues showed that obese children had lower levels of inhibitory control as assessed by a behavioral measure for disinhibition and were more sensitive to reward as assessed by a response preservation measure than leaner children [40]. Above these cross-sectional studies, prospective studies showed that differences in ability to self-regulate were related to weight gain. For example Francis and colleagues showed that children who were less able to self-regulate at ages 3 and 5 years, as measured with behavioral laboratory tasks, had a more rapid weight gain from age 3 to 12 years [51].

Poor self-regulation, as measured with various questionnaires and behavioral measures, has also been shown to predict less weight loss, less weight loss maintenance or more attrition to weight loss programs [27, 28, 30, 40, 53]. For example, those obese children participating in a cognitive behavioral treatment program who showed relatively little inhibitory control lost less weight than those who exhibited higher levels of control [28].

Three decades ago Bonato et al. already suggested that interventions for obese children should aim at improving self-regulation of eating [29]. More recent research indeed indicates that self-regulation of eating can be improved through behavioral treatment. For example, Israel et al. evaluated an intervention for overweight children and their parents that aimed to improve self-regulation in children in order to lose weight. Training components included instructions for goal setting, formulating and implementing a plan to change behavior, self-evaluation, self-reward and training in problem-solving behaviors appropriate for high-risk or tempting situations. The results indicated that improving self-regulation can help to maintain long term weight loss [31]. Bryant et al. also indicated in a review that disinhibition in eating behavior can be successfully diminished through application of behavioral therapy aimed at self-regulation of eating behavior [27].

In sum, relatively poor self-regulation is likely to contribute to the development of obesity as well as to a lower amount of long-term weight loss as a result of treatment. Therefore, studying the role of self-regulation in the effectiveness of weight loss therapy may contribute to the development of more successful interventions [28]. The main objective of this study is to determine whether the ability to self-regulate predicts long-term weight loss in severely obese children and adolescents. To our knowledge, such studies have not been performed in severely obese children and adolescents.

14.1.4 The Potential Moderating Role of other Psychosocial Factors

An additional objective of this study is to identify other psychosocial factors that may modify the relation between the general ability to self-regulate and long-term weight loss in severely obese children and adolescents. Gaining understanding in moderating factors is important as it might help to improve tailoring interventions to children. The following factors that plausibly play an important role will be assessed:

1. Competence, in this study operationalized as general self-efficacy and self-worth.
2. Motivation, in this study operationalized as autonomous motivation.
3. Relatedness, in this study operationalized as interaction between parent and child, peer body size, social competences and social problems, parental feeding style and affect of the parent.
4. Outcome expectations, in this study operationalized as the difference between current and expected own body size.

The selection of these additional psychosocial factors to study, was made based on 1) reviews by Teixeira et al. [26] and Elfhag and Rössner [54], 2) advice by experts in the field of psychological child obesity research and treatment and 3) two prevailing psychological theories: self-determination theory [55] and social cognitive theory [56].

The self-determination theory and the social cognitive theory are general theories of human behavior, but have also been applied to weight control. According to self-determination theory, a theory of human motivation and behavior, three innate psychological needs are the basis for autonomous motivation: 1) competence (i.e. having a feeling of efficacy), 2) autonomy (i.e. perceiving an internal locus of causality; having a feeling of free will) and 3) relatedness (i.e. having a sense of security and belonging) [55]. Conditions in the social context, like positive or negative feedback, can either enhance or hinder the fulfillment of these three basic needs [55]. When satisfied, these psychological needs facilitate autonomous motivation, which is important for behavioral persistence in for example weight-related behaviors [55, 57].

According to social cognitive theory human behavior is a result of a continuous reciprocal interaction between behavior, cognitive and affective personal factors and environmental events [56, 58]. This interaction is influenced by people's beliefs about their capabilities to exercise control over their own level of functioning and over events that affect their lives [56, 59]. These self-efficacy beliefs determine people's level of motivation and the effort they are willing to put in reaching their goals [56, 59]. Self-efficacy influences outcome expectations which has an effect on the motivation to perform: when you expect to succeed that is an incentive to pursue the needed actions [56].

Some of the factors from the self-determination theory and the social cognitive theory are also mentioned in reviews by Teixeira et al. and Elfhag and

Rössner [26, 54] on psychosocial factors that are associated with weight control in adults. These reviews for example show that more autonomous motivation is associated with weight loss maintenance [26, 54]. Other factors that are mentioned are: self-efficacy [26, 54], self-esteem [26], autonomy [26, 54], social support [54], body image [26] and outcome expectations [26, 54].

In sum, the objective of this study is mainly to determine whether the ability to self-regulate predicts long-term weight loss in severely obese children and adolescents and in addition to identify other psychosocial factors that may modify the relation between the general ability to self-regulate and long-term weight loss.

It is hypothesized that having less self-regulating abilities will result in less weight loss and less weight loss maintenance. The following factors are expected to negatively influence the relationship between self-regulation ability and weight loss and weight loss maintenance: less general self-efficacy, lower self-worth, less autonomous motivation, lower quality of the relationship between parent and child, larger body size of peers, less social competences, more social problems, a less adequate parental feeding style, more negative affect of the parent and unrealistic outcome expectations.

14.2 METHODS/DESIGN

14.2.1 Study Design

This study is designed as a prospective observational study of children and adolescents undergoing an intensive combined lifestyle intervention during one year for their severe obesity. The treatment program has either a 2 months or a 6 months inpatient period.

The Medical Ethics Committee of VU University Medical Center Amsterdam has approved the study design, protocols and informed consent procedure. This study is a collaboration with a study that aims to provide insights into the effectiveness and cost-effectiveness of the interventions [60].

14.2.2 Setting

This study is carried out in the childhood obesity clinic Heideheuvel (part of Merem Treatment Centers) in Hilversum, The Netherlands between August 2009 and July 2013.

14.2.3 Study Population

The aim is to include 120 children and adolescents and their parents/caregivers in the study. 80 of the patients will undergo a 2 months inpatient period and 40 a 6 months inpatient period.

Patients (8–19 years of age) are admitted to Heideheuvel for their severe obesity. Inclusion criteria are a SDS-BMI ≥ 3.0 according to the growth curves based on the fourth Dutch National Growth Study of 1997 (this corresponds to the 99.9th percentile) or a SDS-BMI ≥ 2.3 (corresponding to the 99th percentile) with obesity related morbidity (e.g. obstructive sleep apnea syndrome, hyperinsulinemia, diabetes type 2, liver function disorders, dyslipidemia, musculoskeletal problems). Before admission, these children and adolescents have, unsuccessfully, received outpatient obesity care elsewhere. Some patients, who are diagnosed to not be able to profit from outpatient care, are referred directly. All patients are referred by their local pediatrician.

Criteria for exclusion from the study are: syndromal/chromosomal determined obesity, obesity caused by endocrine disorders (e.g. hypothyroidism, Cushing syndrome, primary hyperinsulinemia, pseudohypoparathyroidism, acquired (structural) hypothalamic damage) or use of medication (e.g. antiepileptic drugs, antidepressants), psychiatric disorders (e.g. severe depression, schizophrenia) that may obstruct adequate treatment, presence of eating disorders (binge eating disorder, bulimia nervosa) to such a degree that specific therapeutic attention is needed before starting the intervention, children/adolescents or parents that can or will not give 'informed consent', parents that can or will not participate in the treatment, children/adolescents with an IQ below 75 or attending a school for intellectually challenged children. Written informed consents are obtained from both the participants (from age 12) and their parents.

Participants do not pay for the treatment which is temporarily reimbursed by the Ministry of Health, Welfare and Sports. For their participation in the research they get reimbursed with a 20 Euros gift voucher to cover travel expenses.

14.2.4 Time Schedule

The study period is four years. Since the capacity to treat patients is limited in the clinic, the patients are treated in sequential groups of 10 children (8–13 years) or 10 adolescents (13–19 years). At the end of the fourth year 120 patients will have completed the program and follow up period.

Measurements will be taken at three points in time: at baseline (start of treatment; T0), at the end of treatment (12 months after baseline; T12), at the end of follow-up (24 months after baseline; T24). Besides weight and height, measured at T0, T12 and T24, measurements include (also for the parents of the patients) several questionnaires on psychosocial characteristics: Dutch Eating Behavior Questionnaire for children (administered at T0, T12, T24), General self-efficacy scale (T0, T12, T24), Self-Perception Profile for Children/Adolescents (T0, T12, T24), Treatment Self-Regulation Questionnaire (T0), parent and child version of the Parent–child Interaction Questionnaire (T0), Child Behavior Checklist (T0, T12, T24), Parental Feeding Style Questionnaire (T0, T12, T24), Positive and Negative Affect Schedule (T0), line drawings of silhouettes to choose from (T0, T12, T24). In addition the children's self-regulation abilities are evaluated by two behavioral computer tasks: The Stop Signal Task (T0, T12, T24) and the Balloon Analogue Risk Task (T0, T12, T24). All questionnaires and computer tasks are described in the measurements section below.

14.2.5 Interventions

The treatment is an intensive one year lifestyle intervention program by a multidisciplinary team with emphasis on nutrition, exercise and behavior and implementation of the learned behavior in the home situation. Treatment consists of group treatment as well as individual sessions. For an extensive description of the treatment components, see Makkes et al. [60].

There is active and frequent participation of the parents during the whole treatment because parents have a major influence on their children's weight and weight-related behaviors through modeling and encouraging of appropriate health behaviors, controlling the quality and quantity of the food available in the household, facilitating physical activity, and engaging in appropriate feeding practices. An additional advantage of family-based interventions is that they can improve health behaviors and weight not only in the treated child but also in siblings and adults living in the household [61, 62].

The behavioral part of the treatment program is carried out by psychologists, social workers and group coaches in individual as well as group sessions with children and parents together and separately. The program uses behavior change techniques, e.g. from cognitive behavioral therapy, to improve the general ability to self-regulate. This improvement in general self-regulation abilities is assumed to facilitate the self-regulation of the newly learned healthier behavior. For example, the program teaches patients to delay gratification (I want a cookie now, but I will wait until it is tea time), to plan behavior (e.g. forming if-then plans: if it rains, I will still take my planned thirty minute walk) or to self monitor behavior (keeping a diary of the cookies eaten and the walks taken). The treatment further addresses: disordered eating behaviors, self-worth, self-efficacy, behavioral and emotional problems, autonomous motivation, body image, outcome expectations, mood disorders, eating and exercise behavior, interaction between parent and child, parental feeding styles, relationships with peers, body acceptance and coping. To achieve its aims, the program applies a number of behavior change techniques. These techniques can be specified with a 40-item taxonomy, called CALO-RE, that is developed by Michie et al. [63]. The chief psychologist of the treatment program scored the intervention with this CALO-RE taxonomy, which gives an overview of relevant behavior change techniques for interventions aimed at increasing physical activity and healthy eating [63]. The treatment program uses 27 of the 40 defined behavior change techniques to some extent (number 1–13, 15–16, 19, 21–22, 28–29, 33, 35–40). For example, the program uses goal setting to define a desired behavior that can be related to changes in diet or physical activity. Goal setting is also used to define health outcomes. Another used behavior change technique is prompting generalization of a target behavior from the clinic to the home situation. To learn how to cope with barriers to change the behavior, like certain feelings and desires, the treatment uses barrier identification and problem solving techniques. The treatment also uses modeling of behavior, which involves showing how to perform a certain behavior in for example a role play, by the staff, the peers and the parents. Another applied technique is motivational interviewing in which the staff is trained and that is used to assess and if necessary help change the phase of behavior change the patient is in.

14.2.6 Measurements

14.2.6.1 Outcome Measures

The primary outcome measurement is the gender and age-specific ΔSDS-BMI between baseline (T0) and follow up (T24) indicating total weight loss from baseline to follow up and ΔSDS-BMI between end of treatment (T12) and follow up (T24) indicating weight loss maintenance after treatment.

14.2.6.2 Determinants of Long-term Weight Loss and Weight Loss Maintenance

14.2.6.2.1 Behavioral Measures of General Self-regulation Ability

Our hypothesis is that a primary determinant of (sustained) weight loss is the general ability to self-regulate. We assess two separate aspects of general self-regulation: sensitivity to reward and inhibitory control. Both are measured with two computerized behavioral tasks that are not food related and an objective measure of the general ability to self-regulate: the Stop Signal Task and the Balloon Analogue Risk Task [64, 65].

The Stop Signal Task is a measure of inhibitory control [66] also referred to as executive response inhibition [67]. The task correlates significantly with related measures for self-control [66]. A Dutch adaption of the task by C. Nederkoorn was used [68]. The Stop Signal Task is a computer task consisting of a series of 4x64 trials, preceded by two practice blocks of 8 and 16 trials, in which individuals are exposed to a colored quadrangle on the right or the left side of the screen (the go signal). Individuals have to press the shift button on the side where the quadrangle appears as quick as possible. However, in 25% of the trials respondents hear a tone, after which individuals should inhibit their response to press the shift button. Failing to inhibit the response when the stop signal sounds, indicates lack of self-regulation. At the start of the task the delay between the go signal and the stop signal is set to 250 milliseconds. The computer changes the stop signal delay after every stop signal trial. Following an unsuccessful inhibition the delay is decreased by 50 milliseconds, making the task easier. After a successful inhibition the task is made more difficult by increasing the stop signal delay by 50 milliseconds. This dynamic adjustment results in a stop signal delay that enables the participant to stop on approximately 50% of the stop trials. The main outcome is the stop signal reaction time (SSRT), which is calculated by subtracting the stop signal delay from the mean go signal reaction time, measured in milliseconds. A longer SSRT means that the participant takes longer to inhibit his/her response and indicates less inhibitory control [64]. The Stop Signal Task demonstrated less inhibitory control in children with impulse control problems like ADHD [64, 69] and in obese children [28, 70], making it a valid test to study self-regulation in the present sample as well.

The Balloon Analogue Risk Task (BART) is a measure of sensitivity to reward [65], which has been shown to correlate significantly with related measures of self-control [66] and impulsivity [65]. The BART assesses the willingness to consciously risk long term loss in order to get higher rewards on the short term [67]. A Dutch adaption of the task by C. Nederkoorn was used. This version of the BART is a computer task consisting of a series of 29 trials. In every trial a small red balloon is shown on the computer screen. The participant is instructed to inflate the balloon by pressing a pump button. He or she is warned that the balloon will explode at some point, but that this can happen any time from after the first pump until after the balloon has expanded to fill the whole screen. Every pump produces a gain of 5 points in a temporary bank. As long as the pumping continues, the points go up. However, the balloons all explode at some point, according to a predetermined sequence with the weakest balloon exploding on the first pump and the strongest balloon exploding after 128 pumps. If that happens before the gained points are transferred to the permanent bank, all points for that balloon are lost. Transfer to the permanent bank can be done at any chosen moment by pressing the collect button and results in the next trial with a new uninflated balloon. The total amount of points earned is shown on the computer screen [65]. In deciding whether to make each pump, the participant must balance the potential gain of accruing more money against the potential risk of losing all money accrued for that balloon [71]. Individuals who are more sensitive to rewards will demonstrate a higher number of pumps on each balloon prior to money collection [65]. For analysis of the results the adjusted value is used, defined as the average number of pumps excluding balloons that exploded [65, 72, 73].

14.2.6.2.2 Self-report Measure of Eating Specific Self-regulation Ability

In addition to the computer tasks, self-reported indicators of eating-specific self-regulation are assessed. Hereto, a version specifically adapted to children [74] of the Dutch Eating Behavior Questionnaire (DEBQ), originally developed by Van Strien and colleagues [75], is used. This 33-item questionnaire assesses three eating styles that reflect dysfunctional regulation of food intake: 1) external eating (i.e. the tendency to eat in response to external cues), 2) emotional eating (i.e. the tendency to overeat in response to emotions) and 3) restrained eating (i.e. the tendency to attempt to refrain from eating) [75].

14.2.6.3 Moderators of the Relation between Self-regulation Ability and Weight Loss and Weight Loss Maintenance

As outlined earlier, factors related to competence, motivation, relatedness and outcome expectations will be examined as moderating factors. Hereto, all moderating factors are assessed at baseline and at follow-up examinations. Except for a few moderators that are only measured at T0.

14.2.6.3.1 Competence

Self-efficacy is measured with the Dutch adaptation of the 10-item General self-efficacy (GSE) scale, which assesses one's sense of personal competence to cope across a variety of demanding or novel situations [76].

Self-worth is measured with Dutch adaptations [77, 78] of the Self-Perception Profile for Children (SPPC) and Adolescents (SPPA) developed by Harter [79, 80], which are questionnaires with 36 items (SPPC) or 35 items (SPPA) in six (SPPC) or seven (SPPA) domains: 1) global self-worth, 2) scholastic competence, 3) social acceptance, 4) athletic competence, 5) physical appearance, 6) behavioral conduct, and 7) close friendship (only SSPA).

14.2.6.3.2 Motivation

Motivation to enter a weight loss program is measured with a 18-item version of the Treatment Self-Regulation Questionnaire (TSRQ) that assesses reasons to enter a weight-loss program [81]. The questionnaire was translated into Dutch by two of the authors of this article (JH and EdV) with help from a native English speaker, in which process it was slightly adapted for use with children and adolescents. It assesses to what extent children and adolescents enter a weight-loss program for autonomous (e.g. "I really want to make some changes in my life") and controlled reasons (e.g. "People will like me better when I'm thin") on a 7-point Likert scale ranging from 1 (not at all for this reason) to 7 (totally for this reason).

14.2.6.3.3 Relatedness

Interaction between child and parent is measured with the Dutch version of the Parent–child Interaction Questionnaire—Revised (PACHIQ-R) [82] that assesses how the parent evaluates the relationship with the child (PACHIQ-R Parent version, 21 items) and how the child assesses the relationship with the parent (PACHIQ-R Child versions for mother and father, 25 items). The questionnaire concerns both behavioral interaction and attitudes. It has two subscales: conflict resolution (quality of preventing and solving conflicts) and acceptance (warmth, comfort, protection).

Social competences and social problems as assessed by the parent are measured with the Child Behavior Checklist (CBCL/6-18) [83] that rates children's functioning. We use the Dutch translation [84] of the questionnaire that assesses competences (16 items) and behavioral and emotional problems (120 items) in the past six months. In the present study, only two scales are included: 1) The "Social scale" (this is one of the three competence scales) that comprises 6 questions, which concern group activities and social relationships (e.g.: "Please list any organizations, clubs, teams, or groups your child belongs to"; "About how many close friends does your child have? (Do not include brothers & sisters)"; "Compared to others of his/her age, how well does your child play and work alone?") [83]. 2) The "Social problems scale" (this is one of the five emotional and behavioral problem scales) that consists of 11 items, which concern topics like loneliness, jealousy, getting teased and clumsiness (e.g.: "Clings to adults or too dependent"; "Complains of loneliness"; "Easily jealous"; "Feels others are out to get him/her") [83].

Parental feeding style is measured with a Dutch translation [85] of the 27-item Parental Feeding Style Questionnaire (PFSQ) which asks parents to report the frequency with which they use a number of feeding strategies that are grouped into 1) emotional feeding (i.e. "I give my child something to eat to make him/her feel better when s/he is feeling upset), 2) instrumental feeding (i.e. "I reward my child with something to eat when s/he is well behaved"), 3) prompting/encouragement to eat (i.e. "I praise my child if s/he eats what I give him/her") and 4) overt control over eating (i.e. "I decide how many snacks my child should have") [86].

Affect of the parents is measured with the Dutch translation of the 20-item Positive and Negative Affect Schedule (PANAS) [87, 88], which asks parents to indicate what they currently feel on two scales: 1) positive affect (the extent to which a person feels enthusiastic, active and alert) and 2) negative affect (subjective distress and unpleasurable engagement that subsumes a variety of aversive mood states, including anger, contempt, disgust, guilt, fear and nervousness).

Peer body size is measured by asking children and adolescents to select from a range of line drawings (separate for boys and girls) the silhouette that most closely resembles how their five best same sex friends look. The used drawings are taken from Colleen S.W. Rand [89], who composed the drawings based on drawings by M.E. Collins [90] and T.I.A. Sorensen et al. [91].

14.2.6.3.4 Outcome Expectations

The same silhouette drawings are also used to assess outcome expectations. Children and adolescents are asked to select 1) the silhouette that most closely resembles their current body size and 2) the silhouette that most closely resemble the body size they expect to have after treatment. Outcome expectations are calculated by measuring the difference between these current and expected own body sizes.

14.2.6.4 Covariates

Several covariates will be assessed. It is likely that the intensity and duration of treatment are related to both the ability to self-regulate and ΔSDS-BMI. We will investigate the intensity of the treatment, expressed by the duration of the residential period (2 versus 6 months) as it might explain part of the variation between individual children and adolescents in weight loss and in the ability to self-regulate at the end of treatment (T12). We will also investigate the health care the children and adolescents receive in the period between the end of the treatment at Heideheuvel and the follow up one year later as the prolongation of treatment might influence weight loss maintenance after the first year of treatment. Furthermore we will assess the gender and age-specific ΔSDS-BMI between baseline (T0) and end of treatment (T12) because the amount of weight lost during treatment might be a predictor of weight loss maintenance after treatment. Finally the influence of SDS-BMI at the start of treatment, gender, age and educational level of the children and adolescents on the long-term weight outcome will be assessed.

14.2.7 Statistical Analyses

First we will provide information on the baseline characteristics of the patient group. Secondly, SDS-BMI levels and changes will be described at the three time points, i.e. at baseline (T0), after one-year (T12) and at two-year follow-up

(T24). This allows for the description of total weight loss (computed as ΔSDS-BMI between T0 and T24) and weight loss maintenance (computed as ΔSDS-BMI between T12 and T24). Next, determinants (general and eating-specific self-regulation) and moderators (factors related to competence, motivation, relatedness and outcome expectations) will be described and compared at baseline (T0) and one year later (T12). This enables detailed scrutiny of the variability of the determinants and moderators in this specific target group of severely obese children and adolescents. Furthermore, it will provide insight into the change in determinants and moderators after following a treatment of one year.

Third, the relation between self-regulation and initial weight loss at one-year follow-up and potential moderators of this relation will be tested using hierarchical multiple regression analyses. Linear regression analyses (with ΔSDS-BMI between T0 and T12 as dependent variable) and logistic regression analyses (with a dichotomous variable high versus low weight loss as dependent variable) will be conducted. To discriminate participants with a high and low weight loss a median split in ΔSDS-BMI between T0 and T12 will be conducted. In the first step, other factors will be added (e.g., age, gender, SDS-BMI at T0, treatment intensity). In the second step, the self-regulation indicators (at T0) will be entered simultaneously as independent variables. In the third step, interaction terms between the moderators (at T0) and (the most important) self-regulation indicators will be computed and added to the model. Significant interaction terms will subsequently be decomposed to gain insight into the relation between self-regulation and initial weight loss at high and low levels of the moderator.

Finally, the relation between self-regulation and weight loss maintenance at two year follow-up and potential moderators of this relation will again be examined using hierarchical multiple regression analyses. Linear regression analyses (with ΔSDS-BMI between T12 and T24 as dependent variable) and logistic regression analyses (with a dichotomous variable high versus low maintenance of weight loss as dependent variable) will be conducted. To calculate high versus low maintenance of weight loss a median split in ΔSDS-BMI between T12 and T24 is conducted. The same steps as in the one-year analyses will be conducted, except that for the determinants and most moderators the data collected at T12 will be entered. A few moderators that are only measured at T0, will be entered as assessed at T0.

We will explore the possibility of multiple imputations to deal with missing data. Missing data will be imputed multiple times, using the 'Predictive Mean Matching' (PMM) procedure that runs under the SPSS 20.0 program. All analyses will be performed on the complete case data and on the imputed data. In case of missing item scores, we will explore the possibility of a single imputation technique.

14.3 DISCUSSION

We have identified psychosocial factors predicting weight loss success from studies done in (obese) adults. Whether or not these are also determinants in younger patients suffering from severe obesity, is not known. The present study aims to fill this gap.

This study will provide knowledge about the relation between self-regulation and long-term weight loss after intensive lifestyle interventions in severely obese children and adolescents, a growing but often overlooked patient group. We aim to investigate to what extent (changes in) the general ability to self-regulate predicts weight loss and weight loss maintenance. This study will also contribute to the knowledge on how this association is modified by other psychosocial factors. The results can provide important information about the potential for treatment success according to psychosocial characteristics. This may help professionals to tailor interventions to children. The information can also be used to determine which patients might need more guidance than others in the relapse prevention phase after an intensive intervention.

The study population is severely obese and has not been able to profit sufficiently from previous treatments, which may suggest that these patients are relatively therapy resistant. It remains to be investigated whether this is really the case. If so, the present study might result in a lack of variance in weight loss success and maintenance which would limit the analyses. That the study population belongs to a very specific subgroup of patients also implies that the study results cannot easily be generalized to other treatment populations or other treatment forms. Interpretation of the study results should also be done with caution because the data collection on what happens to the patients in the follow-up year is limited to measurements at the end of follow up. The effect of for example major live events in this period is not included in the analyses.

In addition to these limitations, also some important strengths need to be acknowledged. Studies with a long term follow up are scarce. This study, with a follow up of 2 years, is relatively long. Short-term weight loss is much easier to achieve than longer term weight loss and weight loss maintenance. Our primary endpoint (2 years post-baseline) strikes the balance between following the patients and their parents long enough to assess long-term outcomes with what is feasible within a 4 year study period. The two year time span gives us the opportunity to assess the effects of the therapy after its termination. Moreover it also enables the investigation of maintenance of the attainted ability to self-regulate. Nevertheless we are not able to follow the participants' health and wellbeing for life and the long-term treatment impact remains speculative. They suffer from a chronic condition that can result in various medical, psychological and social difficulties during the course of their lives. In order to make measurements after a longer follow up period possible, all participants in the study are asked during the last measuring moment whether they are willing to participate in future research.

A final issue that needs to be discussed is the use of SDS-BMI and behavioral computer tasks as proxies for change in dietary intake. Generally, instruments to capture dietary intake may not be sufficiently valid. A healthier dietary pattern is assumed to be reflected in a change in SDS-BMI. In a similar vein, improvements in self-regulation abilities (as assessed with the computer tasks) are assumed to echo in improvements in dietary intake. Computer tasks are used because they provide a relatively objective measurement of self-regulation abilities. Both used computer tasks are non-food related. They measure general self-regulation, a supposedly general ability that affects eating behavior. If the results of the computer tasks do not show a relation between self-regulating ability and weight loss maintenance, this might be attributed to the use of these general measuring instruments and does not necessary mean there is no change in self-regulation of eating behavior. If this study does show an association between self-regulation ability and weight loss maintenance, future research could extend on that by demonstrating the causal pathway explaining the association.

14.4 CONCLUSION

To conclude, the present study will provide knowledge about the role of self-regulation abilities in weight loss success and maintenance in severely obese children and adolescents over a two-year period.

REFERENCES

1. Schönbeck Y, Talma H, van Dommelen P, Bakker B, Buitendijk SE, Hirasing RA, van Buuren S: Increase in prevalence of overweight in Dutch children and adolescents: a comparison of nationwide growth studies in 1980, 1997 and 2009. PLoS One. 2011, 6 (11): e27608-10.1371/journal.pone.0027608.

2. Visscher TL, Kromhout D, Seidell JC: Long-term and recent time trends in the prevalence of obesity among Dutch men and women. Int J Obes Relat Metab Disord. 2002, 26 (9): 1218-1224. 10.1038/sj.ijo.0802016.
3. Wang Y: Child Obesity and Health. International Encyclopedia of Public Health. Edited by: Heggenhougen K, Quah SR. 2008, Oxford: Academic Press, 590-604.
4. Dietz WH: Health consequences of obesity in youth: childhood predictors of adult disease. Pediatrics. 1998, 101 (3 Pt 2): 518-525.
5. Ludwig DS: Childhood obesity–the shape of things to come. N Engl J Med. 2007, 357 (23): 2325-2327. 10.1056/NEJMp0706538.
6. Wang G, Dietz WH: Economic burden of obesity in youths aged 6 to 17 years: 1979–1999. Pediatrics. 2002, 109 (5): E81-81. 10.1542/peds.109.5.e81.
7. Falkner NH, Neumark-Sztainer D, Story M, Jeffery RW, Beuhring T, Resnick MD: Social, educational, and psychological correlates of weight status in adolescents. Obes Res. 2001, 9 (1): 32-42. 10.1038/oby.2001.5.
8. Puder JJ, Munsch S: Psychological correlates of childhood obesity. Int J Obes. 2010, 34 (Suppl 2): S37-S43.
9. van Wijnen LG, Boluijt PR, Hoeven-Mulder HB, Bemelmans WJ, Wendel-Vos GC: Weight status, psychological health, suicidal thoughts, and suicide attempts in Dutch adolescents: results from the 2003 E-MOVO project. Obesity. 2010, 18 (5): 1059-1061. 10.1038/oby.2009.334.
10. Puhl RM, Latner JD: Stigma, obesity, and the health of the nation's children. Psychol Bull. 2007, 133 (4): 557-580.
11. Lumeng JC, Forrest P, Appugliese DP, Kaciroti N, Corwyn RF, Bradley RH: Weight status as a predictor of being bullied in third through sixth grades. Pediatrics. 2010, 125 (6): e1301-e1307. 10.1542/peds.2009-0774.
12. Strauss RS, Pollack HA: Social marginalization of overweight children. Arch Pediatr Adolesc Med. 2003, 157 (8): 746-752. 10.1001/archpedi.157.8.746.
13. Gortmaker SL, Must A, Perrin JM, Sobol AM, Dietz WH: Social and economic consequences of overweight in adolescence and young adulthood. N Engl J Med. 1993, 329 (14): 1008-1012. 10.1056/NEJM199309303291406.
14. Schwimmer JB, Burwinkle TM, Varni JW: Health-related quality of life of severely obese children and adolescents. JAMA. 2003, 289 (14): 1813-1819. 10.1001/jama.289.14.1813.
15. Zeller MH, Roehrig HR, Modi AC, Daniels SR, Inge TH: Health-related quality of life and depressive symptoms in adolescents with extreme obesity presenting for bariatric surgery. Pediatrics. 2006, 117 (4): 1155-1161. 10.1542/peds.2005-1141.
16. Krebs NF, Himes JH, Jacobson D, Nicklas TA, Guilday P, Styne D: Assessment of child and adolescent overweight and obesity. Pediatrics. 2007, 120 (Suppl 4): S193-S228.
17. Seidell JC, Halberstadt J, Noordam H, Niemer S: An integrated health care standard for the management and prevention of obesity in the Netherlands. Fam Pract. 2012, 29: i153-i156. 10.1093/fampra/cmr057.
18. Yanovski JA, Yanovski SZ: Treatment of pediatric and adolescent obesity. JAMA. 2003, 289 (14): 1851-1853. 10.1001/jama.289.14.1851.
19. View ArticlePubMed
20. Spear BA, Barlow SE, Ervin C, Ludwig DS, Saelens BE, Schetzina KE, Taveras EM: Recommendations for treatment of child and adolescent overweight and obesity. Pediatrics. 2007, 120 (Suppl 4): S254-S288.

21. Barlow SE: Expert committee recommendations regarding the prevention, assessment, and treatment of child and adolescent overweight and obesity: summary report. Pediatrics. 2007, 120 (Suppl 4): S164-S192.
22. Rossner S, Hammarstrand M, Hemmingsson E, Neovius M, Johansson K: Long-term weight loss and weight-loss maintenance strategies. Obes Rev. 2008, 9 (6): 624-630. 10.1111/j.1467-789X.2008.00516.x.
23. Seidell JC, de Beer JJ, Kuijpers T: [Guideline 'Diagnosis and treatment of obesity in adults and children']. Ned Tijdschr Geneeskd. 2008, 152 (38): 2071-2076.
24. Kelly KP, Kirschenbaum DS: Immersion treatment of childhood and adolescent obesity: the first review of a promising intervention. Obes Rev. 2011, 12 (1): 37-49. 10.1111/j.1467-789X.2009.00710.x.
25. Tsiros MD, Sinn N, Coates AM, Howe PR, Buckley JD: Treatment of adolescent overweight and obesity. Eur J Pediatr. 2008, 167 (1): 9-16.
26. Butryn ML, Wadden TA, Rukstalis MR, Bishop-Gilyard C, Xanthopoulos MS, Louden D, Berkowitz RI: Maintenance of Weight Loss in Adolescents: Current Status and Future Directions. J Obes. 2010, 10.1155/2010/789280.
27. Teixeira PJ, Going SB, Sardinha LB, Lohman TG: A review of psychosocial pre-treatment predictors of weight control. Obes Rev. 2005, 6 (1): 43-65. 10.1111/j.1467-789X.2005.00166.x.
28. Bryant EJ, King NA, Blundell JE: Disinhibition: its effects on appetite and weight regulation. Obes Rev. 2008, 9 (5): 409-419.
29. Nederkoorn C, Jansen E, Mulkens S, Jansen A: Impulsivity predicts treatment outcome in obese children. Behav Res Ther. 2007, 45 (5): 1071-1075. 10.1016/j.brat.2006.05.009.
30. Bonato DP, Boland FJ: Delay of gratification in obese children. Addict Behav. 1983, 8 (1): 71-74. 10.1016/0306-4603(83)90059-X.
31. Cohen EA, Gelfand DM, Dodd DK, Jensen J, Turner C: Self-control practices associated with weight loss maintenance in children and adolescents. Behav Ther. 1980, 11 (1): 26-37. 10.1016/S0005-7894(80)80033-5.
32. Israel AC, Guile CA, Baker JE, Silverman WK: An evaluation of enhanced self-regulation training in the treatment of childhood obesity. J Pediatr Psychol. 1994, 19 (6): 737-749. 10.1093/jpepsy/19.6.737.
33. Crescioni AW, Ehrlinger J, Alquist JL, Conlon KE, Baumeister RF, Schatschneider C, Dutton GR: High trait self-control predicts positive health behaviors and success in weight loss. J Health Psychol. 2011, 16 (5): 750-759. 10.1177/1359105310390247.
34. Volkow ND, Wang GJ, Baler RD: Reward, dopamine and the control of food intake: implications for obesity. Trends Cogn Sci. 2011, 15 (1): 37-46. 10.1016/j.tics.2010.11.001.
35. Sturman DA, Moghaddam B: The neurobiology of adolescence: changes in brain architecture, functional dynamics, and behavioral tendencies. Neurosci Biobehav Rev. 2011, 35 (8): 1704-1712. 10.1016/j.neubiorev.2011.04.003.
36. Birch LL, Davison KK: Family environmental factors influencing the developing behavioral controls of food intake and childhood overweight. Pediatr Clin North Am. 2001, 48 (4): 893-907. 10.1016/S0031-3955(05)70347-3.
37. Baumeister RF, Vohs KD: Handbook of self-regulation: research, theory and applications. 2004, New York: Guilford Press
38. Maes S, Karoly P: Self-regulation assessment and intervention in physical health and illness: a review. Applied Psychology. 2005, 54 (2): 267-299. 10.1111/j.1464-0597.2005.00210.x.

39. De Ridder DTD, De Wit JBF: Self-regulation in health behaviour. 2006, West Sussex: John Wiley & Sons Ltd
40. Baumeister RF, Heatherton TF: Self-regulation failure: an overview. Pschological Inquiry. 1996, 7 (1): 1-15. 10.1207/s15327965pli0701_1.
41. Nederkoorn C, Braet C, Van Eijs Y, Tanghe A, Jansen A: Why obese children cannot resist food: the role of impulsivity. Eat Behav. 2006, 7 (4): 315-322. 10.1016/j.eatbeh.2005.11.005.
42. Graziano PA, Calkins SD, Keane SP: Toddler self-regulation skills predict risk for pediatric obesity. Int J Obes. 2010, 34 (4): 633-641. 10.1038/ijo.2009.288.
43. Epstein LH, Dearing KK, Temple JL, Cavanaugh MD: Food reinforcement and impulsivity in overweight children and their parents. Eat Behav. 2008, 9 (3): 319-327. 10.1016/j.eatbeh.2007.10.007.
44. Appelhans BM, Woolf K, Pagoto SL, Schneider KL, Whited MC, Liebman R: Inhibiting food reward: delay discounting, food reward sensitivity, and palatable food intake in overweight and obese women. Obesity. 2011, 19 (11): 2175-2182. 10.1038/oby.2011.57.
45. Appelhans BM: Neurobehavioral inhibition of reward-driven feeding: implications for dieting and obesity. Obesity. 2009, 17 (4): 640-647. 10.1038/oby.2008.638.
46. Temple JL, Legierski CM, Giacomelli AM, Salvy SJ, Epstein LH: Overweight children find food more reinforcing and consume more energy than do nonoverweight children. Am J Clin Nutr. 2008, 87 (5): 1121-1127.
47. Stice E, Yokum S, Burger KS, Epstein LH, Small DM: Youth at risk for obesity show greater activation of striatal and somatosensory regions to food. J Neurosci. 2011, 31 (12): 4360-4366. 10.1523/JNEUROSCI.6604-10.2011.
48. Braet C, Claus L, Verbeken S, Van Vlierberghe L: Impulsivity in overweight children. Eur Child Adolesc Psychiatry. 2007, 16 (8): 473-483. 10.1007/s00787-007-0623-2.
49. Pauli-Pott U, Albayrak O, Hebebrand J, Pott W: Association between inhibitory control capacity and body weight in overweight and obese children and adolescents: dependence on age and inhibitory control component. Child Neuropsychol. 2010, 16 (6): 592-603. 10.1080/09297049.2010.485980.
50. Johnson WG, Parry W, Drabman RS: The performance of obese and normal size children on a delay of gratification task. Addict Behav. 1978, 3 (3–4): 205-208.
51. Sobhany MS, Rogers CS: External responsiveness to food and non-food cues among obese and non-obese children. Int J Obes. 1985, 9 (2): 99-106.
52. Francis LA, Susman EJ: Self-regulation and rapid weight gain in children from age 3 to 12 years. Arch Pediatr Adolesc Med. 2009, 163 (4): 297-302. 10.1001/archpediatrics.2008.579.
53. Batterink L, Yokum S, Stice E: Body mass correlates inversely with inhibitory control in response to food among adolescent girls: an fMRI study. Neuroimage. 2010, 52 (4): 1696-1703. 10.1016/j.neuroimage.2010.05.059.
54. Hjördis B, Gunnar E: Characteristics of drop-outs from a long-term behavioral treatment program for obesity. Int J of Eating Disorders. 1989, 8 (3): 363-368. 10.1002/1098-108X(198905)8:3<363::AID-EAT2260080311>3.0.CO;2-3.
55. Elfhag K, Rossner S: Who succeeds in maintaining weight loss? A conceptual review of factors associated with weight loss maintenance and weight regain. Obes Rev. 2005, 6 (1): 67-85. 10.1111/j.1467-789X.2005.00170.x.
56. Ryan RM, Deci EL: Self-determination theory and the facilitation of intrinsic motivation, social development, and well-being. Am Psychol. 2000, 55 (1): 68-78.
57. Bandura A: Human agency in social cognitive theory. Am Psychol. 1989, 44 (9): 1175-1184.

58. Teixeira PJ, Silva MN, Mata J, Palmeira AL, Markland D: Motivation, self-determination, and long-term weight control. Int J Behav Nutr Phys Act. 2012, 9: 22-10.1186/1479-5868-9-22.
59. Bandura A: The self system in reciprocal determinism. Am Psychol. 1978, 33 (4): 344-358.
60. Bandura A: Social cognitive theory of self-regulation. Organ Behav Hum Decis Process. 1991, 50 (2): 248-287. 10.1016/0749-5978(91)90022-L.
61. Makkes S, Halberstadt J, Renders CM, Bosmans JE, van der Baan-Slootweg OH, Seidell JC: Cost-effectiveness of intensive inpatient treatments for severely obese children and adolescents in the Netherlands; a randomized controlled trial (HELIOS). BMC Public Health. 2011, 11 (1): 518-10.1186/1471-2458-11-518.
62. Shrewsbury VA, Steinbeck KS, Torvaldsen S, Baur LA: The role of parents in pre-adolescent and adolescent overweight and obesity treatment: a systematic review of clinical recommendations. Obes Rev. 2011, 12 (10): 759-769. 10.1111/j.1467-789X.2011.00882.x.
63. Knowlden AP, Sharma M: Systematic review of family and home-based interventions targeting paediatric overweight and obesity. Obes Rev. 2012, 13: 499-508. 10.1111/j.1467-789X.2011.00976.x.
64. Michie S, Ashford S, Sniehotta FF, Dombrowski SU, Bishop A, French DP: A refined taxonomy of behaviour change techniques to help people change their physical activity and healthy eating behaviours: the CALO-RE taxonomy. Psychol Health. 2011, 26 (11): 1479-1498. 10.1080/08870446.2010.540664.
65. Logan GD, Schachar RJ, Tannock R: Impulsivity and inhibitory control. Psychol Sci. 1997, 8 (1): 60-64. 10.1111/j.1467-9280.1997.tb00545.x.
66. Lejuez CW, Read JP, Kahler CW, Richards JB, Ramsey SE, Stuart GL, Strong DR, Brown RA: Evaluation of a behavioral measure of risk taking: the Balloon Analogue Risk Task (BART). J Exp Psychol Appl. 2002, 8 (2): 75-84.
67. Duckworth AL, Kern ML: A meta-analysis of the convergent validity of self-control measures. Journal of Research in Personality. 2011, 45 (3): 259-268. 10.1016/j.jrp.2011.02.004.
68. Cross CP, Copping LT, Campbell A: Sex differences in impulsivity: a meta-analysis. Psychol Bull. 2011, 137 (1): 97-130.
69. Papachristou H, Nederkoorn C, Havermans R, van der Horst M, Jansen A: Can't stop the craving: the effect of impulsivity on cue-elicited craving for alcohol in heavy and light social drinkers. Psychopharmacology. 2012, 219 (2): 511-518. 10.1007/s00213-011-2240-5.
70. Schachar R, Mota VL, Logan GD, Tannock R, Klim P: Confirmation of an inhibitory control deficit in attention-deficit/hyperactivity disorder. J Abnorm Child Psychol. 2000, 28 (3): 227-235. 10.1023/A:1005140103162.
71. Verbeken S, Braet C, Claus L, Nederkoorn C, Oosterlaan J: Childhood obesity and impulsivity: an investigation with performance-based measures. Behaviour Change. 2009, 26 (3): 153-167. 10.1375/bech.26.3.153.
72. Aklin WM, Lejuez CW, Zvolensky MJ, Kahler CW, Gwadz M: Evaluation of behavioral measures of risk taking propensity with inner city adolescents. Behav Res Ther. 2005, 43 (2): 215-228. 10.1016/j.brat.2003.12.007.
73. Lejuez CW, Aklin WM, Zvolensky MJ, Pedulla CM: Evaluation of the Balloon Analogue Risk Task (BART) as a predictor of adolescent real-world risk-taking behaviours. J Adolesc. 2003, 26 (4): 475-479. 10.1016/S0140-1971(03)00036-8.
74. Lejuez CW, Aklin WM, Jones HA, Richards JB, Strong DR, Kahler CW, Read JP: The Balloon Analogue Risk Task (BART) differentiates smokers and nonsmokers. Exp Clin Psychopharmacol. 2003, 11 (1): 26-33.

75. Braet C, Beyers W, Goossens L, Verbeken S, Moens E: Subtyping children and adolescents who are overweight based on eating pathology and psychopathology. Eur Eat Disord Rev. 2012, 20 (4): 279-286. 10.1002/erv.1151.
76. Van Strien T, Frijters JE, Bergers GP, Defares PB: The Dutch Eating Behavior Questionnaire (DEBQ) for assessment of restrained, emotional, and external eating behavior. Int J Eat Disord. 1986, 5 (2): 295-315.10.1002/1098-108X(198602)5:2<295::AID-EAT2260050209>3.0.CO;2-T.
77. Scholz U, Dona BG, Sud S, Schwarzer R: Is general self-efficacy a universal construct? Psychometric findings from 25 countries. European Journal of Psychological Assessment. 2002, 18 (3): 242-251. 10.1027//1015-5759.18.3.242.
78. Veerman JW, Straathof MAE, Treffers PDA, Van den Bergh BRH, Ten Brink LT: [Manual for the Dutch version of the SPPC]. 2004, Amsterdam: Pearson Assessment and Information B.V.
79. Treffers PDA, Goedhart AW, Van de Bergh BRH, Veerman JW, Ackaert L, De Rycke L: [Manual for the Dutch version of the SPPA]. 2002, Amsterdam: Pearson Assessment and Information B.V.
80. Harter S: Manual for the Self-Perception Profile for Children. 1985, Denver, CO: University of Denver.
81. Harter S: Manual for the Self-Perception Profile for Adolescents. 1988, Denver, CO: University of Denver.
82. Williams GC, Grow VM, Freedman ZR, Ryan RM, Deci EL: Motivational predictors of weight loss and weight-loss maintenance. J Pers Soc Psychol. 1996, 70 (1): 115-126.
83. Lange A, Evers A, Jansen H, Dolan C: The parent child interaction questionnaire–revised. Fam Process. 2002, 41 (4): 709-722. 10.1111/j.1545-5300.2002.00709.x.
84. Achenbach TM, Recorla LA: Manual for the ASEBA School-Age Forms & Profiles. 2001, Burlington, VT: University of Vermont, Research Center for Children, Youth, & Families
85. Verhulst FC, Van der Ende J, Koot HM: [Manual for the CBCL/4-18]. 1996, Rotterdam: Sophia Children's Hospital, Erasmus MC
86. Sleddens EF, Kremers SP, De Vries NK, Thijs C: Relationship between parental feeding styles and eating behaviours of Dutch children aged 6–7. Appetite. 2010, 54 (1): 30-36. 10.1016/j.appet.2009.09.002.
87. Wardle J, Sanderson S, Guthrie CA, Rapoport L, Plomin R: Parental feeding style and the inter-generational transmission of obesity risk. Obes Res. 2002, 10 (6): 453-462. 10.1038/oby.2002.63.
88. Watson D, Clark LA, Tellegen A: Development and validation of brief measures of positive and negative affect: the PANAS scales. J Pers Soc Psychol. 1988, 54 (6): 1063-1070.
89. Peeters FPML, Ponds RWHM, Vermeeren MTG: [Affectivity and self-report of depression and anxiety]. Tijdschr Psychiatr. 1996, 38 (3): 240-250.
90. Rand CSW, Wright BA: Continuity and change in the evaluation of ideal and acceptable body sizes across a wide age span. Int J Eat Disord. 2000, 28 (1): 90-100. 10.1002/(SICI)1098-108X(200007)28:1<90::AID-EAT11>3.0.CO;2-P.
91. Collins ME: Body figure perceptions and preferences among preadolescent children. Int J Eat Disord. 1991, 10 (2): 199-208. 10.1002/1098-108X(199103)10:2<199::AID-EAT2260100209>3.0.CO;2-D.
92. Sorensen TI, Stunkard AJ, Teasdale TW, Higgins MW: The accuracy of reports of weight: children's recall of their parents' weights 15 years earlier. Int J Obes. 1983, 7 (2): 115-122.

CHAPTER 15

Enhancing Self-Regulation as a Strategy for Obesity Prevention in Head Start Preschoolers: The Growing Healthy Study

Alison L. Miller, Mildred A. Horodynski, Holly E. Brophy Herb, Karen E. Peterson, Dawn Contreras, Niko Kaciroti, Julie Staples-Watson, and Julie C. Lumeng

15.1 BACKGROUND

The Institute of Medicine [1] identifies childhood obesity as an urgent problem; nearly 1 in 5 young children are obese and socioeconomic and racial/ethnic disparities in obesity rates appear even during the preschool years [2–4]. Once established, childhood obesity typically persists [5] and predicts health problems including cardiovascular disease and diabetes [6–8]. Preventing obesity is essential, yet few programs for young children have been rigorously tested, and effects are modest [9–11]. The goal of the Growing Healthy trial is to test the effectiveness and feasibility of two obesity prevention interventions. The first intervention is an education curriculum promoting obesity prevention behaviors, and the second intervention places this curriculum in the context of an additional intervention to enhance behavioral self-regulation. Both interventions are delivered to low-income preschoolers and their parents by community-based, nutrition-education specialists partnering with Head Start (HS) staff.

The education curriculum, Preschool Obesity Prevention Series (POPS), is designed to promote empirically-tested obesity prevention behaviors informed by expert recommendations by the American Academy of Pediatrics (AAP) [12] and the American Dietetic Association (ADA; now Academy of Nutrition and Dietetics) guidelines for Pediatric Weight Management [13]. The ADA supports increased fruit and vegetable (FV) intake based on intervention trials that found FV intake associated with reduced adiposity indices [14–16]. Sugar-sweetened beverage (SSB) consumption is consistently associated with body mass index (BMI) and child obesity in prospective studies and intervention trials, [12, 13, 17–21] and inversely associated with milk intake [22]. Dietary variety is related to greater FV intake and dietary quality [23]. The Centers for Disease Control (CDC) [24] and AAP recommend that screen time be limited to less than 2 hours per day, [12] based on intervention trials [25–27] and observational studies [25]. Thus, POPS focuses on increasing FV intake, reducing SSB consumption and eating a diet rich in calcium (following United States Department of Agriculture (USDA) recommendations on low-fat dairy), increasing dietary variety, and reducing screen time. POPS involves both children and parents in learning about obesity prevention behaviors and building skills to enact them, which is critical for a comprehensive approach, yet not common in existing programs.

Improving behavioral self-regulation (i.e., inhibiting impulses, calming down when upset) may also be important for preventing childhood obesity. Stress can lead to increased appetite and a shift in preference to foods high in added sugar and fats [28–30]. Obesity is more common in children who engage in emotional eating, [31, 32] disinhibited eating, [33] or eating in the absence of hunger [34–36]. Children who cannot cope with stress well may engage in such stress-eating patterns as a way to self-regulate emotion and behavior, and over time become obese. The literature supports this impression; children who have difficult temperaments, [37–39] behavior problems, [40] tantrums over food, [41] impulsivity, [14, 42–45] and difficulty delaying gratification [46–51] are more likely than their peers to be obese. The preschool years are an important period for the development of eating behavior, [52] lifelong obesity risk, [53] and self-regulation [54]. Thus, developing effective interventions for children this age that integrate these domains—and, importantly, include parents—could be a promising new direction for obesity prevention.

The Growing Healthy Study tests this novel combined approach to obesity prevention. First, the POPS intervention is designed to provide developmentally appropriate, empirically-validated, and coordinated obesity prevention messages to preschoolers and their parents. Second, we embed POPS within a self-regulation framework by implementing the Incredible Years Series (IYS), an evidence-based program shown to enhance self-regulation in young, low-income children [55–57]. With an emphasis on modeling positive behavioral management techniques and parenting as part of IYS, the IYS + POPS intervention will teach children behavioral self-regulation strategies (e.g., ways to calm down without relying on food), and also give parents new techniques for managing child behavior (e.g., responding to children's tantrums in ways that do not involve food). Thus, the IYS + POPS intervention may not only prevent obesity through directly reducing stress-eating as a form of self-regulation, but also lay the groundwork for better overall 'absorption' of information in the POPS curriculum by enhancing child self-regulation and improved parent–child interactions. Our conceptual model is outlined in Figure 1.

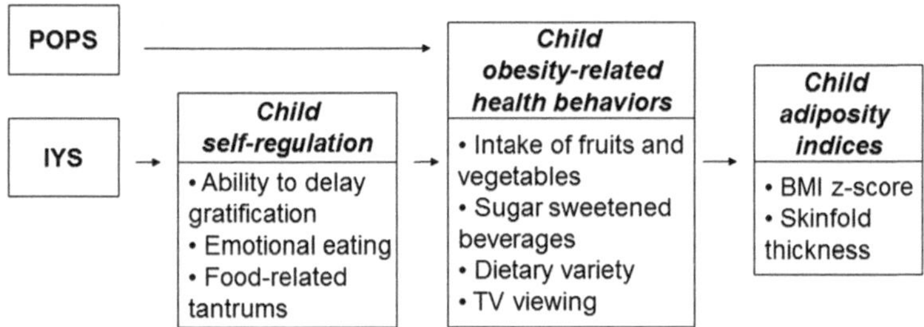

FIGURE 15.1 Conceptual model.

15.1.1 Study Aims and Hypotheses

The primary aim of this study is to examine the effectiveness and feasibility of the two obesity prevention interventions described above: 1) POPS and 2) POPS + IYS, as delivered by community-based nutrition educators and HS staff to low-income preschoolers and their parents. Hypotheses are that across an academic year, compared to Usual HS Exposure: (1) POPS will result in improved obesity-related health behaviors and adiposity indices; (2) POPS + IYS will result in the greatest improvement in obesity-related health behaviors and adiposity indices, and this greater effect will be mediated in part by increased child self-regulatory capacity. A process evaluation to assess the feasibility, fidelity, parental engagement, and educational effectiveness of the POPS and POPS + IYS interventions will also be conducted. This project was funded by the USDA National Institute of Food and Agriculture (NIFA) Agriculture and Food Research Initiative (AFRI) Competitive Grants Program, Childhood Obesity Prevention Challenge Area.

15.2 METHODS/DESIGN

15.2.1 Study Design

The Growing Healthy study is a randomized controlled trial (RCT). Classrooms (n = 75) are randomized through an automated system to one of 3 study arms (200 children per arm): (1) POPS; (2) POPS + IYS; or (3) Usual HS Exposure. Each HS program hosts all 3 study arms, and all children in an individual classroom participate in only one arm. Only one classroom participates per physical school site to prevent cross-contamination across study arms and ensure that participants are blind to group assignments. Families are assigned to study arm as a function of their classroom assignment. Every effort is made to match intervention and comparison classrooms on demographic characteristics in order to minimize differences not due to the intervention (e.g., % minority race/ethnicity, teacher education).

Data are collected pre-intervention (in the fall) and post-intervention (in the spring). Interventions occur between October and April of the academic year. Process implementation data are collected throughout the study. Children are enrolled in each of 4 academic years, with 50 children enrolled into each of the 3 study arms per year. Data collectors are separate from the interventionists, and blinded to the study arm to which participants in a classroom are assigned.

15.2.2 Participants and Recruitment

Participants are from three HS programs in mixed rural and urban areas of Michigan. These programs serve 3,222 children (67% white, 28% black; ethnicity 23% Hispanic; 12.6% English as second language) per year in 184 half-day classrooms. The prevalence of overweight (BMI ≥ 85th percentile and < 95th, based on US Centers for Disease Control (CDC) reference growth curves for age and sex), 16.2%) and obesity (BMI ≥ 95th percentile, 17.0%) in these programs is similar to other HS cohorts [3, 58]. Inclusion criteria are that the child is aged 3 or 4 years at study enrollment. Exclusions are significant developmental disabilities that would preclude participation, child is a foster child, or parent is non-English-speaking. Almost all families in the participating HS programs have annual household incomes below the federal poverty line, as this is an eligibility requirement for 90% of the children enrolled.

Families are told about the study during classroom open houses and through flyers in children's backpacks, and compensated for returning an initial enrollment packet, including a signed written informed consent form. They are then contacted by telephone to review eligibility criteria that they reported in the enrollment packet and to confirm complete understanding of the study and validate informed consent. Next, a data collector (blind to study condition) completes pretest assessments. Appropriate compensation, tokens of appreciation and regular contact from project staff are incorporated to enhance retention.

15.2.3 Research Ethics Approval

This study has been approved by the Institutional Review Boards of both collaborating universities, the University of Michigan Medical School Institutional Review Board (UM-IRBMED) and Michigan State University Social Science/Behavioral Education Review Board (MSU-SIRB). We follow the usual standards of a Data and Safety Monitoring Plan as required by the National Institutes of Health for an RCT. Quality assurance reports are prepared on a monthly basis and reviewed by the Study Directors.

15.2.4 Interventions: POPS and POPS + IYS

15.2.4.1 Preschool Obesity Prevention Series (POPS)

Social Cognitive Theory was the theoretical basis for the curricula that have informed POPS (Healthy Toddlers [59]; Nutrition Education Aimed at Toddlers [60]). POPS also uses an Experiential Learning approach, which emphasizes active learning through the senses. Each lesson provides opportunities to engage with content (e.g., cooking activity), reflect on content through discussion, and apply the new concept (e.g., through goal setting). POPS parent and child sessions include complementary content to reinforce concepts and improve parental knowledge and efficacy to promote specific childhood obesity prevention behaviors. Content of units is summarized in Table 1 (each unit contains more than one lesson).

TABLE 15.1 POPS Units

POPS-Parent	
1	Eating a Rainbow of Fruits and Vegetables
2	Trying New Foods: From Never to Maybe
3	Turning Off the TV and Tuning Into Fun and Family
4	Keeping You and Your Child Naturally Sweet – Limiting Sugar- Sweetened Beverages through Role-Modeling
5	Let's Make Easy and Healthy Meals at Home
6	Eating Together: Family Meals = Better Diets
7	A Healthy Way To Start The Day: Meal Planning
8	Healthy Choices When Eating Out
POPS-Child	
1	Eating the Alphabet
2	I Will Never Not Ever Eat a Tomato
3	The Berenstain Bears and Too Much TV
4	Oliver's Milkshake
5	It's a Sandwich
6	My Amazing Body

The POPS-Parent component consists of eight 75-minute weekly lessons followed by reinforcing telephone contacts after every other lesson. Each lesson offers opportunities for parents to develop and practice skills, and a discussion of strategies to overcome challenges and problem-solving techniques, with an emphasis on building knowledge and self-efficacy about preventing childhood obesity. Recipes and hands-on activities are included in each lesson. Lessons are implemented by community-based, master's level trained Extension Educators from Michigan State University (a land-grant institution). Consistent with the land-grant mission to translate research findings into community-based practices, Extension Educators help people improve their lives through an educational process that applies knowledge to critical issues, needs and opportunities, Extension Educators regularly collaborate with scholars and work with parents, schools and community organizations, and each POPS Educator has extensive experience working with parents in the community on nutrition education issues.

The POPS-Child component uses children's stories with embedded obesity prevention themes related to behavioral goals (e.g., more FV consumption; less screen time). Six lessons are delivered over 12 weeks by the HS teacher and Extension Educators. Activities include classroom cooking experiences, games/activities associated with story themes, and goal setting. "Family Links" and "Parent Pages" are sent home to reinforce content from school to home. Each lesson runs on a two-week cycle in which the classroom teachers read the selected book (featuring one or more of the POPS obesity prevention behaviors) and introduce reinforcing classroom activities. The following week, the Extension Educator revisits the story and implements a hands-on cooking/tasting activity with the children.

15.2.4.2 POPS Training, Quality Control, and Implementation Fidelity

To ensure consistency in the implementation of the curriculum, we conduct a 2-day training for Extension Educators and a shorter training for HS teachers (with booster sessions each year). Training covers curriculum specifics as well as strategies for promoting parent self-efficacy for behavior change and importance of fidelity. Fidelity of POPS delivery in the field is assessed by observing at least one session per group (including classroom activities and parent sessions) and documenting any deviations from the curriculum. Phone support from trainers is also available as needed. Child and parent engagement in POPS classroom and parent sessions, respectively, are documented by extension educators.

15.2.5 Incredible Years Series (IYS)

IYS [56] is a widely-used, evidence-based program that includes Parent, Teacher, and Child components designed to promote self-regulation and prevent behavior problems in children. IYS uses observational learning and reinforcement techniques, and emphasizes behavior change strategies such as descriptive commenting about child behavior, praise, role-plays, and coaching to encourage and model positive behavior for parents and children [61]. Effects are greatest when multiple components (Parent, Child, Classroom) are implemented, [56] which is our approach. IYS has been extensively tested and found to be effective with HS children and families [55, 57]. IYS units are listed in Table 2 (each unit includes multiple lessons).

TABLE 15.2 IYS Units

IYS-Parent (BASIC)	
1	Strengthening Children's Social Skills, Emotional Regulation & School Readiness
2	Using Praise and Incentives to Encourage Cooperative Behavior
3	Positive Discipline – Rules, Routines and Effective Limit Setting
4	Positive Discipline – Handling Misbehavior
IYS-Child (Dinosaur School)	
1	Making Friends and Learning Rules (Apatosaurus)
2	Understanding and Detecting Feelings (Triceratops)
3	How to Do Your Best in School (Iguanodon)
4	Problem-Solving Steps (Stegosaurus)
5	Anger Management (Tyrannosaurus Rex)
6	How to Be Friendly (Allosaurus)
7	How to Talk With Friends (Brachiosaurus)
IYS-Teacher (Classroom Management)	
1	The Importance of Teacher Attention, Encouragement, Praise
2	Motivating Children Through Incentives
3	Preventing Behavior Problems—the Proactive Teacher
4	Decreasing Students' Inappropriate Behaviors
5	Building Positive Relationships With Students, Problem Solving

The IYS-Parent component (12–14 weeks, 2 hours/week) focuses on parenting skills such as using effective praise, incentives, limit-setting, and handling misbehavior. Concepts are discussed using video vignettes about parenting challenges. Parents complete homework and receive follow-up phone calls. IYS-Parent sessions are delivered by master's-level mental health specialists (MHS) (one per HS program, employed by HS).

For the IYS-Child component, sixty 15–20 minute lessons are delivered throughout the year during "Circle Time" in HS classrooms, followed by small group activities. Lessons address self-regulation skills, problem-solving strategies, and prosocial behavior, and use child-size puppets to teach skills and engage children. IYS-Child lessons are delivered by the MHS, and HS teachers direct small group activities after each lesson. Teachers are mentored by MHS in delivering IYS-Child, so that delivery can slowly progress from delivery by MHS, to co-delivery by MHS and teacher, to sole delivery by the teacher over time, which is an effective model for dissemination [62]. MHS and teachers also receive training in classroom management strategies (e.g., handling transitions effectively), which is the IYS-Classroom component.

15.2.6 IYS Training, Quality Control and Implementation Fidelity

MHS and teachers receive extensive training in all components that they deliver, as required by IYS [56]. MHS communicate extensively to share ideas and coordinate efforts across sites, and receive monthly supervision from IYS trainers about their delivery of IYS components, and consultation as needed. MHS also work with teachers within their own site to develop lesson plans and small group activities. Fidelity of IYS intervention delivery is assessed via videotape, and covers the same elements as our POPS fidelity assessment.

15.2.7 Comparison Group: "Usual Head Start Exposure"

In the Usual HS Exposure group, classes are taught by a teacher and teacher's aide. HS performance standards require nutrition and parenting curricula, but not intensive programs like POPS or IYS. Nutrition information is delivered to parents primarily via newsletter and each HS program contracts with a dietitian to review menus and individual child needs; these activities are documented for all programs.

15.2.8 Data Collection Procedures

Data collectors (blind to family intervention status and not involved in implementation) are trained by Study Directors in all protocols. Data collection quality is monitored (e.g., surveys completed fully; child weight/height in appropriate range). Data collectors are trained to respond appropriately with referral information if parents make such requests.

Prior to intervention start in the fall, data collectors make a home visit to measure maternal weight and height, gather questionnaires, and obtain the first of three 24-hour dietary recalls (24HR; remaining 24HR are completed by phone). Children are weighed, measured, and participate in a 15-minute videotaped self-regulation task in a private room at school. Teachers complete questionnaires for each child. In the spring, mothers, children, and teachers repeat the same tasks as post-intervention assessments.

Questionnaires are completed using computer-assisted interviewer administration. Data are saved to a master database after each home visit, or double entered and any data entry errors corrected. Video-recordings of self-regulation tasks (see below) are coded by undergraduates trained to reliability (Cohen's kappa ≥ 0.70) by Study Directors. Data are stored on a password protected server, which is automatically backed up multiple times per day.

15.2.9 Primary Outcome Measures

15.2.9.1 Anthropometry

Individuals are weighed without shoes or heavy clothing using a Detecto Portable Scale Model #DR550C and measured using a Seca 213/217 portable stadiometer. Duplicate measures are taken for both weight and height. Body mass index (BMI) is calculated and child BMI z-score derived (using CDC reference growth curves for age and sex [63]), in order to estimate prevalence of child obesity and overweight (classified per national recommendations [12]). Maternal weight and height are measured using the same methods, and maternal BMI calculated (kg/m^2) for use as a covariate.

Triceps and subscapular skinfolds improve prediction of body fatness and correlate with chronic disease risk in children [64, 65]. Duplicate measures of each skinfold in children are obtained using Lange Calipers (triplicates when tolerance of 2 mm is exceeded) [15, 64].

15.2.9.2 Obesity-related Health Behaviors

Three 24-hour dietary recalls (24HR) are collected from mothers regarding child intake, using the USDA 5-step Automated Multiple Pass Method [66]. The initial 24HR is obtained at the home visit, using food models and handouts showing child-appropriate portion sizes to assist [67–69]. Two additional unannounced 24HR are conducted by phone. The 24HRs generate data on individual foods [70] and food groups, [71] including daily FV and SSB servings, adjusting for energy (kcal) intake [17, 72]. We also assess dietary variety based on these data.

Screen Time is based on maternal report of the child's TV viewing and computer use on weekdays and weekends [27, 67, 73]. Maternal report of usual minutes of outdoor play, a covariate, is assessed with a validated measure for preschoolers [74].

15.2.9.3 *Food-related Self-regulation*

Ability to Delay Gratification (ATDG) is a well-validated measure of self-regulation [75] that tests a child's ability to wait when an appealing food is presented. Videotapes of this task are later coded to assess how long the child waits to eat the treat, and what behaviors they use during the waiting period (e.g., how much they pay attention to the treat vs. ignore it).

Emotional Eating is measured using the Children's Eating Behavior Questionnaire, [76] a validated and reliable maternal-report questionnaire with 8 subscales: Food Responsiveness, Emotional Overeating, Enjoyment of Food, Desire to Drink, Satiety Responsiveness, Slowness in Eating, Emotional Undereating, and Food Fussiness Undereating, and Food Fussiness.

Food-related tantrums are captured with a series of questions used in prior work [41]. Mothers report, during the last 4 weeks, how often (1) the child asked for something to eat; (2) the mother told the child he/she could not have something to eat; (3) the child became upset in response; (4) the child had a tantrum in response.

15.2.9.4 *Parent Knowledge and Self-efficacy*

Change in parent knowledge, self-efficacy, and outcome expectations regarding child nutrition and obesity prevention is assessed using questionnaires specific to POPS, and knowledge and self-efficacy regarding parenting and child behavior is assessed with questionnaires developed by IYS.

15.2.10 Secondary Outcome Measures, Covariates, and Demographics

Additional constructs that may relate to obesity and/or self-regulation (e.g., maternal depression; child temperament) are also assessed. Parents complete the Caregivers' Feeding Styles Questionnaire, [77] Dutch Eating Behavior Questionnaire, [78] USDA Household Food Security Scale, [79] Center for Epidemiologic Studies Depression Scale, [80] Child Behavior

Questionnaire-Short Form, [81] The Parenting Scale, [82] and the Alabama Parenting Questionnaire [83]. Parents and teachers both complete the Eyberg Child Behavior Inventory (Student Behavior Inventory version for teachers) [84] and the Social Competence and Behavior Evaluation [85]. Following ATDG, children participate in Gift Delay—Wait, Bow and Wrap Tasks [86] to assess non-food-related self-regulation, and in brief interviews to assess their emotion knowledge [87], a focus of IYS. Because an element of each intervention is classroom-based and results may reflect classroom-level processes, independent observers also assess the emotional climate of the classroom and teachers' support of children's self-regulation (fall and spring) via the Caregiver Interaction Scale [88] and the Supports for Social-Emotional Growth Assessment [89]. Teachers also report their use of IYS classroom management strategies using the Teacher Strategies Questionnaire [55]. Finally, parents provide demographic data, including child sex, race, ethnicity, maternal education, family income-to-needs ratio, family structure, and child's birth weight and gestational age.

15.2.11 Process Evaluation Measures

Process data is gathered to assess intervention implementation and feasibility. Data include parent attendance at sessions, parent satisfaction with program elements, and reasons for not attending sessions or withdrawing from the study (via exit interviews). Child school attendance and participation in the lessons is also recorded.

In addition to implementation fidelity observations (described above), HS Staff and Extension Educators complete questionnaires regarding intervention buy-in (e.g., perceived need for and interest in the intervention, time devoted to implementation), and are interviewed on a quarterly basis regarding intervention strengths/weaknesses, implementation issues, and challenges of retention.

15.2.12 Sample Size, Power Calculations, and Data Analysis

15.2.12.1 Sample Size and Power Calculations

Enrolling 200 participants per arm, assuming attrition of 25%, will achieve a final sample size of 150 participants per arm. This sample size of 150 per arm will enable detection of small to moderate effect sizes of $f = .16$ (between groups vs. within group variation), with a power of 80%, $\alpha = .05$ and assuming and intraclass correlation $r = .05$. This sample size also provides 80% power with $r = .20$, $\alpha = .05$ to detect an effect size of $f = .185$.

15.2.12.2 Analysis Plan

The primary objective is to determine whether POPS + IYS is more effective, compared to POPS alone or Usual HS Exposure, in reducing adiposity measures (BMI z-score, skinfolds thickness). Additional focal outcomes are dietary intake, TV viewing, ATDG, emotional eating, and food-related tantrums. Baseline comparability of the 3 groups will be assessed. To account for clustering of children within a classroom, Proc Mixed in SAS with a random intercept for classroom will be used to analyze continuous outcomes, and General Estimating Equations (GEE) techniques [90] will be used to compare the prevalence of obesity and overweight across the 3 groups. Analyses will be conducted both with and without adjustment for baseline characteristics such as age, sex, race, and baseline BMI or BMI z-score. All models will incorporate covariates that are related to the outcomes to reduce residual variance and thus help reduce Type II error. Significance will be assessed using a two-sided test at $\alpha = 0.05$.

Analyses will be based on the intention to treat principle where all randomized participants, including dropouts, are included in the analysis based on their randomized intervention group [90]. Given that a substantial portion of participants will likely have only partial adherence to the intervention (e.g., only attend some parent sessions), dose–response analyses will also be performed where dose corresponds to number of sessions attended.

As outlined in the conceptual model (Figure 1), analyses will be conducted to test whether the effect of POPS + IYS on obesity-related health behaviors and adiposity indices is mediated by self-regulation (using parent-reported, teacher-reported, and direct child assessment measures). As a secondary analysis, models will also be examined separately for boys and girls, white and non-white children, and children who are overweight or obese versus non-overweight at baseline.

Finally, process data on recruitment, retention, participant engagement in the intervention, participant and educator satisfaction, and implementation fidelity will be analyzed using descriptive and qualitative approaches, to inform continued collaborations with HS and allow more effective dissemination of findings.

15.3 DISCUSSION

The Growing Healthy study will provide: 1) increased knowledge about self-regulation promotion as a strategy for obesity prevention in preschoolers, which will add to the scientific literature; 2) demonstration of the feasibility of an intervention delivered by HS staff and Extension educators; and 3) a research-based, empirically-tested obesity prevention curriculum product appropriate for use by HS and Extension staff. Thus, the study should advance fundamental science as well as translational research by generating new knowledge of the behavioral factors that influence childhood obesity, and by delivering this science to people who serve children through education and extension efforts.

POPS and POPS + IYS are theory-based, multi-component interventions that have the potential to be sustainable, given that they are being implemented in existing infrastructures and by community-based educators. By providing POPS and IYS in partnership with such agencies, the potential exists to enhance programming nationwide through broad-based dissemination. Analysis of the effective components of the POPS and POPS + IYS interventions may thus have important implications not only for early childhood curricular practices within Head Start but also in other early childhood programs.

REFERENCES

1. Koplan J, Liverman C, Kraak V: Preventing childhood obesity: Health in the balance. Washington, D.C.: National Academies of Science; 2005.
2. Anderson SE, Whitaker RC: Prevalence of obesity among US preschool children in different racial and ethnic groups. Arch Pediatr Adolesc Med 2009, 163:344–348.
3. Feese M, Franklin F, Murdock M, Harrington K, Brown-Binns M, Nicklas T, Hughes S, Morales M: Prevalence of obesity in children in Alabama and Texas participating in social programs. JAMA 2003, 289:1780–1781.
4. Ogden CL, Carroll MD, Curtin LR, Lamb MM, Flegal KM: Prevalence of High Body Mass Index in US Children and Adolescents, 2007–2008. JAMA 2010, 303:242–249.
5. Nader P, O'Brien M, Houts R, Bradley R, Belksy J, Crosnoe R, Friedman S, Mei Z, Susman E: Development NIoCHaHDSoECCaY: Identifying risk for obesity in early childhood. Pediatrics 2006, 118:e594-e601.
6. Dietz WH: Childhood weight affects adult morbidity and mortality. J Nutr 1998, 128:411S.
7. Dietz WH: Health consequences of obesity in youth: childhood predictors of adult disease. Pediatrics 1998, 101:518–525.
8. Freedman D, Khan L, Dietz W, Srinivasan S, Berenson G: Relationship of childhood obesity to coronary heart disease risk factors in adulthood: the bogalusa heart study. Pediatrics 2001, 108:712–718.

9. Summerbell CD, Waters E, Edmunds L, Kelly SAM: Brown T. Campbell KJ: Interventions for preventing obesity in children. Cochrane Database of Systematic Reviews; 2009.
10. Stice E, Shaw H, Marti CN: A meta-analytic review of obesity prevention programs for children and adolescents: The skinny on interventions that work. Psychol Bull 2006, 132:667–691.
11. Bluford DAA, Sherry B, Scanlon KS: Interventions to prevent or treat obesity in preschool children: a review of evaluated programs[ast]. Obesity 2007, 15:1356–1372.
12. Barlow S: Committee atE: Expert Committee Recommendations regarding the prevention, assessment, and treatment of child and adolescent overweight and obesity: Summary report. Pediatrics 2007, 120:S164-S192.
13. Association AD: Pediatric Weight Management: Evidence-Based Nutrition Practice Guideline. Chicago, IL: American Dietetic Association; 2010.
14. Epstein LHBM, Roemmich JN: Increasing healthy eating vs. reducing high energy-dense foods to treat pediatric obesity. Obesity 2008, 16:318–326.
15. Gortmaker S, Peterson K, Wiecha J: Reducing obesity via a school-based interdisciplinary intervention among youth. Arch Pediatr Adolesc Med 1999, 153:409–418.
16. Boynton-Jarett RTT, Peterson KE, Wiecha JL, Gortmaker SL: Impact of television viewing patterns on fruit and vegetable consumption among adolescents. Pediatrics 2003,112(6):1321–1326.
17. Ludwig DS, Peterson KE, Gortmaker SL: Relation between consumption of sugar-sweetened drinks and childhood obesity: a prospective, observational analysis. Lancet 2001, 357:505–508.
18. James JTP, Cavan D, Kerr D: Preventing childhood obesity by reducing consumption of carbonated drinks: Cluster randomized controlled trial. Br Med J 2004,328(7450):1237–1241.
19. Mrdjenovic GLD: Nutritional and energetic consequences of sweetened drink consumption in 6- to 13- year-old children. J Pediatrics 2003, 142:604–610.
20. Striegel-Moore RHTD, Affenito SG, Franko DL, Obarzanek E, Barton BA, et al.: Correlates of beverage intake in adolescent girls: the National Heart, Lung, and Blood Institute Growth and Health Study. J Pediatr 2006,148(2):183–187.
21. Welsh J, Cogswell M, Rogers S, Rockett H, Mei Z, Grummer-Strawn L: Overweight among low-income preschool children associated with consumption of sweet drinks: Missouri 1999–2002. Pediatrics 2005, 115:e223-e229.
22. Harnack LSJ, Story M: Soft drink consumption among US children and adolescents: Nutritional consequences. J Am Diet Assoc 1999,99(4):436–441.
23. Nicklaus S: Development of food variety in children. Appetite 2009, 52:253–255.
24. CDC: PedNSS User's Guide Section 2: Field Definitions, Codes and Edits. Atlanta, GA: Centers for Disease Control and Prevention; 2004.
25. Gortmaker S, Must A, Sobol A, Peterson K, Colditz G, Dietz W: Television viewing as a cause of increasing obesity among children in the United States, 1986–90. Arch Pediatr Adolesc Med 1996, 150:356–362.
26. Robinson TN: Reducing children's television viewing to prevent obesity: a randomized controlled trial. JAMA 1999,282(16):1561–1567.
27. Peterson KEFM: Addressing the epidemic of childhood obesity through school-based interventions: what has been done and where do we go from here? J Law Med Ethics 2007, 35:113–130.

28. Epel E, Lapidus R, McEwen B, Brownell K: Stress may add bite to appetite in women: A laboratory study of stress-induced cortisol and eating behavior. Psychoneuroendocrinol 2001, 26:37–49.
29. Adam T, Epel E: Stress, eating, and the reward system. Physiol Behav 2007, 87:449–458.
30. Zellner D, Loaiza S, Gonzalez Z, Pita J, Morales J, Pecora D, Wolf A: Food selection changes under stress. Physiol Behav 2006, 87:789–793.
31. Jahnke D, Warschburger P: Familial transmission of eating behaviors in preschool-aged children. Obesity 2008, 16:1821–1825.
32. Wardle J, Sanderson S, Guthrie C, Rapoport L, Plomin R: Parental feeding style and intergenerational transmission of obesity risk. Obes Res 2002, 2002:453–462.
33. Francis L, Ventura A, Marini M, Birch L: Parent overweight predicts daughters' increase in BMI and disinhibited overeating from 5 to 13 Years. Obesity 2007, 15:1544–1553.
34. Birch L, Fisher J, Davison K: Learning to overeat: Maternal use of restrictive feeding practices promotes girls' eating in the absence of hunger. Am J Clin Nutr 2003, 78:215–220.
35. Fisher J, Birch L: Restricting access to foods and children's eating. Appetite 1999, 32:405–419.
36. Fisher J, Birch L: Eating in the absence of hunger and overweight in girls from 5 to 7 years of age. Am J Clin Nutr 2002, 76:226–231.
37. Ravaja N, Keltikangas-Jarvinen L: Temperament and metabolic syndrome precursors in children: a three-year follow-up. Prev Med 1995, 24:518–527.
38. Pulkki-Råback L, Elovainio M, Kivimäki M, Raitakari O, Keltikangas-Jarvinen L: Temperament in childhood predicts body mass in adulthood: The cardiovascular risk in young Finns study. Health Psychol 2005, 24:307–315.
39. Carey W, Hegvik R, McDevitt S: Temperamental factors associated with rapid weight gain and obesity in middle childhood. J Dev Behav Pediatr 1988, 9:194–198.
40. Lumeng J, Gannon K, Cabral H, Frank D, Zuckerman B: The association between clinically meaningful behavior problems and overweight in children. Pediatrics 2003, 112:1138–1145.
41. Agras W, Hammer L, McNicholas F, Kraemer H: Risk factors for childhood overweight: A prospective study from birth to 9.5 years. J Pediatr 2004, 145:20–25.
42. Nederkoorn C, Braet C, Eijs YV, Tanghe A, Jansen A: Why obese children cannot resist food: The role of imsulsivity. Eat Behav 2006, 7:315–322.
43. Waring ME, Lapane KL: Overweight in children and adolescents in relation to attention-deficit/hyperactivity disorder: results from a national sample. Pediatrics 2008, 122:e1–6.
44. Agranat-Meged AN, Deitcher C, Goldzweig G, Leibenson L, Stein M, Galili-Weisstub E: Childhood obesity and attention deficit/hyperactivity disorder: A newly described comorbidity in obese hospitalized children. Int J Eat Disorder 2005, 37:357–359.
45. Holtkamp K, Konrad K, Muller B, Heussen N, Herpertz S, Herpertz-Dahlmann B, Hebebrand J: Overweight and obesity in children with Attention-Deficit/Hyperactivity Disorder. Int J Obes Relat Metab Disord 2004, 28:685–689.
46. Seeyave D, Coleman S, Appugliese D, Corwyn R, Bradley R, Davidson N, Kaciroti N, Lumeng J: Ability to delay gratification at age 4 years and risk of overweight at age 11 years. Arch Pediatr Adolesc Med 2009, 163:303–308.
47. Francis LA, Susman EJ: Self-regulation and rapid weight gain in children from Age 3 to 12 Years. Arch Pediatr Adolesc Med 2009, 163:297–302.
48. Bonato DP, Boland FJ: Delay of gratification in obese children. Addict Behav 1983, 8:71–74.

49. Johnson WG, Parry W, Drabman RS: The performance of obese and normal size children on a delay of gratification task. Addict Behav 1978, 3:205–208.
50. Sigal JJ, Lillian A: Motivational effects of hunger on time estimation and delay of gratification in obese and nonobese boys. J Genet Psychol 1976, 128:7–16.
51. Sobhany MSRC: External responsiveness to food and non-food cues among obese and non-obese children. Int J Obesity 1985, 9:99–106.
52. Birch L, Fisher J: Development of eating behaviors among children and adolescents. Pediatrics 1998, 101:539–549.
53. Guo S, Chumlea W: Tracking of body mass index in children in relation to overweight in adulthood. Am J Clin Nutr 1999, 70:145S-148S.
54. Cole PM, Martin SE, Dennis TA: Emotion regulation as a scientific construct: Methodological challenges and directions for child development research. Child Dev 2004, 75:317–333.
55. Webster-Stratton C, Reid JM, Hammond M: Preventing conduct problems, promoting social competence: a parent and teacher training partnership in head start. J Clin Child Psychol 2001, 30:283–302.
56. Webster-Stratton C, Reid MJ: The Incredible Years Parents, Teachers, and Children Training Series: A Multifaceted Treatment Approach for Young Children with Conduct Disorders. In Evidence-based psychotherapies for children and adolescents. 2nd edition. Edited by: Weisz J, Kazdin A. New York: Guilford Publications; 2010.
57. Cybele Raver C, Jones SM, Li-Grining CP, Metzger M, Champione KM, Sardin L: Improving preschool classroom processes: Preliminary findings from a randomized trial implemented in Head Start settings. Early Child Res Q 2008, 23:10–26.
58. Hu W, Foley T, Wilcox R, Kozera R, Morgenstern B, Juhn Y: Childhood obesity among Head Start enrollees in Southeastern Minnesota: Prevalence and risk factors. Ethnic & Dis 2007, 17:23–38.
59. Horodynski M, Baker S, Coleman G, Auld G, Lindau J: The healthy toddlers trial protocol: an intervention to reduce risk factors for childhood obesity in economically and educationally disadvantaged populations. BMC Public Health 2011., 11:
60. Coleman G, Horodynski MA, Contreras D, Hoerr S: 2005. J Nutr Educ Behav 2005, 17:96–97.
61. Webster-Stratton C, Reid MJ: Parents, teachers and therapists using the child-directed play therapy and coaching skills to promote childrne's social and emotional competence and to build positive relatiionships. In Play therapy for preschool children. Edited by: Schaefer CE. Washington DAPA; 2009:245–273.
62. Han S, Weiss B: Sustainability of teacher implementation of school-based mental health programs. J Abnorm Child Psych 2005, 33:665–679.
63. Kuczmarski R, Ogden C, Grummer-Strawn L, Flegal K, Guo S, Wei R: CDC Growth Charts. Adv Data 2000, 314:1–28.
64. Lohman T, Roche A, Martorell R: Anthropometric Standardization Reference Manual. Champaign, IL: Human Kinetics; 1988.
65. Freedman D, Wang J, Ogden C, Thronton J, Mei Z, Pierson R, Dietz W, Horlick M: The prediction of body fatness by BMI and skinfold thicknesses among children and adolescents. Ann Hum Biol 2007, 34:183–194.
66. Conway JMIL, Moshfegh AJ: Accuracy of dietary recall using the USDA five-step multiple-pass method in men: an observational validation study. J Am Diet Assoc 2004, 104 (4): 595–603.

67. Peterson KE FA, Fox MK, Black B, Simon DS, Bosch RV, et al.: Validation of YRBSS Questions on Dietary Behaviors and Physical Activity among Adolescents in Grades 9–12. Prepared for Centers for Disease Control and Prevention, Division of Adolescent and School Health. 1996.
68. Hoerr SL, Horodynski MA, Lee SY, Henry M: Predictors of nutritional adequacy in mother-toddler dyads from rural families. J Am Diet Assoc 2006, 106:1766–1773.
69. Hoerr S, Lee S, Schiffman R, Horodynski MA, McKelvey L: Beverage consumption of mother-toddler dyads in families with limited incomes. J Pediatr Nurs 2006, 21:403–411.
70. University of Minnesota: Nutrition Data System for Research software vNCC. Minneapolis, MN: University of Minnesota;
71. Thompson O, Ballew C, Resnicow K, Gillespie C, Must A, Bandini L: Dietary pattern as a predictor of change in BMI z-score among girls. Int J Obes 2006, 30:176–182.
72. Willett W: Nutrition Epidemiology. 2nd edition. New York: Oxford Press; 1998.
73. Hernandez BGS, Laird NM, Colditz GA, Parra-Cabrera S, Peterson KE: [Validity and reproducibility of a questionnaire on physical activity and non-activity for school children in Mexico City]. Salud Publica Mex 2000,42(4):315–23.
74. Burdette HL WR, Daniels SR: Parental report of outdoor playtime as a measure of physical activity in preschool-aged children. Arch Pediatr Adolesc Med 2004, 158:353–357.
75. Mischel W, Ebbesen EE: Attention in delay of gratification. J Pers Soc Psychol 1970, 16:329–337.
76. Wardle J, Guthrie C, Sanderson S, Rapoport L: Development of the children's eating behaviour questionnaire. J Child Psychol Psychiatry 2001, 42:963–970.
77. Baughcum A, Powers S, Johnson S, Chamberlin L, Deeks C, Jain A, Whitaker R: Maternal feeding practices and beliefs and their relationships to overweight in early childhood. J Dev Behav Pediatr 2001, 22:391–408.
78. Strien TV, Frijters J, Bergers G, Defares P: The dutch eating behavior questionnaire (DEBQ) for assessment of restrained, emotional, and external eating behavior. Int J Eat Disord 1986, 5:295–315.
79. Service ER: US Household Food Security Module: Three-Stage Design with Screeners. Washington, DC: USDA; 2008.
80. Radloff L: The CES-D Scale: A self report depression scale for research in the general population. J Applied Psychol Measurement 1977, 1:385–401.
81. Putnam S, Rothbart M: Development of short and very short forms of the children's behavior questionnaire. J Pers Assess 2006, 87:103–113.
82. David S, Arnold SGOL, Wolff LS, Maureen M: Acker the parenting scale: a measure of dysfunctional parenting in discipline situations. Psychol Assess 1993, 5:137–144.
83. Clerkin SM, Marks DJ, Policaro K, Halperin JM: Psychometric properties of the alabama parenting questionnaire-preschool revision. J Clin Child Adolesc Psychol 2007, 36:19–28.
84. Eyberg SRA: Assessment of child behavior problems: The validation of a new inventory. J Clin Child Adolesc Psychol 1978, 7:113–116.
85. LaFreniere PDJ: Social competence and behavior evaluation in children ages 3 to 6 Years: the short form (SCBE-30). Psychol Assess: J Consult Clin Psych 1996,8(4):369–377.
86. Kochanska G, Aksan N, Penney SJ, Doobay AF: Early positive emotionality as a heterogenous trait: Implications for children's self-regulation. J Pers Soc Psychol 2007, 93:1054–1066.
87. Kusche CA, Beike RL, Greenberg MT: Coding manual for the kusche affective interview-revised. 1988.

88. Arnett J: Caregivers in day-care centers: Does training matter? J Appl Dev Psychol 1989, 10:541–552.
89. Smith S: Pilot of a new classroom assessment instrument: Supports for Social-Emotional Growth. Steinhardt School of Education, Culture, and Human Development, New York University unpublished study 2004.
90. Zeger S, Liang K: Longitudinal data analysis for discrete and continuous outcomes. Biometrics 1986, 42:121–130.

Keywords

- Youth
- Determinants
- Dietary behavior
- Umbrella review
- Summer food service meal program
- Students
- Nutrients
- Food groups
- Food insecurity
- Feeding practices
- Mexican Americans
- Latinos
- Fathers
- Longitudinal
- General parenting
- Parenting style
- Parent behaviors
- Family meals
- Measurement
- Assessment
- Birth order
- Siblings
- Body Mass Index
- Family
- Videotape Recording
- Mothers
- Feeding behaviors
- Adolescents
- BMI

- **Breakfast**
- **Education**
- **Residence**
- **Diet**
- **Eating out**
- **Food**
- **Meals**
- **Restaurant**
- **Socioeconomic**
- **Take-away**
- **Fruit and vegetable consumption**
- **Breakfast consumption**
- **Socio-economic status**
- **Home food environment**
- **Children**
- **Parents**
- **preschool children**
- **nutritional intervention**
- **Childhood obesity**
- **Self-control**
- **Self-regulation**
- **adolescents**
- **body image**
- **overweight**
- **obesity**
- **weight self-control**
- **dieting**
- **exercising**
- **Pediatric**
- **Weight loss**
- **Lifestyle**
- **Psychology**
- **Obesity prevention**

- **Low-income children**
- **Preschoolers**
- **Head start**
- **Incredible years series**
- **Intervention study**

Author Notes

Chapter 1

Acknowledgments
This research was funded by The Netherlands Organization for Health Research and Development, project number 115100008. The authors would like to thank Professor C. de Graaf for his cooperation on this project.

Competing Interests
The authors declare that they have no competing interests.

Authors' Contributions
ES, WK, SK and JB conceptualized the study. EV and PK performed the literature search; ES, WK, EV, LB and SK were involved in the screening process; ES, WK, LK and LB extracted data. ES drafted the manuscript. All authors reviewed draft versions of the manuscript and provided critical feedback. All authors have made a significant contribution to this manuscript, and all authors read and approved the final manuscript.

Chapter 2

Acknowledgments
This work is a publication of the USDA/ARS Children's Nutrition Research Center, Department of Pediatrics, Baylor College of Medicine, Houston, Texas. This project has been funded in part by federal funds from the USDA/ARS under Cooperative Agreements No. 143-3AEL-2-80121 and 58-6250-6001. The contents of this publication do not necessarily reflect the views or policies of the USDA, nor does mention of trade names, commercial products, or organizations imply endorsement by the U.S. Government.

Chapter 3

Acknowledgements
This research was support by grant R01 HL084404 from the National Heart, Lung and Blood Institute awarded to J.M. Tschann. We thank Jennifer Cho,

Irene Takahashi, and the Kaiser Foundation Research Institute, which provided access to members of Kaiser.

Competing Interests

The authors declare that they have no competing interests.

Authors' Contributions

All authors were involved in all parts of the study, contributed to conceptualization of the manuscript, participated in questionnaire development, and approved the final manuscript. JT was responsible for the study design and drafted the manuscript. SM and CdG performed statistical analyses, SG provided guidance on statistical analyses, and SM wrote much of the statistical analysis section. CP was responsible for overseeing the translation of the questionnaire and the study implementation. LP, EF, NB, and JD contributed to the writing, interpretation of the results, and finalizing of the manuscript. LG provided access to participants and obtained ethics approval.

Chapter 4

Acknowledgements

We are grateful to the staff at the Weight Control and Diabetes Research Center (RI) and the Center for Healthy Eating and Activity Research (CA) who participated in data collection and the families who participated in the study. This research was supported by grant number K23HD057299 from the Eunice Kennedy Shriver National Institute of Child Health and Human Development awarded to KR.

Competing Interests

The authors declare that they have no competing interests.

Authors' Contributions

KR conceived of and designed the study, obtained funding for the study, acquired and analysed the data, and drafted the manuscript. SD participated in the design of the study, analysis of the data, and manuscript revision. EJ participated in the design of the study, collection of data, and manuscript revision. KB participated in the collection of data and manuscript revision. RS participated in the design of the study and manuscript revision. RW contributed to the design of the study and manuscript revision. All authors read and approved the final manuscript.

Chapter 5

Acknowledgments
This study was supported by NIH grant 5R01HD06135.

Competing Interest
The authors declare that they have no competing interests.

Authors' Contributions
RM designed the study, analyzed the data, and drafted the initial manuscript. JL, AM, and KR designed the data collection instruments, coordinated and supervised data collection, and critically reviewed the manuscript. NK, KP, and AB provided input on the analysis plan and critically reviewed the manuscript. All authors have approved the final manuscript as submitted.

Chapter 6

Acknowledgements
This paper presents independent research funded by the National Institute for Health Research (NIHR)'s School for Public Health Research (SPHR) with support from Durham and Newcastle Universities, and the NIHR Collaboration for Leadership in Applied Health Research and Care of the South West Peninsula (PenCLAHRC). The views expressed are those of the author(s) and not necessarily those of the NHS, the NIHR or the Department of Health.

The School for Public Health Research (SPHR) is funded by the National Institute for Health Research (NIHR). SPHR is a partnership between the Universities of Sheffield, Bristol, Cambridge, UCL; The London School for Hygiene and Tropical Medicine; The Peninsula College of Medicine and Dentistry; the LiLaC collaboration between the Universities of Liverpool and Lancaster and Fuse; The Centre for Translational Research in Public Health, a collaboration between Newcastle, Durham, Northumbria, Sunderland and Teesside Universities.

AJA is director, CS is a senior investigator and JA and AAL are members of staff in Fuse, the Centre for Translational Research in Public Health, a UKCRC Public Health Research Centre of Excellence. Funding for Fuse from the British Heart Foundation, Cancer Research UK, Economic and Social Research Council, Medical Research Council, the National Institute for Health Research, under the auspices of the UK Clinical Research Collaboration, is gratefully acknowledged.

Competing Interests
The authors declare that they have no competing interests.

Authors' Contributions
JA conceived the idea for the analysis. All authors contributed to methods development. LG and JA performed the analysis. All authors contributed to data interpretation. JA drafted the manuscript. All authors provided critical comments on the manuscript. All authors read and approved the final manuscript.

Chapter 7

Acknowledgements
This research was supported by funds from the United States Department of Agriculture, Grants No. 2006-55215-16695 and No. 2011-68001-30009. This work is a publication of the United States Department of Agriculture (USDA/ARS) Children's Nutrition Research Center, Department of Pediatrics, Baylor College of Medicine, Houston, Texas, and has been funded in part with federal funds from the USDA/ARS under Cooperative Agreement No. 58-6250-0-008. The contents of this publication do not necessarily reflect the views or policies of the USDA, nor does mention of trade names, commercial products, or organizations imply endorsement from the U.S. government. The authors have no financial relationships relevant to this article to disclose.

The researchers thank the following individuals for their help in data coding and analysis: Gabriela Barbosa, Jennifer L. Edgar, Whitney Rose, and Elijah Oliveros-Rosen.

Competing Interests
The authors declare that they have no competing interests.

Authors' Contributions
TGP: Power helped conceptualize and design the coding system and the study, helped train the videotape coders, analyzed the data, drafted the original manuscript, and approved the final manuscript as written. SOH: Hughes helped conceptualize and design the coding system and the study, coordinated the recruitment of subjects and data collection, helped interpret the data, reviewed and revised the manuscript, and approved the final manuscript as submitted. LSG and SLJ: Goodell and Johnson helped conceptualize and design the coding system and the study, helped develop the plans for data analysis, helped interpret the data, helped place the findings in the context of the larger

literature, reviewed and revised the manuscript, and approved the final manuscript as submitted. JAJD: Ms. Duran helped conceptualize and design the coding system and the study, trained and supervised the videotape coders, coded videotapes, assisted in data analysis, helped interpret the data, reviewed and revised the manuscript, and approved the final manuscript as submitted. KW: Ms. Williams helped revise the coding system, coded videotapes, assisted in data analysis, helped interpret the data, reviewed and revised the manuscript, and approved the final manuscript as submitted. ADE: Ms. Eaton helped analyze the data, helped interpret the data, reviewed and revised the manuscript, and approved the final manuscript as submitted. LAF: Dr. Frankel helped interpret the data, helped place the findings in the context of the larger literature, reviewed and revised the manuscript, and approved the final manuscript as submitted.

Chapter 8

Acknowledgements

The Italian HBSC 2010 Group: National coordinators HBSC 2010: Franco Cavallo, Patrizia Lemma, Paola Dalmasso, Paola Berchialla, Sabina Colombini, Alessio Zambon, Lorena Charrier, Alberto Borraccino (University of Turin—Department of Public Health and Microbiology); Mariano Giacchi, Giacomo Lazzeri, Valentina Pilato, Stefania Rossi, Andrea Pammolli (University of Siena—Centre of Research for Health Education and Promotion—CREPS); Massimo Santinello, Alessio Vieno, Francesca Chieco, Michela Lenzi (University of Padua—Department of Developmental Psychology and Socialization Process LIRIPAC); Angela Spinelli, Giovanni Baglio, Anna Lamberti, Paola Nardone (National Institute of Health—National Center for Epidemiology, Surveillance and Health Promotion); Daniela Galeone, Lorenzo Spizzichino, Maria Teresa Menzano, Maria Teresa Scotti (Ministry of Health).

National coordinators of the regional school offices: Maria Teresa Silani, Silvana Teti (Regional School Office in Lazio); Regional coordinators: Antonio Ciglia, Manuela Di Giacomo, Silvia Spinosa (Abruzzo), Giuseppina Ammirati, Gabriella Cauzillo, Gerardina Sorrentino (Basilicata), Caterina Azzarito, Marina La Rocca (Calabria), Renato Pizzuti, Gianfranco Mazzarella (Campania), Emanuela Di Martino, Paola Angelini, Marina Fridel (Emilia Romagna), Alessandro Bavcar (FriuliVenezia Giulia), Giulia Cairella, Esmeralda Castronuovo (Lazio), Federica Pascali (Liguria), Corrado Celata, Marco Tosi, Veronica Velasco, Marina Bonfanti, Liliana Coppola (Lombardia), Giordano Giostra (Marche), Maria Letizia Ciallella (Molise), Marcello Caputo

(Piemonte), Elisabetta Viesti, Giovanna Rosa, Savino Anelli (Puglia), Serena Meloni, M. Letizia

Senis, Rita Masala (Sardegna), Achille Cernigliaro, Simonetta Rizzo (Sicilia), Mariano Giacchi, Anna Maria Giannoni (Toscana), Marco Cristofori (Umbria), Anna Maria Covarino, Giovanni D'Alessandro (Valle D'Aosta/Vallée D'Aoste), Silvano Piffer (Trento), Antonio Fanolla, Sabine Weiss (Bolzano).

We thank all students who completed the questionnaires. Special thanks to the school head teachers and teachers who actively participated in the implementation of the initiative: their contribution has been crucial to the success of the data collection.

We thank all the Regional and Local Health Units coordinators and the health workers for their fundamental contribution to the project. We gratefully acknowledge Barbara De Mei, Chiara Cattaneo and Ilaria Giovannelli of the Centre of Epidemiology, Surveillance and Health Promotion (National Institute of Health), for their important contribution to develop the communication materials and train the staff.

The Italian HBSC 2010 study was funded by the Italian Ministry of Health/ Centre for Disease Prevention and Control (Chapter 4393/2005—CCM).

Competing Interests

The authors declare that they have no competing interests.

Authors' Contributions

GL conceptualized the study, interpreted the results, wrote manuscript and approved the final manuscript as submitted. MG drafted the initial manuscript, critically reviewed the manuscript and approved the final manuscript as submitted. AS and FC conceptualized and designed the study, interpreted study results, drafted the initial manuscript, and approved the final manuscript as submitted. PD and AP carried out the statistical analyses. AL and PN coordinated and supervised data collection, reviewed and revised the manuscript, and approved the final manuscript as submitted. All authors have read and approved the final manuscript.

Chapter 9

Authors' Contribution

WJCvA, CTMS and DvdM were involved in the design of this study. WJCvA was responsible for data collection, performed the statistical analyses and drafted the manuscript. CTMS was the daily supervisor of the project. CTMS,

DvdM and GR helped with the interpretation of the data. GR revised the manuscript. CTMS and DvdM helped to draft the manuscript. All authors read and approved the final manuscript.

Acknowledgements
The authors thank V. Dam, S. de Schepper, I. de Vlieger, Y. Pierik, S. Pooyé and R. Roubehie-Fissa for their help in the data collection. This project was financed by the Netherlands Organisation for Health Research and Development (ZonMw; project no. 115100004).

Competing Interests
The authors declare that they have no competing interests.

Chapter 10

Acknowledgments
This study was funded by a grant for the Sid Richardson Foundation. Thanks to Christina Keeney, Nutrition Services Specialist for Cen-Tex Family Services, Inc., for her help with the data collection. Thanks also to the teachers and director of Cen-Tex Family Services, Inc. for their cooperation during the project. And thanks to Mohammed Hassan Rajab for the data analysis.

Conflict of Interest
The author declares no conflict of interest.

Chapter 11

Disclosure
Veronika Dolar is the coauthor.

Conflict of Interests
The authors declare that there is no conflict of interests regarding the publication of this paper.

Acknowledgments
The authors would like to thank the children and staff at the boys and girls club for supporting this research project. A big thank-you is also extended to the undergraduate nutrition student volunteers from Long Island University for their time, hard work, and dedication to improvement of the health of children.

Chapter 13

Author Contributions

JT, MB, AP, and JP conceived, designed, devised and supervised the study. MB, JP, and JT collected and supervised the samples. MB, AP, and JT analyzed the data and JP, MB, and JT wrote the manuscript. AP and JT obtained funding. All authors read and approved the final manuscript. The study sponsor had no role in study design.

Conflict of Interest Statement

The authors declare that the research was conducted in the absence of any commercial or financial relationships that could be construed as a potential conflict of interest.

Acknowledgments

The study was supported by the Spanish Ministry of Health and Consumption Affairs (Program of Promotion of Biomedical Research and Health Sciences, Projects 05/1276, 08/1259, 11/01791, and PI14/00636, Red Predimed-RETIC RD06/0045/1004, and CIBEROBN CB12/03/30038), Grant of support to research groups no. 35/2011 (Balearic Islands Gov. and EU FEDER funds), Spanish Ministry of Education and Science (FPU Program, Ph.D. fellowship to MB). The Research Group on Community Nutrition and Oxidative Stress, University of the Balearic Islands, belong to the Centre Català de la Nutrició (IEC) and Exernet Network.

Chapter 14

Acknowledgements

We acknowledge the assistance of Caroline Braet, Colleen Doak, Miranda Fredriks, Martijn Heymans, Lisa Numann, Anita Planje, Pedro J. Teixeira and Ottelien van Weelden. The study is funded by The Netherlands Organization for Health Research and Development (ZonMw).

Competing Interests

OHBS is affiliated with the treatment program as pediatrician. Other than that the authors declare no competing interests.

Authors' Contributions

All authors made substantial contributions to the conception and design of the study. JH, EV and JCS drafted the manuscript. All authors were involved in revising the manuscript critically for important intellectual content. All authors read and approved the final manuscript.

Chapter 15

Acknowledgements
The authors thank the participating Head Start agencies and the Extension staff from Michigan State University for their participation. We also thank the research teams and students from the University of Michigan and Michigan State University, and the participating families. This study was funded by the United States Department of Agriculture (USDA) / National Institute of Food and Agriculture/Agriculture and Food Research Initiative (NIFA/AFRI) Grant # 2011-68001-30089, PI J. Lumeng.

Source of External Federal Funding
United States Department of Agriculture (USDA) / National Institute of Food and Agriculture/Agriculture and Food Research Initiative (NIFA/AFRI) Grant # 2011-68001-30089.

Competing Interests
The authors declare that they have no competing interests.

Authors' Contributions
ALM, JCL, MAH, HBH, KEP, and DC conceived the project, contributed to the development of the study design and obtained funding, developed the interventions and conceived of the study design, and drafted the manuscript. NK carried out the statistical analyses and design and revised the manuscript. JSW managed the project and monitored recruitment and intervention procedures. All authors read and approved the final manuscript.

Index

E

F

G

H

I

K

L

Q

R

S

Y

Z

T - #0823 - 101024 - C358 - 229/152/16 - PB - 9781774636862 - Gloss Lamination